A Cure Too Far

The struggle to end HIV/AIDS

Fountain Publishers
P.O. Box 488
Kampala
E-mail: sales@fountainpublishers.co.ug
          publishing@fountainpublishers.co.ug
Website: www.fountainpublishers.co.ug

Distributed in Europe and Commonwealth countries outside Africa by:
African Books Collective Ltd,
P.O. Box 721,
Oxford OX1 9EN, UK.
Tel/Fax: +44(0) 1869 349110
E-mail: orders@africanbookscollective.com
Website: www.africanbookscollective.com

ISBN 978-9970-25-149-0

Cover Photo: By New Vision and Background by Janet Derbyshire

A Cure Too Far

The struggle to end HIV/AIDS

Peter Mugyenyi

FOUNTAIN PUBLISHERS
www.fountainpublishers.co.ug

Dedication

In memory of my late wife Christine Mugyenyi; my parents Rev. Canon Semu Ndimbirwe and Yudesi Ndimbirwe my late siblings Eleanor Kurubeija, Jonathan Byamugisha, James Muhumuza, Godfrey Ndimbirwe, and Benon Mugabe and my late brothers-in-law Philip Kurubeija and Eric Kazarwa.

Contents

Privacy policy

Careful consideration has been given to safeguard individual privacy. Accordingly, unless the information was already in public domain or voluntary consent had been obtained, no real names or specific identities of patients or affected people alive or dead have been used. Also, some details of events that could lead to public identification of individuals have been changed without altering the essential facts of the story. In addition, some of the dialogues have been reconstructed for better communication.

Preamble

Budomola and Twenty Corpses

The buzzword in town was *budomola*. And virtually everyone in Kampala had heard of it.

Budomola was the weapon that spearheaded one of the most unbelievable *coups d'état* that ousted the long-established professionals, dislodging them from their esteemed and powerful position in society. However, unlike the swift and bloody coups that Africa had witnessed since the 1960s, this creepy takeover was bloodless and ironic.

For almost a decade the doctors' dominance of disease management had been slipping away from their tight grip, as it emerged increasingly that they had nothing to offer to a mounting number of their sick and dying patients. By 1990, faith in them was all but gone as they were evidently impotent in the face of the outbreak of a newly identified disease that had turned into a rampant killer of the community's mothers, fathers and children. Therefore, doctors were unable to put up any credible resistance against the rise of a ragtag army of cocky herbalists, who claimed confidently to have a cure. Their alleged cure was budomola.

The word *budomola* (singular *akadomola*) is a Ugandan generic name adapted from the Swahili language for any synthetic fluid containers, usually made of plastic material. But in the era of HIV/AIDS it had taken on a brand-new meaning. It referred to the one to two and half litre fluid containers in which a variety of AIDS herbal medicines were commonly dispensed to throngs of patients by an ever-increasing number of herbalists. Budomola and AIDS medicine became almost synonymous — so much so that anyone seen with *akadomola* was thought to have AIDS.

Budomola business was brisk, the demand was high and growing all the time. As a result more and more amateur herbalists sprang up in all corners of the country on an almost daily basis. Herbal clinics with fancy names advertised by attention-grabbing signposts suddenly mushroomed everywhere. Claims of discoveries of new herbal cures were frequently advertised on radio, in print media and by word of mouth. Not to be outdone, witchdoctors revived their flagging practices. Some built new shrines in which they practised a mixture of traditional medicine and a brand of witchcraft rituals targeting AIDS victims.

Faced with stiff competition some herbalists developed new strategies to help them capture the lucrative new trade. Some opened mobile clinic businesses and took to the highways, stopping at towns and markets on the way to sell their products. Others roamed the major towns in old vehicles with sound amplifiers mounted on their roofs—blaring out adverts for their concoctions in multiple languages. I later found out that Ugandan herbalists and witchdoctors were not the only ones who claimed "breakthrough" AIDS cures. Trails of such claims extended far and wide on the African continent and beyond.

Later –much later – when their AIDS treatment businesses flopped, some herbalists and witchdoctors turned their shrines to other gruesome uses. It is perhaps no coincidence that child sacrifice and ritual murders linked to witchcraft increased at the time when AIDS patients, who previously constituted a highly lucrative source of income for the witchdoctors abandoned witchdoctors' cures for the evidently more effective antiretroviral (ARV) treatment. Other quacks just changed tactics and embarked on the biggest promotion and advertisement of their herbal medicines Uganda had ever seen. They advertised widely in virtually all print media, taking particular advantage of vernacular newspapers, where their wild claims were least likely to be challenged or noticed by national drugs regulatory authorities. They sponsored expensive primetime programmes on TV and numerous local language FM radio stations, to promote their quack cures for virtually all real or imagined physical diseases and a variety of social conditions.

From the early 1980s up to the mid 1990s, when Uganda was the AIDS epicentre in Africa, the country became the focus and a prime target of anyone who claimed to have an AIDS therapy. More sophisticated foreign quacks with high-sounding titles and dubious letters after their names, laden with US dollars to set themselves up, citing pseudo-scientific data, targeting high government officials and those in elite circles came rushing in. Among those claiming a cure who swarmed in from many corners of the world included one I will call Johannes Gasket, who jetted in from Georgia, USA, in 1989. He quickly set up a clinic in a suburb of Kampala called Half London, where he started admitting seriously ill AIDS patients. He soon started making claims of incredible success. On 22 October 1990 he wrote an urgent memo to the government. "We have been using my method of ultraviolet exposure of small amounts of blood of HIV infected people (a process he dubbed photo-oxidation), which is then returned to the patients' bloodstream for over a year. Hundreds of patients have been treated with impressive results. We have been so inspired by clinical response that we have asked for help from an Arab nation known for their generosity in dealing with medical problems," Gasket reported.

But the so called photo-oxidation was not the only treatment technique he used. With pomp, he announced yet another one of his discoveries. He claimed to have developed a special procedure of completely cleansing the blood of AIDS sufferers by "bathing" it in hydrogen peroxide and ozone gas. It consisted of draining some blood from patients, flushing bubbling gas through it and then transfusing the bubbly blood back into the patients. "I have cured many AIDS cases in USA using my revolutionary therapy," Gasket proclaimed boastfully, as he addressed a select group of awestruck senior government and Ministry of Health officials.

He proposed three phases for what he described as effective, affordable and sustainable treatment of AIDS in Uganda. The first one was the introduction of treatment that was to last six months, followed by the training of five doctors and thirty nurses, and the third would be treatment of 50,000 patients within one year. "Uganda spends about $6 million dollars on ineffective treatment of AIDS," Gasket wrote. "We strongly recommend that government spends only $ 1,815,000 of that money on my programme."

Among those listening to Gasket was an astute doctor I call Solomon Bugezi, who was assigned the duty of checking out Gasket's "high tech" cure. In subsequent private correspondence to government which Bugezi has kept to this day, Gasket issued a stern warning. "The entire programme has to be kept secret until the end when we shall surprise the world with our announcement that AIDS can be treated." Gasket also pointed out other benefits that Uganda would derive from his initiative. "Uganda's image on the international scene has been so negative, because of AIDS — treating it effectively is the one thing that we think can help us change that image. As a result, Uganda will gain respect, and consequently attract tourists and investors to rebuild her decimated economy."

"He talked with such showiness and confidence, using rather strange scientific-sounding phrases about his discovery, that a number of top state officials and I, who heard him speak, were won over," Bugezi said to me, as he recalled, with some degree of embarrassed hindsight on how Gasket had fooled them all. "It now appears ridiculous, but at that bleak time, we jostled to refer our bedridden friends and relatives to him for treatment. It was like a mini-stampede."

Obligingly, Gasket made them an offer which they thought they had no other alternative but to accept. "I will treat only 20 patients free of charge just for demonstration purposes," Gasket announced, "just to reassure you that my treatment cures AIDS. But the rest will have to pay," he added, dimming the hope of many very poor patients. Gasket had made it clear right from the beginning that he was not on a charity mission — and that his treatment would not come cheaply.

"Following the pronouncement, many rushed to have their relatives included among the lucky twenty," Bugezi recalled. The number was realised in one day, leaving many unsuccessful people with their sick relatives in tears — some of them attributing their failure to corruption of health officials.

Gasket, who often interspersed his promises of a cure with undisguised threats to anyone who dared question his unorthodox therapy, had further demands. "As this is patented therapy, I will treat all patients in strict privacy. And this will remain my method of work until such time when I will be ready to announce my breakthrough discovery to the world." Of course, no one dared to disagree with him openly, just in case he became annoyed and walked out.

Intimidation is commonly employed by peddlers of fake therapies, and in the multi-billion dollar "complementary" or "alternative" medicine industry. These products on the worldwide market include widely publicised special health foods, herbal cures often dubbed "natural cures," vegetables claimed to treat cancer and AIDS among other diseases, various kinds of food supplements, antioxidants, and some homeopathic remedies—diluted multi-trillion times and still claimed to be effective on the pretext that "water molecules have memory", among other implausible explanations. When challenged to provide scientific evidence to substantiate their claims, some proprietors and sellers of such products either fail to provide solid scientific substantiation, or respond with less than customary civility, as Dr Ben Goldacre, a British medical doctor turned journalist and author of *Bad Science*, found out the hard way when he explained in his highly acclaimed book that "debunks such medical nonsense":

> They get angry, they threaten to sue, they scream and shout at you... they complain spuriously and with ludicrous misrepresentations—time-consuming to expose, of course, but that's the point of harassment........they send hate mails,.... They bully, they smear to the absolute top of the profession, and they do anything they can in a desperate bid to shut you up, and avoid having a discussion about the evidence. They have even been known to threaten violence...

Gasket, evidently one of such characters, had his way. He went ahead and admitted the twenty "lucky" AIDS patients in his makeshift clinic that he had hurriedly set up in a rented residential house in Nakasero, a Kampala upper-class suburb. No visitors, however closely related to the patients, were allowed.

The end result of his demonstration treatment was twenty corpses.

Following the botched therapy, "Dr" Gasket sneaked out of the country, leaving the relatives of the dead to clean up after him. No apologies—of course!

"It is outrageous that you allowed this crook to get away with it," I railed at Bugezi.

"Wise up man," he responded coolly. "Those were desperate times and the situation was much more complex than you imagine. Who, for instance, would even have admitted that their relatives had AIDS?" At the time, the fate of every AIDS patient was death. Guaranteed! And everyone knew it. Therefore there was nothing unusual about twenty of those who were destined to die —dying. After all, many more than that were dying daily."

"Except that these particular ones died too soon — they were murdered," I interjected swiftly.

"I'm not so sure of that," he snapped, "because I spent some time with Gasket. He was so animated and convincing. At the time, I mistakenly thought he believed in his treatment. He seemed to mean no harm – and I still wonder whether it was really his treatment that killed them. All were terminal cases, and they would have died anyway." Bugezi explained. "However, six months or so later I considered changing my mind," Bugezi added as an afterthought. "When I visited the USA I was astonished to find pamphlets published by the same old Gasket. He was still unrepentant. Unbelievably, he claimed that his therapy had cured ten thousand Ugandans of AIDS!" Bugezi scratched his bald head. "I was so angry, but there was nothing I could do," he added.

Things were getting worse. Hardly had another six months passed when three Nigerian nationals clad in black suits, sporting dark glasses, and smelling of expensive aftershave lotion, arrived in Uganda. They made a beeline for the office of the vice president (VP), and introduced themselves as UK-based AIDS researchers. Pills, research protocols, letters of recommendation, purportedly from top British scientists – name it – they had it all, complete with a prominent London street address on their letterheads. Their credentials seemed impeccable.

"We are very concerned about the AIDS bloodbath in Uganda," their leader whom I will call Banjo, reportedly said to the VP who had a private hospital filled with AIDS patients. "We work with leading scientists in the UK, where effective AIDS treatment has already been developed. Unfortunately, it is too expensive for poor countries like Uganda. But in the sprit of African solidarity, we are here to rescue your country from this dilemma," Banjo announced convincingly. "First of all, we shall treat three patients within your hospital for three weeks to demonstrate the effectiveness of our novel but still secret treatment. We already successfully treated over 500 AIDS patients in Malawi in 1989," they claimed though without volunteering any evidence to confirm it.

"We also plan to set up an AIDS victims' charity in Uganda, through which we shall donate laboratory equipment, X-ray machines, and fax machines. However, our first and most urgent mission is to help you to stop the deaths by providing Uganda with the latest AIDS treatment," Banjo clarified further. "AIDS treatment costs millions of pounds in Europe, but we are ready to transfer the technology to Uganda so that it can be cheaply manufactured here. In the meantime, we need only £170,000 Sterling plus £60,000 to cover personal expenses, to start."

The evidently very impressed VP promised them his unequivocal support. And they almost got away with it. Their smooth run was ruined by the same Solomon Bugezi. He had been asked, once again, to investigate the claims of their treatment and offers of donations.

Backed and empowered by the VP, the Nigerians arrived at Bugezi's office teeming with confidence. "They appeared to fit the role," Bugezi recalled, "but they were let down by a couple of things. First they appeared to be in too much of a hurry and secondly they made some unreasonable demands. They requested diplomatic status, unrestricted licence to practise medicine in Uganda, and first-class air travel. I took a good long look at them and became awfully sceptical of their claims, especially as they failed to produce evidence of their past experience," Bugezi recalls. He asked to have a look at their travel documents, and was surprised to find that they were travelling on Ghanaian passports. He asked a few basic medical questions and found their answers lacking the kind of depth expected of researchers on the cutting edge of science. As a safeguard, he insisted that they first present their research findings to a select group of top Ugandan doctors and scientists before they would receive their cheque.

However, some senior government officials strongly opposed Bugezi's handling of the matter on the ground that he was delaying the rescue of many suffering AIDS patients. But Bugezi stood his ground. The unanticipated hurdle to their hitherto smooth act ruffled the gang of three. They reacted by trying to arrange what they described as a "cosy chat" but Bugezi declined their invitation. "The bottom line remains," Bugezi insisted, "no presentation of your treatment to Ugandan doctors — no deal."

"Only a few hours earlier the big prize had seemed within reach," Bugezi told me, "but now they must have feared that it was being snatched away from them". Something needed to be done quickly. The brazen fellows rushed back to where they had started — the office of the VP to mobilise support. However, they could not shake off the tenacious doctor. Besides blocking their access to the bank (which Bugezi suspected to have been the reason for requesting diplomatic status, so that they could get away scot-free with their loot), he kept asking questions. The more questions he asked, the clearer it must have become that the prize was slipping further away from their grasp. Then, all of a sudden, they agreed to do the presentation.

"They ran the risk of their cover being completely blown," Bugezi explained their sudden change of mind. "They must have gone back to work on plan B." They requested for first-class return tickets to London, ostensibly to fetch their research data, promising to be back within a week to present it. With their refundable tickets safely in their briefcases, they melted into thin air."

It was not long that my turn came to scientifically verify claims of similar claimants identify and expose the quacks among them. In the course of my work I followed up numerous alleged cures, to places as far away as America, Europe and the Far East. There, I met with an amazing array of unforgettable characters, ranging from genuine humanitarian donors to unrepentant crooks. Each encounter had its unique and sometimes surprising facet. I was urged on by the growing number of worried patients who besieged my clinic daily and equally concerned authorities trying to find a way out of the national crisis.

The long search brought me face to face with peddlers of dubious concoctions and drugs of questionable efficacy. For instance, December 1992 found me in Beijing, heading a Ugandan delegation on the trail of a much-hyped "breakthrough" Chinese AIDS drug. It was however not the rigours of the mission at hand that troubled me, but an irate member of my own team who had suddenly turned against me, and almost ruined our assignment. Over to Bonn, then the capital of West Germany, I had the pleasure of meeting a beautiful female doctor who captivated me with stories of the perfect AIDS cure that she had discovered as we savoured the rich aroma of freshly brewed coffee. The search also took me to picturesque rural France. There, I breakfasted in an ancient castle close to the Belgian border with a brilliant, but rather eccentric scientist with a strange phobia, who taught me how to manufacture AIDS drugs.

I must briefly mention the case of a very polite and soft-spoken Japanese entrepreneur who, one day in 1993, turned up in my office loaded with woody mushrooms. He bowed twice, Japanese style, and then placed the mushrooms on my desk. "These can be processed into a drug to treat AIDS," he explained. "And incidentally, they can be grown locally." He was right about the latter because I have since found similar mushrooms growing wild near my home town. He also had samples of the processed products which he left with me. I never found out whether his claimed cure worked or not. We heard later that he had been run over by a car in South America. We were told that he had been on his way to the Amazon jungle to find out whether the legendary rain forest held a cure for AIDS. For almost a decade, I kept one of the woody mushrooms in my office as a memento.

Drama once unfolded in my office as an entrancing witchdoctor demonstrated how his amazing implements would finish off AIDS. A remarkable American caused pandemonium at Entebbe Airport customs section, where he landed with a strange cargo that he declared to be an AIDS cure for Uganda. Yet, as narrated below, these are just a sample of the many incidents and characters of many nationalities that I met as I tried to find a solution for a horrific disease that was literally annihilating our people.

The search for treatment was not the only challenge. When it came to finding a vaccine, totally unexpected controversies emerged. In the absence of a cure, one would think that effective preventive measures would be universally welcomed. Instead, it raised much debate. While these controversies unfolded, hundreds of thousands suffered, not only from AIDS but also from stigma, denial and other complications associated with it.

The experiences of HIV/AIDS-infected and affected people who suffered and responded to their plight in different ways emphasise the imperative of the continuing search for an AIDS cure.

1

Denial

Not Really Alive

Relatives of people suffering from AIDS almost routinely drew me aside to whisper in my ear. "Doctor, the situation does not look good." This was almost always a gross understatement. "Should we prepare for the worst?" Virtually everyone who asked knew the answer, but they asked anyway. Their fear was understandable, because the 1990s was a gloomy decade for many families in Uganda and many parts of Africa.

Then there was the acrimonious controversy about calling sufferers victims, to which many HIV-infected people took strong exception. "It is highly stigmatising," they complained. The obvious alternative was to refer to the sufferers by the long established and generally acceptable name of patients. Yet HIV had a very long incubation period. It could be up to eight years and not infrequently longer before symptoms of AIDS appeared. Until it did, many infected people remained healthy, looked good, felt well, and went about their lives unaware that the treacherous bug was insidiously wearing them down.

"Look, we are not sick," those who had not come down with the fully blown disease yet would plead. "We are as fit as anyone else." But the clock was ticking.

At the time, after two decades of medical practice on three continents, I had never encountered anyone who had any objection to the word patient. The search for a non-stigmatising description of people living with HIV was imperative. In an attempt to remain transparent, some hospitals started referring to AIDS patients as clients. But doctors had never had 'customers'! Perhaps it was accurate, as all that an HIV-infected person got from a hospital, if anything at all, was counselling – provided by a new cadre of mainly lay healthcare providers. Other than treating a few opportunistic infections, doctors had nothing to offer. However, soon whispers that clients in hospitals were AIDS patients started and the previously neutral word became negative.

What HIV/AIDS sufferers really needed was a benign description that could not be readily linked to AIDS, but still imply AIDS, indirectly—merely hint. Eventually a solution that was initially thought to be trouble-free was found. HIV-infected people came to be known by the general description, People Living with AIDS. There were two positive words: People and Living. This was uplifting. For a short time, it became the official label. But, there was a disconcerting side to it too—the word AIDS. It was too ominous to be acceptable. Happily – so it seemed – a way out was found. People Living with AIDS was abbreviated to PLWA. In speeches, in seminars and conferences, PLWA was always used. Though it avoided mention of the negative word, PLWA, besides being a tongue twister, begged for an explanation. Neither was it correct to imply that all HIV-infected people were living with AIDS. It was back to the drawing board. The term was refined to People Living with HIV/AIDS, abbreviated as PLWHA or PLWHIV. Still, not everyone was happy. What was really needed was not merely a name, but a cure. Anyway, the name stuck, especially in professional circles.

In the meantime, patients, clients, PLWHIV or whatever other aliases, were advised by counsellors to try and live one day at a time. By doing this, they would not dwell too much on the future, or worry too much about the inevitable that tomorrow would bring.

In the absence of a cure, PLWHIV prayed that they would at least be treated with dignity, not be shunned, discriminated against or stigmatised. They needed to be described in a positive way. Just like the counsellors advised—live positively. However, the slogan was easier chanted than practised. For instance, at moments when one was alone, it was hard to live positively.

As the health of the PLWHIV inevitably deteriorated, I noted that they often fell into one of two main camps. There were those who accepted the reality that no cure existed, came to terms with their situation and meekly accepted their fate, and others who recoiled in denial.

Not infrequently, I was called to the bedside of a patient far beyond the possibility of even temporary resuscitation. I went not just for the patient, but also for his or her family, relatives and especially the children. They needed to know that people cared, even though I had no medicine to offer them. I never wanted it whispered afterwards that "If only the doctor had come...."

Whenever I visited patients, it was mainly the entry into the house that I found difficult. I would try to project an aura of calmness. But I am not sure if I was always successful. I would do all I could to avoid pointless rush, try to control my body language to avoid arousing either a state of panic or false hope. Above all, I took care to avoid looking like a stereotypical doctor – the type you see in films, with a stethoscope around the neck, rushing in to administer a life-saving injection. As I entered, drained eyes would painfully lift and fix on me. Weary mouths, long short of anything inspirational to say, would open and utter some words in various degrees of desperation.

I recall one incident involving a woman who was nursing her sick husband. I was dragged out of my clinic by the woman's panic-stricken sister who said she had a desperate emergency at home. She had a taxi waiting outside. At her urging, the driver whisked us across the city at breakneck speed. She shepherded me into a poorly-lit room.

"Hurry doctor! There he is," she said agitatedly pointing to a dark corner with her head turned aside. She nudged me forward while retreating towards the door. It took moments for my eyes to adjust to the dark room that smelled of insecticide and air freshener. Then I saw a woman seated in an old wooden chair with a broken armrest by the bedside. There was an open bible on a side table which also held a variety of bottles containing fluids of various colours, which I suspected to be herbal concoctions and juices. She was in a sort of catatonic state, hardly moving, just staring straight ahead expressionlessly.

In the bed I made out the outline of a still, long thin figure that could have been easily mistaken for a banana stem covered with a blanket. At the top end, propped on a thin pillow was what could be called a face, but it was so emaciated that it looked more like a skull with paper-thin, dark, pockmarked skin stretched over it. Prominent were exposed teeth and eyes deeply sunken in their sockets. The woman seemed unaware of my presence. I stood there in respectful silence, waiting for a gesture or some sort of invitation to examine the patient. After a while, without looking up, she said to me in an impassive quiet voice, *Otambira enkoko agitambira n'ekirasya*—a Runyankole language expression meaning that time to save her husband had long run out.

But not all families allowed me to enter through the front door. Not infrequently, I was smuggled in through the back door. I could clearly see that they desperately needed me to see (read "cure") their ill-fated relatives. I understood that it was a mixture of fear and stigma that lead many to take such extraordinary measures to ensure that I was well hidden from the neighbours and other prying eyes. And they had good reason for taking such extraordinary measures—I was well known as an AIDS doctor.

Sometimes the relatives of a patient would take the extraordinary measure of evacuating visitors from the house so that I could enter unnoticed. One of the most successful improvisations to get everyone out of the way was to invite them to attend prayers in a discret place. This almost always succeeded as everyone wished to be seen praying for the sick. Often, the prayers would be extended to cover my exit as well. Sometimes the patient would be moved to an isolated place to which I would be taken to see him or her.

Many of the poverty-stricken patients that I encountered had just one or two rooms, and therefore no means of achieving privacy. I recall a family of four living in a crowded slum area of Kampala. It was headed by a terminally sick woman in her early thirties who shared a single room with her two children aged seven and four, and a 13-year old orphan girl who had come to live with them because she had nowhere to go, and who ended up serving as a provider and caretaker. I was summoned by the woman's cousin. As I entered the small, dark and damp room with a crumbling roof that looked as if it could cave in anytime, stigma was not an issue. It was only bewilderment that I saw. Indeed, I came across many people suffering double jeopardy of AIDS and extreme poverty. To them, stigma was a "luxury" they could not afford to entertain.

Dishearteningly, but fortunately rarely, some people, in their frustration would become either hostile or rude, blaming me for my failure to cure their loved ones.

"Doctor, are you really unable to do anything?" some said to me, wondering why a supposed AIDS specialist was so powerless to act at the very critical time of their most desperate need. "Doctors are useless these days. They have no cure for modern-day diseases," some others would say without caring whether I was within hearing range.

Indeed, without any effective medicine I frequently felt frustrated and utterly powerless.

Especially haunting were the puzzled looks of children of dying parents as they stared at everybody around them trying to understand what was going on. Initially the poor children would trust that Mum or Dad, who in the eyes of children had solutions to all problems, would somehow revive. Some could not believe it when it actually happened. I recall a child, too young to understand death, running to a relative who had just arrived for the funeral. "Dad is sleeping too much — come, see auntie; he hasn't woken up for two days now."

Some children after their parents' death, had nowhere to go. I was told by an auntie of a girl of six who had fought tooth and nail to prevent her three-year-old brother being taken away by a relative as the orphaned children were "shared" out among relatives, and how she sobbed for weeks when she lost the battle. The auntie said that even as an adult, her niece was troubled by the forced separation. Though the two children frequently saw each other, they never quite bonded as siblings.

I also witnessed heroic battles of survival bravely fought by some AIDS patients who never gave up. At least, not right away. They included one single mother of six. She moonlighted on several manual-labour jobs even as she weakened physically, in a futile effort to pay for the unaffordable AIDS drugs while she fed and schooled her children. I watched powerlessly as she gradually lost the fight, despite my efforts to marshal some assistance for her. The drugs were just too expensive. However, almost up to the end, her fighting spirit lingered on as she hoped against hope for a miracle. She became religious, like many other sufferers. She prayed incessantly, but her prayers like those of others in similar situation were not answered, or if they were, it was in mysterious ways. Then realising that no miracle was forthcoming, she snapped. Finally, she lapsed into depression - sobbing all the time, eventually sinking into apathy and resignation.

Sadly, I also met the opposite reaction including some horrid people who shamelessly abandoned their AIDS dependants for ideological or selfish motives in their hour of critical need — like the case of Petwa described later on. I once attended a funeral where an extremist evangelical man accused his deceased sister of sinning, adding that she got no less than what she properly deserved. In his pseudo-puritan view, he equated AIDS to sin – to be judged mercilessly and deserving punishment by God. Worse still, I saw predatory people waiting rather impatiently for AIDS patients to die so that they could grab their property, take over their jobs, business, or political office and benefit in one way or another. Since the condition had no cure, they were always sure that their waiting would pay dividends. However the sequence of events did not always unfold according to their plots.

The hopelessness of the situation led the people of south-western Uganda to coin a saying that captured the prevalent mood of the times well. *Noriho, tariho* roughly translated "Even those who are alive now, are not really alive." Many desperate people, whether infected or not, had lost hope of survival. Many were just marking time. This was because few knew or wished to know whether they were infected or not. To paraphrase Hamlet's words, in the contest of testing for HIV without a cure, to know or not to know, was the question.

HIV testing was initially only done by one United States Agency for International Development (USAID) supported clinic in Bauman House in central Kampala. It was free. Yet the very act of walking in the direction of the AIDS testing clinic and, worse still, to enter Bauman House required extreme bravery. Understandably, the grim reality of being handed a positive HIV test result was like being presented with an execution order – without the possibility of appeal. As there was no cure anyway, many preferred to avoid the Russian (or should we call it Bauman?) roulette-like exercise. At the time the only treatment available for anyone who tested positive was counselling and herbs. Clearly, by the early 1990s, AIDS, in one way or the other, was impacting on many of the day-to-day social, economic and, to some extent, political issues in the country negatively. Not many would at the time have disagreed with the dictum *noriho tariho*.

The utter bleakness of the situation caused some despondent folks to squander their scanty assets and savings. Some spent it on bogus treatments and useless herbal concoctions, while others used it all up saying a prolonged farewell to the world. However, the "farewell parties" were never declared as such. Those who survived the year would celebrate each New Year's Day with exuberant abandon, like it was their very last! And for some it was. In elite clubs in and around Kampala, in the overflowing bars and drinking joints to which people flocked to seek solace, with noriho tariho ringing threateningly in their ears, it was not uncommon to hear singing:

In heaven there is no beer! That's why we drink it here …

And as the alcohol took effect, transforming the aura of despair and melancholy into an artificial temporary mood of euphoria, the song would become louder and louder as it progressed to a crescendo.

..and when we get to heaven, we shall only worship the Lord there.

But one by one the merry singers vanished.

Others of a more spiritual inclination flocked to the numerous places of worship that sprang up to sing and make peace with their maker — and prepare for paradise. However, not all the places of worship that sprang up had an agenda of saving the souls of soon-to-depart brethren. Many were there to ensure that the departed left all their worldly possessions, or as much of it as possible, in their "safe" custody.

However, not all who were so scared were infected with HIV. A good number of them, to their surprise, lived on and on, with decreasing assets and means to support themselves and their families. In fact I know of some relatively well-off people who became impoverished or alcoholics because of their fear of AIDS. I know of a few people who explicitly admit that the sheer terror of AIDS did them in.

"I could see no point in saving money or making long-term plans when I would soon be dead," one man who sold his farm and small-scale business said to me. Later, when everything was gone, he discovered he was not HIV infected.

I also witnessed some uplifting actions of people and organisations that had been started to support AIDS sufferers. They included Philly Lutaaya, who composed songs about AIDS and traversed the country warning the youth about the dangers of AIDS using himself as a living example (though he had a short time to carry out his mission). Noreen Kalebu started The AIDS Support Organisation (TASO), which gave AIDS a face. She stood by dejected patients, bestowing hope where none was apparent, providing for them materially when their fatigued friends and relatives had long given up, and caring for them until the very end. Another organisation that has played a major role is the Joint Clinical Research Centre (JCRC), which I had the honour to head. The Centre led the struggle to find a cure and in the process saved numerous AIDS patients from a variety of conmen. JCRC developed

AIDS care and treatment best practices that came in handy when life-saving therapy eventually became available.

AIDS brought out the good, the bad and the ugly in people.

Enlisting

I had become used to the hustle and bustle of Mulago Hospital, although the high death rate of children on my ward unnerved me everyday. I was all set for a long, busy stay, determined to dedicate the rest of my professional career to our top referral hospital, when the post of the director of the newly commissioned JCRC was advertised in 1992. As I was already deeply engrossed in my job of a paediatrician, I did not pay any attention to it.

Though highly challenging, my post at Mulago was getting me more involved in some other interesting activities including teaching at the Medical School. I could clearly see that the grossly understaffed Hospital – overwhelmed with patients – needed my services. There were also some special opportunities that Mulago Hospital offered regarding my career advancement. While working abroad, I had become interested in children's kidney diseases, but Mulago Hospital had no specialised children's kidney clinic. I had started one, and successfully convinced one bright postgraduate medical student to take an interest in paediatric nephrology (children's kidney diseases) and make it his area of specialisation, so that he would later join me in training others and make the burgeoning clinic a success. In addition, the head of my department had asked me to take charge of the acute-care clinic that was then poorly equipped and run down, at a time when the numbers of acutely sick children had risen sharply. The miserable circumstances inevitably forced me to take an interest in HIV/AIDS, as it was obviously the main cause of death on my ward and the main reason why the number of children in the acute-care unit had soared.

A professional colleague advised me to apply for the advertised position, on the grounds that it would offer better opportunities to fight HIV/AIDS. I agonised over the prospects of leaving all the programmes that were beginning to take shape, and the auspices of a well-established national referral hospital for a small poorly-facilitated new centre that had to be started from scratch. JCRC initially appeared to me to be the least likely base from which to tackle the most sophisticated disease in recent medical history. However, in coming to a decision I took into account the fact that AIDS was the leading cause of morbidity and mortality in Uganda. I hoped that the new centre would provide a more conducive environment, free of bureaucratic impediments, to facilitate expedited AIDS research.

As I started on my new job at the JCRC, my board members left no doubt in my mind that what they really expected of me was nothing short of finding an AIDS cure. The pittance that was offered as facilitation and the sheer odds against a successful outcome should have served as a red flag. If I had the foresight to see the formidable challenges that lay ahead I would have gone straight back to Mulago to resume my paediatrics practice. On the other hand, I suppose I would have taken it on regardless, not least because I shared my board members' concerns about AIDS, the sense of urgency and the need to do something about it.

However, undertaking one of the toughest medical assignments without sufficient funds still bothered me. The imperative nature of the undertaking was underscored by the fact that the board chairman of the JCRC was none other than the president of Uganda. Other board members were senior cabinet ministers and Manfred Dietrich, a German professor of medicine. Clearly, high-profile and well informed eyes were focussed on me and the cash-starved centre, expecting us to come up with a cure or show cause why not.

On my first day at the Centre, I discovered that the situation at the JCRC was even more dismal than I had anticipated. I was taken aback when I realised that my entire task force consisted of just one junior doctor, an administrative official without any management background, a finance manager with hardly any funds to manage and a handful of paramedical personnel. Clearly, we lacked the firepower to fight the century's most hideous epidemic successfully.

The very first issue that my skeleton staff notified me about, in my new capacity as the director, was the precarious financial state of JCRC. USAID had agreed to help the Centre to start off using funds obtained from food-aid programme returns. But soon, Uganda was declared to be self-sufficient in food and the fund was discontinued. As a result, even the basic monthly salaries of the staff were not secured. The government stepped in and started providing a small fraction of the basic budget. But it was grossly inadequate. Apparently it was up to me to find the funds to top up staff salaries and facilitate the centre's research agenda. The problem was that I did not know how or where to start looking for funds. I had never before in my career had to raise funds. I did not know whether it was just a question of passing the hat around or knocking at the banks' doors. I now understood why many of my colleagues had rejected the job.

Nevertheless, I still fantasised that the elusive cure was somewhere out there just waiting to be found. Even if we failed to find a cure, we could hope to, at least, alleviate the agony caused by AIDS. Therefore, whenever I worried that the exercise may be futile, as happened frequently, I would consider the alternative – the sheer horror and carnage of doing nothing. Therefore throwing in the towel, was never going to be an option. At least I knew where to start. As *budomola* was virtually the only AIDS "medicine" in widespread use, it was inevitable that the first tasks of the newly inaugurated JCRC, which was specifically set up to carry out research on AIDS, would include determining the effectiveness of *budomola*.

It did not take me long to realise that HIV/AIDS was not the only disease that needed a cure. I soon learnt that HIV had created a situation that extended far beyond a mere syndrome to a multifaceted condition, which I call "AIDS complex" (AIDS-C). As the details of AIDS-C unfolded, I was continually surprised by the various twists and turns it took and by its sheer magnitude. For instance, I had never quite imagined the full extent of AIDS-triggered conditions which included betrayal, orphan creation, broken marriages, alcohol abuse, suicides and disruption of culture and traditional customs, that affected individuals, families and society. As the selected cases and individual stories of sufferers will indicate, it was for the entire complex that a cure was needed.

2

Where there is no Cure

My Sister's Keeper

In addition to millions of deaths, many other associated complications, including physical, psychological and social disasters, would be avoided if AIDS had a cure. By the mid-1980s, AIDS was generating headline bad news in Uganda. The situation was deteriorating faster than peoples' ability to make the necessary emotional, mental and cultural adjustments to cope. In many cases, individual and social reactions were unpredictable and often difficult to understand.

It has been said that the first casualty of war is the truth. The same can be said of HIV/AIDS, for which denial is usually the first reaction. The most emotionally debilitating part of AIDS is stigma — a mixture of intense fear and shame that leads to denial and blame, which often transforms into anger and despair. The dilemma was that many people did not know how to cope with their infected mothers, fathers and children.

Barbra (not real name) told me of her family's ordeal which was not unique by any means. "I am still ashamed by the way my family treated my sister," Barbra, who kept referring to herself as "the survivor", recalled.

Her sister was 22-year-old. Her name was Perepetwa, better known to family and friends as Petwa.

"It's not that my family was callous or anything of that sort — everyone was just overwhelmed by fear."

In a long conversation I had with Barbra, the survivor, part of which I have endeavoured to reconstruct, she described her sister Petwa as having been "a jolly, outgoing and a good-looking girl".

"She was a bit of a rebel," Barbra added. "But to be fair to her, she was just like many others who, in the pre-AIDS era, got away with risky youthful frolics and later on became responsible adults unscathed," she said in defense of her sister.

11

"Well, you can't really blame anyone," I said to her by way of support. "At the time, no one knew that a treacherous intruder had crept in to put a spanner in the usual human maturation works."

"She was a handful to our parents," Barbra went on, "She dropped out of school at 17, when she became pregnant. The man - or rather boy – responsible for her pregnancy was another 17-year-old named James. Then she left home, leaving behind her baby boy with our parents."

Petwa's parents, Paulo and Eudia Waiswa, were well known pastors in their community in eastern Uganda. Petwa's elder sister Grace – a stunning woman - had fallen into money through marriage to a rich foreigner who was suspected of having acquired his vast wealth through clandestine business dealings. However, their union was, to speak, not made in heaven. Their stormy marriage came to a sudden end in 1982, when the estranged husband died in circumstances that, according to Barbra, were "as mysterious as his business".

Grace suddenly found herself with a sizeable fortune and the freedom to enjoy it. She became a merry widow who rapidly climbed the social ladder, ending up amidst Kampala's most exclusive elite. In the process she discovered her hitherto latent business acumen. In her exciting new role as a business guru, Grace became the darling of her parents and she helped her grateful siblings to improve their standard of living to levels that would otherwise have been impossible.

In mid-1987, disaster struck the Waiswa family. Initially, it did not appear to be a serious problem. It started with Petwa's unexpected home-coming. She was not well.

"Even today, I still remember the day that she returned. She could hardly stand. She was so drained. I hardly recognised her," Barbra said. From her emotions, betrayed by the tears, I could see that time had not healed the pain.

Petwa told the family that she suffered diarrhoea that had lasted months, fever and a persistent irritating cough that failed to respond to therapy. She had recently been discharged from the hospital, where she had been admitted without the knowledge of her parents. The doctor had informed her that her disease had no cure, and that there was nothing more he could offer her. He advised her to go home and continue with what he described as home-based care, and to live positively. "You are better off in the caring arms of your parents," the doctor reportedly said to her.

"Petwa's homecoming was emotional, as Mum welcomed her with hugs," Barbra recalled. The family rallied around, promising her all the care and support she needed. Mum fussed endlessly over her beloved daughter complaining that she had been starved, wherever she had been. However, this fuss did not last. Only a few days later, Petwa was thrown out of the family home by her parents. She was bluntly warned that she should never attempt to come back. Grace, her uptown sister, was the cause of Petwa's rejection. Grace somehow deduced that the cause of her sister's illness was AIDS. On learning the disgraceful news, a horrified Grace had rushed home to save her family's honour.

"People later gossiped that Grace's main concern had been her newly acquired social status. She wanted to distance herself from the scandal of AIDS in the family. She must have feared the reaction of her celebrated friends and business consorts," Barbra explained. The parents, especially their mother were shocked. They too had their own reasons for the shame that they felt. What their congregation found out that their very devout family harboured a fornicator who got AIDS as a result? Would they be able to be credible pastors?

"Whenever our parents talked about AIDS or Petwa," Barbra remembered. "they always talked in whispers. We were petrified, unable to believe that this was happening in our family!"

Petwa, of course, knew that she had the dreaded AIDS, but as she later told Barbra, she never breathed a word of it to her family for fear of rejection. She suffered alone with the grim knowledge that the clock was ticking. When she lost her family's support, it appeared that the end would come sooner rather than later.

Petwa was dumped at the desolate village bus station and given a little money for bus fare to "nowhere". Grace's parting words of farewell to her bewildered sister were neither endearing nor reassuring: "Just get lost," she reportedly said, before she drove off. The two never met again. Describing her ordeal later, Petwa told Barbra that when the tears dried, she pondered her bleak future, wondering where to go. She could not think of anyone who would welcome her. She felt dirty. Eventually she thought of James the father of her child, whom she knew also shared the "shame" of living with AIDS. All the other men whom she had dated before had, of course, long been scared away.

James was living as a squatter, in a Kampala suburb. Petwa's arrival was a surprise but he offered her temporary shelter. The friends and relatives she approached for help went deaf as soon as AIDS was mentioned or suspected, and she struggled to find a place to stay permanently. Finally, she stumbled across a good Samaritan called Muwereza, whom I also interviewed. He offered Petwa refuge. He apologised that he feared for his young children being close to an AIDS "victim" and would only offer his servant's quarters which was a "safe" distance away from the main house. Under the circumstances Petwa would have been grateful even if it had been a kraal.

Muwereza was one of the few good Samaritans, who tend to emerge in all tragedies. He rose above fear, stigma and personal safety concerns to carry out a humanitarian act. It was not for any reward, religious or ideological ends, but because he felt obuntu (humanism). People like him filled in the gaps for the overwhelmed hospitals which were forced to send away many helpless patients. People like Muwereza provided sanctuary for the ostracised ones and comforted the heartbroken. They eased their pain, and held them in their arms when they died. Thus in the unfolding apocalypse, the legendary African compassion which was beginning to be weakened by the AIDS stigma, showed through in spite of unprecedented challenges.

Barbra traced her sister to Muwereza's home. Without informing her parents, she visited her sister frequently and helped as far as she could. As Petwa weakened, the highlight of her day was a warm bath, which she was too weak to do on her own. "Initially I was scared to bathe her. I feared that I would somehow catch the disease," Barbra recalled. "But she was so insistent, and desperate to rid herself of the stench. She had always been a clean girl. She was so emaciated, it was like bathing a skeleton."

The Muwereza family, their self-evident kindness notwithstanding, were not totally free of prejudice. They made sure that Petwa was kept well hidden, but otherwise saw to it that she was as comfortable as possible. Muwereza found a volunteer doctor to take care of her in her dark nook. The doctor once found Barbra bathing her sister and warned her that she too could get infected. When she explained that she was the only person who could help her sister, the doctor provided her with one pair of surgical gloves. But the doctor couldn't do much; all he could do was to provide palliative treatment, increasing the dose of painkillers to alleviate the pain as Petwa weakened. One day, the doctor took Muwereza and Barbra aside. "This disease is worse than cancer," he explained to them. "It has no cure. Prepare for the funeral." Within a matter of days, he was proven right.

The Waiswa family did not announce Petwa's death, and made sure that her funeral was a hush-hush affair. As usual, no mention of AIDS was made during the funeral eulogies, but this did not stop the whispers.

In time, the devout family once again settled down and continued their evangelical work while Grace continued to prosper as her business enterprises expanded. However, the relative peace was short-lived.

It all started rather insidiously when Eudia, the late Petwa's mother, started complaining of vague pains all over her body. Grace sent a doctor to treat her mother but she failed to respond to therapy. She deteriorated quickly, surprising her doctor, who had failed to make a definite diagnosis. Because of her rather advanced age, religious fanaticism, and the fact that her husband was well and healthy, AIDS seemed out of question and an HIV test was not considered. Nevertheless, the ever-vigilant village grapevines speculated about AIDS as a distinct possibility. The symptoms and signs, as far as the alarmed villagers could discern, were not unlike those of other people in their village who had died of AIDS. At Eudia's funeral it was announced that she had died of a mysterious illness.

Three years later there was no doubt, however, about the illness that afflicted Grace. She was pregnant, and perhaps this was the cause of the rapid progression of the disease. Unlike Petwa, the Waiswa family and especially Grace's father were all in full attendance at her bedside to comfort and support her. After the birth of a sickly baby girl, Grace's health improved but only for a while. After a year of deteriorating health, it was confirmed that the cause of her frailty was AIDS. Six months after the diagnosis, Grace, accompanied by several members of her family, travelled to America to seek advanced therapy. Six weeks later, Grace's body was returned in a coffin marked Danger! Highly infectious! Do not open. In contrast to the usual practice in Uganda, the diagnosis of AIDS was clearly written on the death certificate. The family ensured that no mention of it was made publicly.

As the epidemic hit harder, the Waiswas were to lose to AIDS most of their family members, leaving only one out of eight siblings,

Barbra, to tell the tale. However, the Waiswa family was not the most devastated by AIDS, some families were wiped out completely.

Beyond Endurance

The Schmitt family and I will never forget the events that started unfolding one Monday in August 1996. I was in an important meeting when the telephone rang. On the line was the whispering voice of Alice, our telephone exchange operator, which rather startled me because I had left clear instructions that I was not to be disturbed except under exceptional circumstances.

"I am sorry to break into your meeting," she apologised, as members stared at me sensing my concern. "But I have a woman with a European accent who insists that she must talk to you urgently."

Hardly had the connection been made, than an agitated Jeanne Schmitt, wife of Dieter, a German expatriate, working with German Technical Services (GTZ), said that she was calling about their gardener, James Jamuronge, whom she suspected of suffering from HIV. The sociable Schmitt family was well known to me, and I felt I had to address Jeanne's apparent alarm immediately.

"Don't worry, you can't catch AIDS from casual contact with your worker," I said trying to allay her anxiety, thinking that she was probably one of many people living with ignorance, fear and misconception about AIDS.

"Excuse me, Doctor, I am not that uninformed about AIDS," she retorted. "I am not really worried about catching AIDS. My husband and I would like to help this poor man, for he has been so good to us, and we do not like to see him suffer or die a horrific death," she explained. "We want to do something for him urgently, before it is too late." The kind-hearted Mrs Schmitt could not have possibly imagined that her concern for the welfare of her employee would, within a few days, take a horrible twist.

"Your gardener could be scared of being stigmatised especially by his employers. Therefore you will need a tactful approach," I said. "Bring him to the clinic when he is ready," I advised. Experience had taught me that fear of stigma was almost inevitable.

I learned later, that Jeanne and her husband Dieter, a middle-aged easy-going and pleasant man, called in their long time and dependable gardener, better known to the family and most of his friends as JJ, to the big house that evening for a cup of tea, and what they made appear like a chat. They liked JJ because he was very neat. He kept the compound finely mowed, trees well pruned, and his room in the servants' quarters always looked like it was ready for a military inspection. The Schmitts were proud of having found such an excellent domestic help. That evening, the topic of an AIDS test was casually and gently brought up by the Schmitts, who took special care not to unnerve JJ. However, they need not have bothered as James was not unduly perturbed. When he was asked how he would feel about taking an HIV test he replied that he would have no problem at all. This encouraged Jeanne to carry on with what they had all along planned as the main topic of the evening.

"As a matter of fact," Jeanne said, "we have for quite some time now been rather concerned about your recurrent illnesses and deteriorating health. Since AIDS can be treated, I suggest that you consider undertaking an HIV test just to be sure."

They were pleasantly surprised to find him calm and receptive. They had prepared for a long, drawn-out process of explanations and persuading. "It was like an anticlimax," Jeanne told me later. Surprisingly, far from worrying about HIV, JJ instead expressed thanks and appreciation to the Schmitts for the generous offer to pay for his test, which would otherwise have taken a considerable chunk out of his salary.

The following morning Dieter drove JJ to my clinic for testing. JJ was dressed in spotless casuals, and was apparently in his late twenties or early thirties, slender five-foot-eleven-inches tall. He looked well, except for a mild skin rash on his face and hands. He told me that he was a Luo by tribe from the town of Tororo in Eastern Uganda, but did not seem ready to disclose more about his family background, and I did not press him.

"I recently lost a bit of weight, and I have a slight problem of persistent diarrhoea," JJ reported serenely in answer to my inquiry about his state of health. "Otherwise, I feel fine, except perhaps my itchy skin and general weakness", he added.

"There are many possible causes for your problems," I explained while I took a good look at him to get an idea of the kind of patient JJ was. I could not detect any obvious signs of anxiety, which was usual among those presenting themselves for their first HIV test.

"I am not sure what the cause could be until I carry out some tests." This was one of my usual introductory remarks to a counselling and pre-testing session with new patients.

"I think it is AIDS," JJ interjected. "Doctor, I am ready for the test. I am not afraid." JJ looked unperturbed and rather too casual about the dreadful AIDS that was such a nightmare to so many. Indeed, a rather unconvincing smile betrayed some underlying uncertainty. This meant that JJ was either uneducated about AIDS or was in serious denial. Either condition required careful professional handling; otherwise it could conceal deep-seated anxiety or intense stigma. I therefore recommended further counselling and referred him to Alice Akola our AIDS specialist counsellor.

I requested Alice to spend a little more time than usual educating JJ about AIDS, in addition to explaining the whole procedure and implications of undertaking an HIV test. He initially declined the counselling, arguing that he was psychologically prepared for the test and did not see the need for the lengthy procedure. "Counselling is not just about allaying anxiety," I explained to the rather unconvinced JJ. "It includes sharing and learning more about AIDS. It empowers one to approach issues related to AIDS from a position of knowledge. The counsellor has more time than me to talk to you at length, and will also answer any questions you might have," I added, hoping that this would convince him to accept and attend the counselling session. "At the end of it all, it gives you a chance to finally decide whether you like to proceed with the HIV test or not," I explained further, in an effort to make it very clear that HIV testing was voluntary. Repeated nods signalled his acceptance.

After about an hour and half, in a series of counselling sessions, a more cheerful JJ was back with a report that said he was ready for the test. A blood sample was taken, and he was told to return for results in a few days' time. At the time we did not have the rapid testing kits that provide same-day results That evening a much calmer Mrs Schmitt called to thank me for seeing JJ and wanting to know when the results would be out.

"How is he taking it?" I enquired.

"I think it was good that he got it all off his chest. He is much happier than I have seen him in a long time," Jeanne reported enthusiastically. "He is right now in his room, singing which I have not heard him do in a long time."

When JJ reported for his HIV test results, he thought it was just a matter of picking up the results, but was surprised that the process involved another intensive counselling session. However, he sailed through the session flawlessly. The report said he answered all the assessment questions very well and even asked a few constructive ones of his own. Then he was passed as ready and presented with his HIV blood test results. He was HIV positive.

He received the bad news calmly – almost emotionlessly. Another session of counselling started immediately. The counsellor took time to help him over the usually traumatic post test period. This part is known as "post-test counselling" and involves telling shattered people that there was life after a positive HIV test. It involves both individual and group counselling sessions. Group counselling helps people newly diagnosed with HIV immensely. They look around and see others suffering the same blow, and realise that they are not alone. Most people need all the help they can get to adjust to a new way of life. I have seen many people when faced with positive HIV results, break down and cry like babies. Yet those whose tears flow readily and freely are not necessarily the weak ones. I have known many with obvious manifestation of AIDS in absolute denial, hoping against hope or just deluding themselves that the symptoms are due to some other less ominous disease. I have witnessed people who flatly refuse to accept positive results, blaming laboratory errors, even if different laboratories confirmed the results. I have also seen people reacting in anger, blame and depression, while others accept the bad news with meek resignation or indifference. JJ seemed to fall in this last category.

Following the post-test counselling session with Alice, I once again met with JJ and explained his future ARV treatment and reassured him that he would be fine. He was given an appointment for further tests and possible treatment initiation. The unfretted JJ even managed a smile - a smile of relief, I presumed—as I explained that AIDS no longer meant a death sentence because highly effective drugs were increasingly becoming available. Though the AIDS drugs were very expensive, Dieter had reassured him of his job security, and promised to pay for his treatment. JJ appeared reassured.

After dropping JJ off at home Dieter returned to his job. JJ picked up his gardening tools, seemingly to resume his own work. However, an hour or so after leaving home Dieter received a hysterical call from his housemaid.

"Sir, something terrible has happened!" the maid said. "JJ has shot himself!" the terrified maid said hysterically. Apparently JJ had tricked the police guard and used his gun to kill himself.

As soon as I got the shocking news, I felt obliged to go to the Schmitt's house immediately to help them cope with the catastrophe, and to assist with the police and the crowd that would inevitably gather. I considered it a failure on our part that we did not counsel JJ well enough and take other measures to prevent the tragedy — though I could not immediately see how we could have done it any differently. I arrived at the scene just before the police. I took the opportunity to peep into the servant's room, where JJ's body lay. The now lifeless body of JJ, who only that very morning had been a model patient calmly receiving bad news and promising to live positively, was now unrecognisable. There was something else which was rather odd about the scene that I did not immediately take in. Then I saw it. It was the newspapers most of which were now blood soaked that had been spread everywhere. Apparently, even as he prepared for his death, the neat JJ had lived up to his reputation. He had taken extraordinary care to minimise the mess. I later learned from the housemaid that he had put on his Sunday-best suit and tie, polished his shoes and wrapped his head in a towel to minimise the splash of blood and scatter of flesh. After a scribbling note of farewell in his native Luo language, JJ apparently squatted in the corner, used a chair to steady the gun and pulled the trigger.

The police who arrived at scene immediately arrested their colleague, the hapless guard whose gun JJ had used. I felt sorry for the poor man. They then bundled JJ's body in the back of their truck, covered it with his blanket and a sheet of plastic and drove away. They promised to return later and interrogate the Schmitts.

As the news of the suicide spread, an irate mob consisting of JJ's relatives and curious passersby unaware of the circumstances surrounding the tragedy gathered. They soon constituted an unruly mob that quickly filled the narrow corridor outside the Schmitt's gate. Gossip was rife among the crowd, with all sorts of imagined and exaggerated details of the catastrophe. I learned that some whispered that it was the "hungry and angry white man who, in a rage, had shot his African cook because his lunch was late." In reaction some gullible thugs among them hurled insults at the bewildered Schmitts, accusing them of murder. Morose and reflective, I remained with them for most of the afternoon doing my best to help cool the tempers of the incensed relatives. When this did not succeed, we called the police who dispersed the irate crowd. A few more composed relatives remained to negotiate JJ's terminal benefits with the shell-shocked Schmitts.

During the negotiations, the puzzled Schmitts could not make out who JJ's real next of kin were. Everyone referred to him as a "son" or a "brother", as is common in African extended family traditions. However, the discussion once again took a startling turn when a woman with a young baby suddenly turned up claiming to be JJ's wife.

"I didn't know JJ was even married," the flushed Jeanne exclaimed.

"James never talked about a wife. That's unbelievable," Dieter uttered in amazement.

On the contrary, none of JJ's relatives seemed in the least surprised by this development.

"In fact there is another wife at home with children," the elder who was leading the negotiations remarked casually, and proceeded to request that any money due to JJ be paid to him and not the wife.

"What about the child?" Jeanne asked with increasing incredulity.

"That's for us to sort out," the elder replied.

As soon as I got back to the JCRC, I summoned Alice, the counsellor, to explain and go over the details of her counselling session with JJ. The counsellor was stunned to learn of his suicide and frantically sprang to the defensive, pleading that she had done nothing wrong.

"I followed the counselling procedure strictly and felt sure that he fulfilled the criteria for proceeding to the test," Alice pleaded in apparent despair.

"This is not a court of law," I said gently to reassure her. "All I am trying to do is to find out whether we can learn something from this tragedy so that the next HIV positive test does not end in the same way."

Alice and I went over the preceding events and carefully reviewed the methodology employed in counselling JJ. I found that the counsellor, consistent with her training, had concentrated on the recommended "Prevention and Living Positively" approach without discussing the life-saving antiretroviral treatment in detail. However, I found myself unable to fault her with regard to her conclusion that he was psychologically ready for voluntary counselling and testing. Indeed, when I had seen JJ briefly, soon after his test, he had appeared to have understood what a positive HIV test meant. When I had asked whether the options available to an HIV positive person had been discussed with him he had answered in the affirmative. Indeed, he had appeared to me to have come to terms with his condition. His calm face, gentle manner and great desire to please had masked his real state of mind. But then again, he had also managed to conceal his polygamous family from the Schmitts, despite living and working with them for a number of years.

This incident brought into focus counselling standards and issues surrounding AIDS. JJ died at the time when ARVs capable of transforming AIDS from a death sentence to a life sentence of living with HIV, had just been discovered. The first generation of counsellors in Uganda were trained to help patients to endure pain until death ended their misery. They were trained to guide patients into accepting the inevitability of death and to help them die a "dignified death". Counselling was more like guiding patients to die quietly, to somehow attenuate the stark reality that the slogan "live positively" shrouded. And for those who could see through the futility of it, alternative slogans were coined including, "death is for us all" and "dying with dignity is great," but in reality all AIDS slogans spelt nothing but doom.

Unlike in rich countries, at the time there were no prospects of AIDS drugs ever being the standard of care in Uganda or in other poor countries. The training syllabus for counsellors, almost exclusively funded by donors and external agencies or NGOs, had not been updated to incorporate new recommendations based on the latest scientific advances. Thus counsellors continued to be trained only to attenuate the anxiety associated with AIDS during the painful tottering towards death, instead of preparing patients for new effective drugs that would keep them alive and well. Meanwhile, in rich countries, AIDS was rapidly being transformed from a terminal illness to a manageable chronic disease. In Africa this message was muted. It was almost taboo to mention the new drugs to donors because it was alleged that their use was unfeasible to Africa. The old message that always projected AIDS as a death waiting to happen continued to be broadcast. Yet the scientific reality was different. This was the situation throughout the 1990s, until President George W. Bush announced the President's Emergency Program for AIDS Relief (PEPFAR) in January 2003.

The basic educational standard of many of the original AIDS counsellors was also generally rudimentary, as they were not really expected to accomplish much. Virtually anyone could become an AIDS counsellor irrespective of educational background or, more often, lack of it. In rich Western countries, hospital counsellors are qualified psychosocial support professionals specialising in human psychology and sociology and are able to carry out sophisticated patient assessment and tailor the best scientifically derived intervention. Such professionals did not exist in sufficient numbers and it would be unrealistic in the short term to expect this cadre of counsellors to emerge in a poor country like Uganda. However, the standards and training syllabus of counsellors should have been updated progressively in line with new advances.

When ARVs were introduced, they were initially accessible only to a tiny minority of AIDS patients. Counsellors then faced a tricky situation. Would they inform patients about life-saving AIDS drugs when they were generally inaccessible or would they continue to say that AIDS had no treatment? Would they continue to help patients to die peacefully, or switch to preparing them to live well and long? They had to be careful not to raise their clients' expectations yet at the same time, they had to inform the very few that could afford the exorbitant cost of ARV therapy that it saved lives. This was a delicate balancing act.

To metamorphose from a counsellor who prepared a patient for death to one who helped a patient to live a long and productive life was not easy. The new role required reasonable understanding of the new and sophisticated science of the HIV virus and ARV therapy. Yet it was difficult to convince either the counsellors or their trainers that the tables had been turned and that it was time for change. No-one initially pushed it too hard because in poor countries notorious for acute shortages of human resource it implied the necessity of recruiting and training new people for the new role. Secondly, the then existing counsellors were already comfortably ensconced in their roles and would not take kindly to a suggestion that they had to be replaced by better educated counsellors.

For far too long, the public was told that AIDS had no treatment or cure. In view of the new developments in AIDS care and treatment, it was necessary to go back and explain that AIDS still had no cure but could now be treated. It could be difficult to explain the difference between cure and treatment to lay persons. Partly because of inequitable access to ARVs, and concern that some people, who would confuse treatment with a cure, would engage in high-risk behaviour, some advocated that patients be kept ignorant of ARVs. Some donors expressed fear and concern that patients, once they realised how effective the new drugs were, would demand immediate access to the therapy. Some concerned public-sector workers agreed arguing that creation of a demand that could not be met would be problematic. Their logic was that if people were kept in the dark with regard to Antiretroviral Therapy (ART), then they would not miss it.

They were wrong.

The Rise of the Joter

Absence of AIDS treatment caused a cultural revolution in many African communities. HIV, as JJ's case demonstrates, has overthrown or changed thousands of years of established traditional practices of African tribes.

Although JJ died in Kampala the aftermath of his death was most severely felt almost 200 kilometres away, in the eastern Ugandan district of Tororo, bordering Kenya. Tororo is inhabited mainly by the Luo tribe that lives as far as the Western Nyanza region of Kenya along the shores of Lake Victoria. The Luo people are now world famous because of President Obama, whose father was a prominent member of this tribe.

As per Luo custom, JJ's body was transported to his home village in Tororo for burial. As the funeral got under way, the fate of his family, namely two wives and children came into sharp focus. What would become of them now that the breadwinner had died? The ancient Luo tradition prescribed that as soon as JJ's burial was over his two wives should be inherited by one of JJ's brothers. And if none was available, then the mantle would be passed on to one of the cousins.

Even before his burial, JJ's brothers would be expected to prepare for their new responsibilities. However, recently some changes with regard to such duties had emerged, to the chagrin of some diehard traditionalists. I gathered that according to Luo tradition, one of the first duties of the successful inheritor was to perform the traditional inaugural cleansing sexual intercourse that some inheritors in the past competed for and, when they won, very much looked forward to.

Widow inheritance, or *ter* as it is known in JJ's language, is an ancient tradition of his tribe, but it was facing great challenges in the era of AIDS. Many women were losing their husbands to AIDS, and were therefore likely to be infected too. This put their new inherited husbands at a high risk of HIV infection. In polygamous relationships this had a multiplier effect – a mechanism for spreading HIV. For that reason the practice of widow inheritance faced severe criticism and condemnation by the national AIDS control programmes in Uganda and throughout the region. Even the would-be inheritors who used to engage in competition to win the prized widows were becoming scared, so much so that some resorted to delegating their cultural duties to a *joter* – a sort of mercenary or commercial inheritor, who was willing to undertake the risky but otherwise usually pleasurable cleansing function on their behalf for a fee.

However, widow inheritance was not all about sex. Its main values were to be found in the stability and other important services it provided to the extended family and the community. The practice ensured that the bereaved widow and her family, especially young children, were cared for and provided for. It also kept the family together; the children would be brought up by a blood relative. JJ's wives and children would have a new husband and father to step in his shoes and maintain the family, despite the tragedy.

There were differing opinions, including that of Professor Ocholla Ayayo, an anthropologist at the University of Nairobi, who expressed his rather novel, if not controversial, views regarding this cultural practice. In a special report by Oscar Obonyo published in the Kenyan *Sunday Nation* newspaper in January 2006, Ayayo surprised many when he argued that far from being a conduit for the spread of AIDS, widow inheritance actually helped to prevent the spread of HIV infection.

"If a widow who is HIV positive gets a new husband as per tradition, she will only kill one man and probably his other wife if the inheritor is already married." In the Luo tribe, like many other African tribes, polygamy used to be the norm, though this had changed among various ethnic groups.

"Though an absurd philosophy, I think society should not mind one person being sacrificed for the sake of hundreds of others," the professor was quoted to have said. "The logic of this according to Ayayo, himself a Luo, who has studied widow inheritance and HIV/AIDS, is to have the "dangerous woman" confined," Oscar reported; a sort of quarantine.

At the time when the AIDS mortality rate was 100% and the hopelessness of the situation apparently worsening and no end to the carnage in sight, exploration of any options that could somehow help to alleviate the scourge – however strange – could not be dismissed readily. It seemed a desperate measure for a desperate situation. However, Ayayo's assessment was based on his tribe's culture, which was facing serious challenges because of a killer disease that was in the process of destroying an ancient cultural practice. Some people, perhaps a little too hastily, reportedly dismissed such views as based merely on selfish interests of "cultural warriors". However, his point was that some of the infected widows at large would put more lives at risk if they were forced by economic hardships to either become prostitutes or have multiple sexual relations with unsuspecting men.

Whatever line of argument one takes, one issue was abundantly clear. Without an AIDS cure, the age-old culture of widow inheritance predominant in many African cultures was being dealt a devastating blow from which it may never recover. Therefore many widows and families, previously guaranteed security and continuity within their extended families, faced an uncertain future.

Something to Believe in

Everybody wanna go to heaven, but nobody wanna die– Curtis Mayfield

My impromptu meeting with Richard Egadu, way back in 1997, lives lucidly in my mind. Right away, within a few minutes of our first meeting Richard made it clear that he was determined to do all that it would take to avoid what was obviously a hovering death threat, though I could clearly see that death was defiantly and inexorably heading his way.

Richard, aged about 45 years, was a successful lawyer. As I later gathered, his law practice was popular, as evidenced by a wide clientele including high-profile personalities and upmarket businesses. He had an excellent reputation for winning high-court cases. But law was not all that occupied him. He was also a successful businessman, with considerable investments and expertise in farming.

Like many busy workaholics, when he started falling sick, his immediate concern was not his health but his work and daily chores. As was often the case, AIDS had crept up on him insidiously and, all of a sudden, aggravated and struck him down — like a leopard trailing and finally pouncing on its prey. Initially he had not taken the illness seriously. In any case, all he could see were a few painless discoloured pimples on his skin. By the time he realised there was a problem serious enough to warrant consulting a doctor, it was far too late. Indeed, at that stage, he would have perhaps have done just as well to see a priest instead.

He told me that his illness had started with easy fatigability, but he attributed it to his heavy load of work. This was followed by progressive weight loss, but Richard explained it away to his increasingly concerned family and friends as merely due to erratic meals during the long hours he spent at work. He only allowed himself short, irregular breaks in between for hurried snacks. When he started feeling sleepy in his office he ascribed this to the late nights as he planned for the next day's activities. When he developed an itchy skin rash associated with dark-blue papules on his skin, he thought it was just a minor skin irritation that would soon clear. Finally, when he developed a high fever that necessitated hospitalisation, he thought it was just a simple case of malaria, requiring only a few days' bed rest before he would bounce back. Sadly, he was wrong.

Three days later the fever, having failed to improve led to his being admitted to Mulago Hospital. His doctor ordered a chest X-ray. This was rather unnerving because Richard realised that a chest X-ray was not a routine diagnostic test for a malaria attack. However, after exhaustive tests and examination, the doctors finally cracked the diagnosis. But it was worse news for Richard. The lung infiltrations found on X-ray examination were traced back to his skin's dark-blue bumps and to be sure, a biopsy confirmed the doctors' worst fears. Richard had Kaposi's sarcoma, an HIV-related cancer in advanced disseminated stage.

Richard hatched a plot to escape from hospital. As he was too weak to leave on his own, he involved his sister. She arranged for a taxi, which whisked him out of the hospital and brought him to my clinic, complete with an intravenous line in situ and an infusion bottle dangling by the side. As the anxious taxi driver parked by the entrance, his sister lifted the bottle and Richard mobilised all his remaining energy and staggered inside. No detailed examination was really necessary to ascertain that the new arrival was a critically sick man. Indeed, other waiting patients came to the same conclusion, and forgetting their own pain immediately made way for him to be seen first. He obviously needed emergency hospital readmission. It was also apparent that he was in great pain, but was just holding on by sheer grit.

Lifting his eyes with laboured efforts, he focussed on me. "I take it that you are Dr Mugyenyi," he whimpered wearily.

"Yes, but don't exert your efforts talking," I advised wondering why a patient in such a state was being rushed to a day clinic that was not equipped to handle casualties or very sick emergency cases. But he seemed to suddenly come back to life, his eyes lighting up.

"Are you Dr Mugyenyi?" He obviously wanted to be sure whom he was dealing with. This was a good sign, as it indicated that at least his faculties were still intact. "Yes," I answered as I helped him to lie down on the couch, and readjusted his intravenous fluid line to start it running again. "I have been trying to find you," he said.

After a few deep breaths, he painfully brought himself to a sitting position, and did something that neither his sister nor I, thought was possible. He smiled!

"Dr Mugyenyi, if this is really you, then I am sure I can't die," he said with a wide grin that exposed a dark nodule on the inner side of his lower lip. "I can't die!" he repeated, "because I know you have a cure." Obviously, throbs of pain had overwhelmed his courage, but failed to completely wipe out an apparent expression of hope — that the nightmare would soon be all over. But hope was transformed to disbelief when I advised him to return to hospital and continue with his treatment there. He refused outright. Of course I could understand his plight. All he could remember about being in hospital was getting worse. His chances of survival in Mulago, where they had no treatment for AIDS, must have appeared to him to be utterly hopeless.

"Over my dead body," he swore, as he slumped back on the couch with unconcealed disappointment. "It is AIDS that is killing me," he pleaded. "And I know you are the only person who can cure AIDS!" he added imploringly.

I was in a fix. I realised that I had to spend a little more time with the new patient, trying to understand his problem so that I could find a way of helping him. The session lasted longer than I had planned as he took me by surprise by what he wanted to get off his chest. I was concerned about the other patients waiting to see me but he seemed to go on and on trying to explicate what would be at stake if he died.

"If I die lots of things will go wrong," he started his explanation, interspersed with barely audible groans of pain. "You must therefore do everything in your power to prevent this threatening death," he concluded in a progressively weakening voice. It was as if AIDS, the relentless killer of everyone it attacked, could somehow be persuaded to make him an exception – if only he presented his special case well.

Despite the pain, Richard surprised me further by his insistence on ruminating over some of the highlights of his eventful life, almost oblivious to the stark odds against him. It was like he did not want the story to die with him. I was to be his insurance. He was adamant that he had to narrate it to me, despite my rising impatience to hurry through the session and rush him back to hospital. His breathing was a little laboured and I worried it could get worse. I kept him a little longer so that I could stabilise him before accompanying him back to Mulago Hospital.

During the time I spent with him at the clinic and taking him back to hospital, Richard never stopped talking. He talked of his marriage to his childhood sweetheart, with whom he had five children. Apologetically, he explained that he had initially been faithful to her, but circumstances changed when he became prosperous and found that younger girls were attracted to him, or more likely to "my bank account", as he explained jokingly. I would have loved to meet this man when he was still in good health. I am sure I would have enjoyed listening to his jokes. "One thing led to another," he explained, "and whether by design or accident, one of my girlfriends found that she was pregnant. And as I could afford it I felt obliged to take her up as a second wife. Was I wrong to do this, Doctor?" I did not reply. My job was to ease his pain.

His second wife was pregnant again, expecting their second baby. Richard was not sure how he got infected with HIV but suspected one of his past girlfriends, who had died a few years earlier, following a lengthy relationship with him.

On yet another sentimental and emotional note, he talked about his old and frail mother back in the village in eastern Uganda. "To me, my mother is a special hero," he said. "We are all most indebted to our mothers," I interjected, trying without success to cut the conversation short so that I could get him back to hospital quickly. "My father died when I was little. In fact I don't remember anything about him. Yet my peasant mother who never remarried purely for my sake, brought me up with my sister single-handedly, and sacrificed so much to educate us," he said. "Now that I have some resources, this illness wants to rob me of a chance to show my appreciation to my mother. I had planned a special treat for her, so that she could at least spend her last years in some sort of comfort to compensate her for the long years of scratching the earth for my sake," he sobbed.

Composed once more, he talked briefly of a farm that he owned, 20 km outside Kampala and worried that if he died no one would take care of his farm animals as well as he did. Perhaps it was the lawyer in him that made him talk as if death could be deterred if he pleaded extenuating circumstances or advanced some imperative reasons why it should be kept at bay. Oh, how Egadu wanted to ward off the rude spoiler!

As soon as I could get in a word in, I explained to him that of the two diseases, cancer treatment took priority over AIDS therapy because cancer posed a more immediate threat to his life. I informed him that unless the evidently advanced cancer was treated first or concurrently with AIDS, there was little chance for recovery and the sooner he resumed treatment the better. He seemed to get the point and ultimately accepted my advice, though half-heartedly. He resigned himself to being readmitted to hospital. I stayed with him until he was readmitted in the private medical ward, and promised to keep checking on him.

The next day, I woke up worried about him. I was planning a follow-up visit to the hospital to see him, when I was jolted by a death announcement on one of Kampala's FM radio stations. Though he had been very sick I had not expect, him to die so soon — at least not that very night. Reflecting on his death later brought memories of so many other shattered dreams and the human resources with great potential that were being lost to AIDS daily. I gathered later from the grapevine that Richard had also harboured some political ambitions. Some people talked about an aura of excitement that had built up in his home village as news of his impending candidature for a political office filtered through. His fellow tribesmen expected much of him and his death had wider implications. Two young women lost a husband and six children (and one on the way) had just become orphaned, to add to over one million others in the country. Loss of a father would drastically change the children's lives and greatly impact on their future achievements. A devoted sister had lost a brother, while an ailing mother had lost her only son and provider. The village lost a promising politician who would have possibly introduced developmental programmes in his constituency aimed at breaking the poverty trap. A brilliant lawyer was lost to the profession.

Richard's untimely death was just one of the millions of losses to Uganda and the African continent. His death also reminded me of the many other valuable people including some leading intellectuals and academics. The carnage swallowed Ugandan pioneer journalists, seasoned generals, civil servants, and even the clergy. I recall a distressed eulogy by one bewildered man at the funeral of one prominent academic. "Oh God! Why are you doing this to us? Why do you select only our very best," he lamented. "We have among us some really bad characters and rogues, yet you persistently sidestep them and take those we so desperately need like this one. If at all you do not know who the bad guys are, we are ready to point them out to you," he concluded as he scanned the mammoth crowd of mourners as if to start the identification of the rascals who should have died instead.

Without a cure or life-prolonging medicine, the end to the carnage was nowhere in sight. To further underscore the magnitude of the disaster with respect to the extent of the loss of much-needed trained people, I once asked a Makerere University graduate of the class of 1979 to tell me how many of his 65 or so classmates had died of presumed AIDS by the year 2005, when they would have been expected to be at their productive peak. Fast and furious, he started rattling off names of the dead he could immediately recall. Then, suddenly, catching his breath, he stopped. "Let's just put it the other way round," he finally said after a rather lengthy meditative pause. "I am not suggesting that I know the exact whereabouts of everyone, but right now I can only account for only five of us – alive!"

Confusing the Bug

Brian Bwoba's contemporaries at university – those who were still alive – were in agreement that he was a character they all loved to hate. They remembered him with awe as a brilliant student who was not shy to openly brag about his achievements. One of his classmates, struggling to maintain the high academic standards set by the college, recalls an occasion when Bwoba taunted the class saying that everyone else needed to burn the midnight oil. "You are all far behind my standards, and I don't like to pass the examinations alone," he boasted. "At least, I need a few classmates to liven up the graduation celebrations," Bwoba rubbed it in.

True to his word, Bwoba sailed through the exacting Veterinary School programme with flying colours and looked set for greater things professionally, possibly ending up as a highly successful specialist. Indeed, for the first five years following his graduation, Bwoba's career promised to fulfil his peers' predictions. Within two years after graduation, he married a well-educated woman from a prominent family. He seemed ready to settle down and concentrate on his career. However, tides of unforeseen events were to first swing him high and then low over the subsequent fifteen years, finally leaving him in an unimaginable situation.

I learned later that his change of fortune could be traced back to a time in mid-1984, when his long-standing mistress died of what was whispered to be AIDS. As Bwoba later confessed, her untimely death scared him and paralysed him in a nightmarish limbo for a long time. Despite his macho profile, Bwoba had a soft side too. Although he cheated on her, he still cared for his wife. "But at the same time I feared the worst," he said.

What appeared to be confirmation of his worst fears came only a few months after the death of his mistress, in the form of a vague febrile illness characterised by a skin rash, diarrhoea and fever. Although all indications were that he had malaria, Bwoba, whose veterinary training made it easier for him to understand human diseases, noted that diarrhoea and skin rash were not typically associated with malaria, but were more commonly the presenting symptoms of the dreaded AIDS. This, on top of his past exposure, had left him in no doubt as to his fate.

Polygamy or keeping a concubine besides a wife was a common practice, especially among the well-to-do like Bwoba, who could afford the cost of maintaining two homes. In fact, in Uganda, significant numbers of the early cases of AIDS outside the epicentre of Rakai were among the professionals and the well-to-do who had the wherewithal to support promiscuous lifestyles.

After the shock of his mistress's death, Brian started to view his precarious situation differently. He did not want his family to be part of it. It was his cross for him to carry alone. He reasoned that his continued marriage would serve no useful purpose and that his best chance for survival was to go it alone. "I had to be cruel in order to be kind to my wife," he explained. He therefore abandoned the wife, and started a long solo battle of self-preservation. As a prelude to the separation, it was alleged that he spread a clandestine rumour that his wife had not been faithful during their marriage. However, it is more likely that he assumed that she would inevitably also be infected with HIV. Badmouthing her, if the whispers were to be believed, could merely have been his mean premeditated alibi to absolve him of any blame if she came down with fully blown AIDS in the future.

Many of Bwoba's friends complained about his loose tongue; he became notorious for disclosing his friends' secrets. But it eventually backfired, and could have been a factor in the downward fortunes of his business enterprise. One specific case I was told about concerned a man who confided in him after being diagnosed with HIV. Later that same evening, Bwoba met a relative of the man at a beer party and leaked the story. The man who had confided in him had planned and practised how to break the bad news to his wife gently, but he found total pandemonium at home. The wife was sobbing inconsolably. She already knew the diagnosis!

Without a known cure for AIDS, Bwoba developed a unique survival strategy and adopted a regimented lifestyle aimed at "defeating the bug", as he liked to put it. The counsellors had advised him to adopt a healthy lifestyle so as to strengthen his immunity and keep him healthy for as long as possible. Bwoba saw this as a lifeline. But he probably pushed it to the extreme. First of all, he gave up alcohol and partying even though he enjoyed drinking. He started on measured daily exercises, and set out a timetable for regular special meals. He designed a special supplemental therapeutic diet consisting of raw cabbages, carrots, spinach, tomatoes and cucumbers, which he liquefied and homogenised in a blender and drank liberally several times a day. The former South African health minister who earned the nickname of Dr Beetroot, for promoting vegetables as AIDS treatment, would have been impressed. The concoction did not exactly taste great but, then again, it was a medicine that had to be tolerated as long as it provided the vital vitamins and antioxidants to help his body to fight the feared virus in the blood. Indeed, his recipe seemed to work well for him. He felt stronger and healthier and this encouraged him to persist with the therapy. In fact he started recommending it to other people living with HIV/AIDS. But, to his disappointment, none of them did as well as he did. He attributed this to poor adherence as many who tried the insipid health drink found it virtually impossible to maintain.

Bwoba kept his ears to the ground, keenly following new and emerging scientific advances in the treatment of AIDS. Three major developments had a great effect on him. The first was the discovery of Zidovudine, or AZT as it became to be more widely known in the late 1980s. Bwoba became one of the first Ugandans to access this very first and novel ARV drug. The new treatment made many people feel fine in the short term but worse in the long term. After a brief period of improvement, many would feel lethargic, followed by muscle aches and then they go on to develop constant headache. The worst scenario was severe anaemia, which was often life threatening. It is not clear whether Bwoba suffered these side effects but toxic effects of high-dose AZT, and the discovery that the drug did not by itself prolong life, left many patients including Bwoba disappointed but without a substitute.

The second remedy that Bwoba embraced enthusiastically was an interferon-based drug claimed by a Kenyan doctor to be an AIDS cure. It was named aptly Kemron, with *Ke* standing for Kenya. President Moi reportedly celebrated the Kenyan discovery, but warned the people not to overindulge in sex because of the breakthrough. Other than flu-like symptoms, this drug turned out to be much better tolerated than AZT, and indeed Bwoba had no problems when he started taking it. Besides using the drug for his own treatment, Bwoba became one of the agents of the company that supplied the "wonder drug" to wealthy AIDS-infected Ugandans. On the business side, Kemron turned into a money spinner and Bwoba became a wealthy man. He often confided in his friends how the drug had saved his life. His example encouraged many to dig deeper in their pockets to pay for the pricey drug. Bwoba believed at the time that Kemron was effective against AIDS. However, he was at a loss to explain the apparent lack of improvement among the patients of the doctors to whom he supplied it. The only plausible explanation he could think of was, again, poor adherence. The drug was so expensive that many patients had to interrupt therapy as they raised funds or sold their possessions to pay for it.

One woman who lost several of her sisters to AIDS told me of her family's experience with Kemron. Her sister who had lost a husband to AIDS was desperately sick. Her doctor prescribed Kemron, and advised her to buy it from Bwoba's pharmacy. She had to sell household items until there was nothing left in the home to sell except the family car. Early 1990s cars were very expensive. But within a couple of months the money was all finished and yet the patient's condition was worse. Soon after, she died. The reason why this woman and other AIDS patients who used Kemron never improved was discovered in 1992, when results of research sponsored by the World Health Organisation carried out at Mulago Hospital to determine its efficacy were released.

The study coordinator was Prof Elly Katabira and the independent data and safety monitoring team, which was based in London included Prof Janet Derbyshire. The study was blinded to ensure that neither the researchers nor study monitors knew to which arm of the study any individual participant belonged. Half of the participants were randomly distributed to a group that received Kemron and the other to another arm that received a placebo — tablets that looked like the real Kemrom tablets but without any active ingredient, to serve as a control.

As the study progressed, the monitoring team observed that some of the study participants were showing evidence of improvement, but it was just marginal. They let the study run its course because at the time there was no alternative therapy and any little effect suspected to be a result of a test drug was always considered worth examining further. Secondly there were no serious side effects to worry about. However, when the results were finally un-blinded by revealing the patients' randomisation code, it was found that those showing the occasional improvement were mainly among those who had received the placebo! It was therefore clear that Kemron was totally useless. But the producers and peddlers of the hopeless drug had already ripped off thousands of desperate AIDS patients. This study was also memorable for another wrong reason. It became politicised. As Kenya claimed that their scientist discovered it, it was seen as the first African AIDS drug discovery. Some overzealous activists claimed that European vested interests were out to sabotage an innovative discovery simply because it had been discovered by an African.

From the early 1990s new ARV drugs were developed and Bwoba tried them all as soon as they appeared on the market. Then, in 1995 when triple therapy or Highly Active Antiretroviral Therapy (HAART) which was to revolutionise AIDS therapy, was discovered, Bwoba was again one of the very first Ugandans to access the new therapy. As it was at the time extremely expensive, it was Bwoba's turn to put his properties up for sale. Soon his entire Kemron boom was no more. By the end of five years of therapy he was a bankrupt, sick man. However, the ever-resourceful Bwoba devised his own way out of the dilemma. He developed his own treatment regime that he called a strategy to "confuse the virus". All three drugs were recommended to be taken together but Bwoba did something stupid instead. He used them in series as a cost-saving measure.

"I don't care what anyone says," he rationalised his unorthodox method of treatment, "just imagine the bug, meeting a different kind of enemy every day for three days and then the cycle starts all over again."

As far as was known at the time, this was a disastrous way to use ARVs, as resistance would quickly develop and render all the component drugs ineffective. Sheer terror and desperation drove Bwoba to this weird reasoning. Even with this bizarre strategy the drugs remained too costly, and Bwoba resorted to borrowing money from family and friends. When news spread that he was not paying his debts these sources dried up too.

Finally, by 1998, Bwoba had exhausted all the options he could think of. It appeared to be the end of the road for him after 15 years of "heroic" struggle. For the first time since the unfortunate events had started, he stared defeat in the face. He started thinking the unthinkable – the real possibility of death. AIDS was finally winning but it had been a good fight. In retrospect, he found it ironic that he had lost the battle at the time when effective therapy was finally available. Now he had nowhere to turn, his energy drained, his physical condition at its worst ever, and his fighting spirit numbed. It was time to prepare to meet his maker, but before that Bwoba had one more card to play — the last card.

In March 1999 Bwoba, in desperation approached me for help. He narrated his long valiant fight against AIDS and how he had outwitted death by keeping it at bay for so long, and in the process outliving so many. He was apparently proud of his prowess that had made it possible for him to achieve the unachievable. He lamented that he could have lived on but impoverishment had finally done him in. He claimed that his situation was now looking up and that he had a business deal in the pipeline that would soon solve his financial crisis. So all he wanted was some very short-term help with drugs to keep him going for a little while. I scrambled for some funds to assist him temporarily while he sorted out his crisis.

As Bwoba had confessed to improper use of the drugs in the past, I needed to know the state of his latest laboratory tests including CD4 cells and viral load so that I could advise him on the best drugs combination and the proper way to use them.

"I don't know my CD4," he replied.

"When was the last time you had the tests done?" I asked.

"I've never done any," he answered as I stared at him, flabbergasted.

Sensing my surprise he hastened to add, "As you know, although I am not a medical doctor we study more or less the same in veterinary medicine.

I am a good vet clinician," he laboured to explain, "and I have all this time relied on clinical judgement and signs for my own hitherto successful therapy for over fifteen years," he bragged.

"My own therapy has done wonders for me. All those who got infected at the same time as I did are dead."

"At least you must have done the Elisa," I said, just to pull his leg.

"No," he replied casually.

"What!" I exclaimed, stunned.

Elisa is the very first test done to determine whether someone is infected with HIV. Incredibly, Bwoba had never undergone a basic HIV test! He had simply diagnosed himself to be HIV-infected, based on some vague symptoms that he suspected to be HIV-related, and had gone on to treat himself for almost fifteen years!

"I cannot give you any more AIDS drugs unless I have documented evidence of a positive HIV test," I mumbled, trying to control my rising fury. "Furthermore, without CD4 and viral load tests you may be wasting your money by taking drugs that may no longer be working for you," I went on to admonish him.

Basically, a CD4 test helps the doctor to monitor the progress of the patient. A desirable treatment outcome is a steady rise in CD4. On the other hand, the viral load test measures the suppression of virus copies in blood. The optimum outcome is a level below detection. Treatment failure is associated with the reverse outcome, whereby CD4 declines, and a rise in HIV viral copies in the blood. Treatment failure may mean that drug resistance has set in. If failure is detected in good time, the drugs are changed and replaced with effective ones. Delay in diagnosing treatment failure may result in such severe drug resistance that future drugs may be ineffective. As this is basic AIDS care, I really did not expect this level of incompetence from a scientist.

"Everyone told me how brilliant you were at school. What's happened to you, man? You talked of confusing the bug, but I can now see that you confused yourself instead," I cajoled him. "Anyway, the bottom line is this: no tests, no drugs. With no plausible explanation forthcoming, I asked him to undergo all HIV tests, so that I could start with him from a new beginning, and ensure that he got proper treatment.

Bwoba underwent all the tests, including the Elisa test, Western Blot and the more sophisticated state-of-the art Polymerase Chain Reaction (PCR), otherwise known as viral load.

All the test results returned with a unanimous verdict: Bwoba had never been infected with HIV!

His Lordship's Mistress

The telephone call from Deogratious Bafara (not his real name), the mayor of an upcountry town, found me in the midst of mid-morning rush time at work, but he insisted that he had to talk to me, because the matter was of the utmost urgency. Besides, he explained "it would only take a minute". Apparently, the matter was too confidential to discuss over the phone. I asked him whether the subject matter was medical or not. "It's a bit of both," he replied.

When I met him that evening, he was accompanied by an attractive, fashionably-dressed woman in her late twenties or early thirties. She was composed and rather talkative. Mayor Bafara, more commonly known as Deo, explained his predicament briefly. His mistress and companion, whom I shall call Vicki Mukuzi, was pregnant. But their main concern was that at a routine antenatal screening carried out the previous day, Vicki had been found to be HIV positive. This kind of situation was very common in my practice. Almost instinctively I started explaining the current options, available to a pregnant HIV-infected woman.

"First of all Vicki needs to have a confirmatory HIV test. Secondly we shall need to plan for the safety of the baby on the way," I explained, trying to keep my explanations as simple as possible. I recommended to her the Prevention of Mother to Child Transmission (PMTCT) treatment, which uses ARV drugs to reduce chances of passing on HIV infection from mother to her baby. "This preventive intervention has almost eliminated the transmission of HIV to babies in rich countries," I added enthusiastically. "Since you can afford it, you have an excellent chance of giving birth to an HIV-free baby," I concluded, trying to be as reassuring as possible.

I had thought that the prospect of an uninfected baby would cheer them up. However, to my dismay, neither Deo nor Vicki seemed interested in what I was trying to explain to them. I had presumed that they had talked matters over and had come to some understanding. However, I could sense that the atmosphere was one of unease and, quite evidently, communication between the two and between them and me was not flowing well.

"Could I see you alone?" Vicki finally broke the silence, as she signalled to Deo to leave the room. As soon as the door closed behind him, the reasons for the frosty atmosphere became apparent. She burst out in a harangue of bitterness and venom, exposing the extent of her ill feelings towards her partner.

"This man is evil! Evil! Evil!" she said, as tears flowed freely down her cheeks. "My friends told me that he has infected so many women with HIV, that he qualifies to be called a mass murderer!" she said between sobs. "Now I have become his latest victim." She then dashed to the door to make sure that it was locked securely for extra privacy.

"Now, however, his killing spree is over." she said on her way back. "He has finally met his match — and I have extra hands too," she added as she patted her chest for emphasis. "You know new elections are due next year and his political opponents have heard of my plight, and are working with me to finish him off – first politically and then legally in courts of law," she said, with unconcealed hatred. "I have a cousin who lives in Europe who was also infected by him. When Deo got to know about it, he just dumped her. She is back in the country on holiday and will be one of the witnesses who will give evidence against him."

Evidently, the flamboyant mayor was in trouble. I did not know what to make of his lover's allegations. But, first and foremost, my duty as a doctor was to attend to a patient in distress. The woman needed psychological support so that she could handle the complex situation and make informed decisions. Accordingly, I advised that she needed to give priority to issues of her immediate concern –her pregnancy - and come to terms with her HIV positive sero-status. She had to start to learn to "live positively" with the virus permanently integrated into her body and start planning for the baby on the way.

"Involving people with a political vendetta and mixing it with personal medical and psychological issues, could make things worse," I counselled.

However, the irate Vicki was neither in the mood nor state of mind for lectures. "Give me a break, Doctor! Don't you see that this man is evil? I will avenge my ruined future and the suffering of many other women," she fumed, leaving me in no doubt that her resolve was resolute. I tried to calm her down without success. On the contrary, whatever I said about Deo seemed to infuriate her more.

"Deo is only helping me until I have an abortion, after that he will be off. It is his name that he is concerned about, his reputation, he says. What about mine? What about that of the many other victims? How long can his deadly misadventures be allowed to go on?"

Vicki was sobbing uncontrollably. Considering the circumstances, I could understand her feelings, and I allowed her time to work through her emotional outburst. Suddenly she seemed to get an idea that appeared to restore her composure a little.

"You said that I needed to have another test, didn't you, Doctor? I want him tested too. Right here and together with me. I want his results, and once I have them in my hands I will take hold of him by his AIDS-nested balls and feed him to the hyenas," she said as she dashed to the door, her face contorted by anger.

She was back in a flash with the hapless His Lordship Deo in tow – but what a transformation! Vicki was all smiles, her face fully restored to its natural beauty. "Darling, the doctor wants us to take a test together so that he can help both of us," Vicki said sweetly. This double-crossing schemer was trying to compromise my professional independence and transform me into her accomplice. I was having none of it.

"Look, Vicki, testing is voluntary and results are confidential to the individual unless he chooses otherwise," I admonished her.

"Do we have secrets between us Deo darling?"

Deo, on the other hand, seemed totally resigned to his fate. "What's the point of the test?" Deo asked emotionlessly. "If you are infected, then I am infected too," he said to Vicki.

"I think that Vicki is right in this case," I interjected. "Both of you need to be tested but each one of you has to decide whether you share the results or not," I advised conscious of Vicki's scheme. But she was insistent.

"Darling, we have to stick together at this difficult time," she said. Clearly, I had a dilemma. While patients were entitled to their privacy, I too had my rights, as a doctor and as an individual, which I had to protect. I could therefore not allow Vicki to exploit me for her nefarious ends. I needed to maintain a balanced position. I explained to both of them the advantages and possible pitfalls of testing and getting results together. "Usually I recommend that couples who test together, get their results together," I said. Then I brought up the issue of possible blame, but Vicki said that it would not happen in their case. "You trust me, don't you Deo?" she asked seductively. "Absolutely," Deo answered.

"It still remains my duty to inform you that before you commit yourselves to sharing results you need to be absolutely sure that you are prepared for any eventualities and that you can handle any public exposure by your partner," I said to Deo in anticipation of the looming crisis. "Before I proceed with the tests, I would like both of you to see a professional counsellor. This is a routine practice that ensures that all aspects of HIV/AIDS are fully understood." Initially they both refused to see the counsellor but I finally prevailed on them to accept.

When it came to doing their HIV test, I insisted, despite Vicki's protestations, that I would give out the results to each one individually and it would be left to them to decide whether to share or not, or even come in together to discuss the results with me. The arrangement was agreed, blood samples were taken, coded in their presence and dispatched to the laboratory. An appointment for the next day was made and the couple left hand in hand, like newlyweds in love on their way to their honeymoon. I was to learn later from Vicki that they spent that night together, and made love without a condom.

The next evening they were early for their appointment and much more relaxed than they had been the previous chaotic evening. Was this the sexual healing often talked about? When it came to getting results it was decided among the two that it would be ladies first. Vicki made sure the door was securely locked and then sat down calmly. The first impression that the couple had kissed and made up was soon wiped out of my mind. Vicki was not concerned about her results, which in fact confirmed that she was indeed HIV infected, but had only hatred and revenge on her mind.

"I've an interview with the newspaper to expose Deo today," she said. "Give me his results," she demanded menacingly. "I need to announce it to the press!" she added.

"Please don't draw me into your ugly wrangles," I pleaded with her. "Exposing him means exposing yourself as well. Besides, it may not go entirely according to your plans. It may even backfire on you," I counselled despairingly, as it was clear that absolutely nothing I could do would change the unwavering Vicki's determination. "This action in itself does not solve the other problems," I persisted, trying to get her to put her wisdom above her emotions. "Now that you are HIV positive you will be positive for the rest of your life, and this is not the way to begin to come to terms with a lifetime condition," I added, hoping that these facts would somehow open her stubborn mind to the reality.

"Lifetime, you said? What about the one who gave me the life sentence? I presume you would like me to say thanks to him instead," she retorted with sarcastic bitterness.

"These days we have good medicines that greatly reduce the chances of your baby being born with HIV," I said, once more trying to give her something positive to think about.

"Don't be absurd," she interjected. "I can't carry his bastard. I've an appointment for an abortion this evening," she confided.

"I strongly advise you against abortion. I tell you, you can get an uninfected baby."

"I want his results. Have you seen them?" she asked, ignoring my unsolicited advice and sticking to her guns.

"No they are still sealed, just like yours were, and I can only open them in his presence, alone, as we agreed."

"Well he is stinking sick anyway. This was a waste of your testing chemicals. The brute has been infecting women for over ten years now, and remains unrepentant," she spat. "Though it is too late for me, I will at least save the lives of other unsuspecting women by having him locked up," she added.

"I would like you to see the counsellor again," I said to her, hoping that the counsellor would help her to better understand her situation and take informed decisions. "No! I am through with counsellors," she said.

"Well, if he had any doubt about his status, why did he sleep with me last night without protection, fully aware that I had tested positive?" she asked rhetorically. This surprised me too, but it was not an entirely new situation to me. I had encountered quite a few men who would do exactly the same without blinking. Not infrequently some would get away with it, because not every sexual encounter with an infected person results in HIV transmission to the uninfected partner.

"Look here Doctor, I have lived a disciplined life. I have, over the years been having regular medical checkups and each time testing negative, until this man came into my life. I will wait for him outside while you give him his results," she announced finally after a brief uneasy silence. "But keep your eyes open, you will see sparks - promise!"

On that note Vicki marched out, slamming the door behind her and leaving me totally bemused. A frightened and humbled Deo staggered in and slumped into the chair. There was a lingering smell of stale alcohol in his breath and his eyes were red and tired, indicating paucity of sleep. Over the last 24 hours Deo had aged noticeably. The fiery mayor had no fight left in him. If only his town residents could see their "indomitable" mayor who harangued his opponents on the campaign trails in this state, they would not believe their eyes. Vicki was now in total control and could get out of Deo whatever she needed.

But Deo believed he still had one more card up his sleeve left to play. Even at this late hour, the renowned womaniser still hoped that he would charm his way out of Vicki's web.

"I will take her out a couple of times, and give her a special treat," Deo announced his nifty plan aimed at disarming his treacherous lover, "I am sure this will cool her down. You know how women are."

However, from the little I had seen of Vicki's spleen, I remained unconvinced that Deo's prowess with women, however legendary, would triumph on this occasion.

I had made it a routine practice to open HIV results envelopes in the presence of patients, after careful verification of the code number and crosschecking to confirm the identity in order to minimise the possibility of any doubt that sometimes arises afterwards. Human nature is often tilted towards optimism even in totally hopeless situations. Perhaps, it is some sort of survival instinct. Experience had taught me to appreciate that people needed all the help they could get to come to terms with HIV-positive results. To see is to believe. I found that participating in opening an HIV results envelope is part of an effective counselling strategy.

Deo's HIV results were negative!

Deo and I stared at the laboratory report and then back at each other with disbelief. After all that had been said and done! Surely, there was a mistake somewhere. Occasionally, laboratory results get mixed up, and sometimes false negatives are reported. I carefully went over the report with a fine tooth comb, checking the date, the time when the sample was taken and the clinic registration number. There was nothing amiss. The results definitely belonged to Deo. Meanwhile Deo, as if in a trance, stared fixedly into space seemingly detached from his surroundings.

"It looks like, we have a slight problem here," I said, but successfully jolting him to attention. "I mean, the negative results may not mean a negative result." I attempted to explain, hoping that the bemused Deo could somehow understand this rather ambiguous, if not garbled talk. This raised his eyebrows, begging for an explanation. "Even if this is a true negative, it refers to your sero-status as of yesterday," I said as I tried to look for a sign that Deo was taking in my explanation, but he appeared to be in a daze.

"Well Doctor," he said at length, "there must be a mistake somewhere. After all this exposure, including last night, I believe I am infected."

"There is what we call discordant couples, whereby one partner can remain uninfected for a long time despite frequent sexual exposure," I explained, "and in your case this seems to be the situation."

At that juncture, the door burst open. It was Vicki! We had been too absorbed in discussion about the intricate matter at hand to keep track of time.

"What is taking you so long Doctor? Giving Deo a shoulder to cry on— eh? He can't really be surprised by his result…"

"Vicki, we have a slight problem," I quickly chipped in, trying to prepare her for the full explanation. During my discussion with Deo, he had insisted that I be the one to break the news to Vicki and I had agreed. After all it was my job, even though it was not always pleasant. The situation I faced was based on the people's mistaken belief that having sex with an HIV-infected person inevitably resulted in transmission of the disease. Deo and Vicki needed professional explanation to unravel their sticky situation. I had to make sure that Vicki understood, but somehow, I botched it.

"About Deo's HIV test," I plodded on, tentatively, but Vicki cut me short.

"You knew what the result would be, didn't you Doctor? Why are you pretending to be surprised?"

"Yes, but …" I tried to get a word in, but she interrupted me again.

Vicki was so sure that Deo's test would be positive, she couldn't understand why I was hesitating. Then she realised something was amiss.

"What are you trying to tell me?" she shrieked. She did not give me a chance to explain any further.

"You fake Doctor," she shouted, "you conspired with this crook to doctor the results. Is that what you are trying to tell me?" she shouted as she banged her bag on the table. Turning to Deo she said, "As for you, I have bad news. I have already taken the matter to the Criminal Investigation Department (CID) of the Police. No tricks will save you this time."

"Just listen to me for a moment Vicki, I beg you," I said. The word "beg" must have done the trick.

"Why don't you have the tests repeated in other laboratories so that you are absolutely sure?" Vicki pondered the issue.

"All right" she agreed, sensing the advantage. "Deo, let's go and get tested from a reputable laboratory," she said as she gave him a light shove. The battered Deo, who appeared hesitant, glanced in my direction with beseeching eyes. I nodded reassuringly. He slowly arose from the chair as if the act pained him. Vicki led the crestfallen mayor out of my clinic like a dog on a leash.

It was the last time I saw Vicki, but I was to witness her fireworks – or "sparks", as she had promised - unfold against Deo in the print media. But as I had warned, it did not all go entirely according to her design. Deo visited the next day to inform me that the second test was also negative. He blamed me for not having been clear in explaining to Vicki that he was not HIV infected.

"You left room for doubt in your explanation. If you had been emphatic, very strongly emphatic, it would have saved me this entire predicament," he complained. "She has dragged me to the CID, and I am now under intensive investigation. They have ordered more HIV tests and we are going for them tomorrow," Deo said in a sorry voice.

"Your lady never gave me a chance to explain." I pleaded in self-defence. "And the fact that she is proceeding with the case despite the second negative test means that whatever I said would not have made any difference." Deo seemed to agree with this line of reasoning, as evidenced by his nod. But at the back of my mind I kept wondering whether there could have been some other, better way of handling her.

"Anyway, at the moment no one can say for sure that you are not infected," I explained, as Deo suddenly shifted to the edge of the chair apparently rattled by the unexpected comment. He had obviously started to believe that he was home and dry, only to get a rude awakening. "Since you had unprotected sex only the other day, it will take up to three months before I can say for sure that you are not infected." Deo stared at me. "Provided also, that you do not get any more exposures in the meantime," I added.

After a meditative pause, Deo seemed to gather courage to accept the reality. This appeared to finally settle this issue, at least for a while. With a worried expression, Deo left to sit out the time.

Three months later, a visibly slimmed-down Deo was back for his final test to determine his HIV status. He confessed that the three months of waiting had felt more like a decade. The CID had mercilessly interrogated him over and over again and demanded laboratory tests after tests. His political opponents pursued him relentlessly. With Vicki's help his opponents had produced a number of women of dubious repute some of whom Deo had never set eyes on, all claiming to have had affairs and been infected by him.

I asked Deo whether he had had any sexual exposure during the three months of waiting. "Absolutely not," he answered nervously. "In fact, I've lost my libido completely," he added.

The next day he was back for his results. His final test was also negative. This caused the very first smile I had seen on his face since the whole saga started. Also back was his libido. But Deo swore that he would only be assuaging his yearning with his wife. Hopefully, I thought, because memories can be short and, old habits die hard.

But Deo's problems were not yet over. A young journalist who had been hired by Vicki and his political rivals to publish an exclusive on him saw a potential of a great story that could make his name. The thwarted reporter, faced with contradictory evidence but not wanting to give up entirely came out with a watered-down version that had no chance of making headlines. The more reputable papers would not accept this story, not even for their gossip pages. It was eventually picked up by a tabloid that carefully edited out the more controversial parts to avoid litigation.

But the CID still had some unfinished business with Deo. With so many women swearing that he had infected them with HIV, they concluded that the horny and "crafty" politician had somehow managed to bribe all the laboratories in town to falsify the results (like some politicians habitually do to get elected). The CID insisted on more and more tests, in diverse and randomly selected laboratories, to which Deo's blood samples were sent anonymously.

Six months after the saga started, after numerous HIV tests done at a variety of laboratories all returned a unanimous verdict and his political opponents' knives were safely back in their sheaths; with all the vengeful women scattered and Vicki's pregnancy terminated, the badly battered Deo reckoned he had won and returned to his politicking.

Terror Weapon

Not all people living with AIDS were meek sufferers of the cureless scourge, as a 40-year-old receptionist I call Pricilla and her boss, Nathan Mukubwa, working in the eastern Ugandan town of Tororo, found out the hard way.

Pricilla became an unfortunate victim of AIDS-related harassment inflicted on her by a male workmate living with HIV in the early 1990s. Pricilla, a quiet, timorous and rather emotional woman, appeared to be scared of many things in life, and mainly AIDS. She had watched in horror as two of her workmates died and feared suffering the same fate. She resigned her job as a medical laboratory assistant because the samples she handled every day were mainly from AIDS patients. She was so scared of being infected that she often wore two pairs of gloves. After a long search, she finally found a less-well-paid job as an office receptionist with a non-governmental organisation (NGO). There she felt secure in the knowledge that her work did not involve daily exposure to AIDS patients or their potentially infectious specimens.

Inevitably, even in her new job at the front desk welcoming clients, she would occasionally come across people with signs suggestive of AIDS, which her medical background had taught her to recognise. She would try to avoid getting close to them, but if she was forced to shake hands she would soon after rush to the bathroom and scrub her hands. Initially she tried to keep her phobia secret, but she was not doing a good job of it.

Across her desk, at the entrance, a sly security guard whom I will call Coporo Matoto, was stationed. Under the regime of Idi Amin he had been trained as a surveillance detective, and was rumoured to have been behind the disappearances of a number of Ugandans suspected of being Amin's adversaries. He was briefly detained after Amin's fall, but nothing incriminating was proved against him, and he was set free.

Coporo was living with HIV, which he had been forced to declare to the administration to explain his frequent days of sick leave. Apparently, Coporo's old skills and habits of nosing into other people's affairs had persisted long after his former job had ended. Within a short time he had noticed Pricilla's nervousness whenever he came close to her. It did not take him long to conclude that she was scared of him because he had HIV.

Pricilla was not the only one frightened of HIV, and Coporo was not surprised by her reaction. In fact, he had learned to use his HIV-positive status as a scare "weapon", in almost the same way as he had used his State Research identity card to scare people during his secret service days. He exploited Pricilla's AIDS phobia to menace and haunt her. Initially he tried to flirt with her but his mere approach sent Pricilla into a panic close to frenzy. Coporo, found this pleasurable. Taking advantage of her vulnerability he closed in for the kill.

He resorted to overt sexual harassment. He frequently pestered her for sex, and threatened to rape her if she refused. He would warn her that if she came willingly he would use a condom; otherwise he threatened to give her a vampire kiss, spit in her eyes or bite her and still transmit HIV to her. The well-trained Coporo would only make the threats after making absolutely sure that there were no witnesses, but was ever prepared to stop promptly — ready to deny any wrongdoing if anyone entered the room. He had left Pricilla no escape route.

It did not take long for Pricilla to reach a state of panic. Her work deteriorated so badly that her supervisor contemplated dismissing her. She became so paranoid that she dreaded using the office bathroom for fear of contracting AIDS from toilet seats. She was also terrified of being left alone in a room. Coporo stood back, taking in all of these developments and, according to Pricilla, often giggled in delight as she suffered.

In time Pricilla could not take it anymore and one day she burst into Mukubwa's office and reported Coporo. After doing all that he could to calm her down, he ordered an immediate internal investigation into the matter. Coporo denied any wrongdoing, pointing out that he had recently been very concerned about Pricilla's mental state. He said he had observed her behaving in an odd manner and at times appearing to be close to a nervous breakdown. Coporo said that he suspected the cause to be marital problems. Indeed, he had sniffed out some disharmony between Pricilla and her husband, which he sought to exploit. He even produced a number of staff members as witnesses. The selected witnesses had no idea of the background to Pricilla's plight. They too had noticed that her behaviour had changed, and readily collaborated Coporo's story. Pricilla, not so expressive of her feelings and obviously upset, did not do justice to her side of the story and the investigation concluded that Coporo was the wronged party. She was outraged.

Pricilla rushed to a prominent lawyer saying that she wanted to sue Coporo even if it cost a fortune — which she did not have. The lawyer was shocked by the details of the case and volunteered to help her free of charge. However, because of her agitated state he wondered whether Pricilla was stable. He called her boss to seek his thoughts on the matter and especially whether Coporo was the kind of man to subject a person to this kind of inhumane harassment. Mukubwa told him that in his presence Coporo Matoto was always as polite as a monk and well mannered, though he also suspected that he harboured some sadistic tendencies. He added that he would not put it past him to put up a show. However, when Mukubwa got to know the details it was clear that there was no way Pricilla could have imagined it all. But nothing could be proved against Coporo. He had covered his tracks very well. Therefore the NGO's human resource officer wrote to Pricilla asking her to retract her accusations against Coporo, and tried to get the two to reconcile and work together again. When this did not work the human resource officer contacted the JCRC and asked for our help. I asked one of our counsellors to follow up the case. Meanwhile, Mukubwa also tried his best to counsel Pricilla and to reassure her that everything possible including regular checks on her to ensure that she was protected from any harassment, was being done. Despite our counsellor's intervention, Pricilla resigned her job. She said that nightmares about Coporo frequently woke her up at night.

"I wake up relieved that I had only been tormented by a bad dream only to encounter him in the flesh the next morning at work," she said. However, our counsellor, who tried to help Coporo too, witnessed some worrying developments in the organisation and ended up counselling Mukubwa as well.

Coporo now knew that Mukubwa, at the very least, had some questions about his behaviour and would be observing him very carefully. This worried Coporo and he started plotting to get rid of Mukubwa. Coporo was all over his unsuspecting boss, offering to run errands for him. His loyalty appeared to be beyond reproach. Ever so polite but scheming clandestinely, Coporo gathered all kinds of details about Mukubwa, including about his leisure activities. He scouted all the properties that Mukubwa owned, and gathered titbits of information about him down to what he had for supper at home; he recorded everything in a file. Over time the file swelled; but it was mainly boring stuff as Mukubwa's busy routine did not leave him with enough time to indulge in the kind of exciting adventures that Coporo wished for. This left him with no other alternative but to use his imagination to fake his records and embellish some of the events to project a more vivid report to suit his malevolent plot.

As fate would have it, just before he could strike, Coporo was taken ill with a serious chest infection that turned out to be TB. Nathan Mukubwa arranged for his treatment in a private clinic. But soon after his recovery, there followed complaints from the clinic that Coporo had attacked a member of their staff, the clinic dispenser. While she was giving Coporo his TB drugs someone whom Coporo knew entered the room. He launched a ferocious verbal attack on the dispenser for not concealing his drugs fast enough. Thereafter, the dispenser devised a method of concealing his drugs by always dispensing them in containers marked Paracetamol. Nevertheless, Coporo continued to torment the hapless dispenser for months until Mukubwa intervened. When Coporo was advised to start on ARVs which he could not afford, Mukubwa once again came to his rescue and paid for the treatment.

However as soon as his health improved, he resumed his vendetta to bring down Mukubwa. Mukubwa was stunned to find that Coporo had reported him to the CID, alleging that he was corrupt. Unfortunately for Coporo, he reported these spurious allegations to an ethical CID officer, one of the few that had been recruited after the purges of Idi Amin. Coporo presented a huge file of years of surveillance on Mukubwa, including obscure personal details unrelated to his work. The CID officer told Coporo that he was dismayed by his actions, which were illegal and a breach of individual privacy. He warned him that this was a criminal offence instigated by malice. But Coporo appealed, alleging that the CID officer had been compromised by Mukubwa. A team of other officers took up the case.

A distressing year-long investigation followed, during which Mukubwa was subjected to long hours of interrogation and searches. At the end of it all he was exonerated. All that Mukubwa had to say when I inquired about his ordeal was *Gwowonya egele yalikusambya*, meaning that one good turn does not always result in another. "But I would help Coporo again if the need arose," he hastened to add.

Coporo Matoto, for his part, unremorsefully walked away scot free.

3

Marriage in the Times of the Incurable Plague

Virginity Betrayed

One morning in mid-1993, the office messenger burst into my office to report that there was a young man outside sobbing uncontrollably. I bolted out to find out what the tears were about. When I managed to calm the sobbing man down a little, he told me he wanted to see me privately. I felt I had no alternative but to invite him in.

That is how I first met the 28-year-old man I will call Saul Musoke. Saul told me how he had been just a month away from fulfilling his childhood dream of marrying his sweetheart, Violet, when he suffered a devastating heartbreak. Theirs had been a long and disciplined romance. They had known each other since their primary school days and had become engaged while they were both freshers at Makerere University. He explained how they had vowed to abstain from sex and to remain faithful to each other until marriage. Against all odds, especially peer pressure, they had succeeded where the vast majority of their age mates faltered.

"It was the power of the Holy Spirit that gave us the resilience to succeed," he said. At long last, their self-denial, was about to reward them with the fulfilment of their goal which they had looked forward to for years — the marriage of two virgins.

Both were born-again Christians and always attended evening Bible study and Sunday church services together. The vicar often invoked their ideal relationship in his sermons as an example to be emulated by other youths. The charismatic preacher had promised that he would personally wed them, and said that he looked forward to delivering a special sermon exalting the virtues of their model relationship. But just as the preparations were complete and everything seemed to be on course for the wedding, things fell apart.

Saul said that 2 years had passed since he had walked hand in hand with Violet to get their HIV test results from a Kampala clinic. The vicar had established a rule that all couples marrying in his church had to have an HIV test. But in their case, he had an additional reason why he needed the results. He planned to use it in his sermon to demonstrate to the congregation that abstinence from sex was the "only" guaranteed protection against HIV. But that was not to be. The doctor had stammered as he explained their discordant results, Saul recalled.

I thought two years would have been sufficient time for him to have healed. The tears should have dried by now. I inquired how he had coped since he tested positive. He narrated the story with strong emotions, as if it just happened a day before

"I have been fine, but I saw her today with a baby," he started sobbing again. "That baby should have been mine," he said fighting back the tears. "You see, Doctor, she married someone else and swore never to speak to me again for causing her such an embarrassment. I could see she has never forgotten or forgiven me. When I met her she ignored me as if she has never set eyes on me before." In a tremulous voice, Saul looked back at that painful period that time had failed to heal. "She called me 'a good actor' and it hurt me so much. She said I pretended to be a born-again Christian when in reality I was just a dirty, scheming sinner out to kill her." His composure kept improving progressively as he talked. "But this is not true because I was a virgin then. And I am still a virgin now," he joined his hands as if in prayer. "No one believes me Doctor, and I can see you don't believe me either!"

"Oh, no! I promise you that I trust all my patients," I said to him reassuringly. "Of course there are other ways to acquire HIV, including blood transfusion and contaminated needles. And in some cases there are those infected with a type of HIV disease that progresses slowly, especially among those who acquired the infection at birth. A small number among them would never know that they were infected until they were teenagers."

"None of those apply to me Doctor, and that's why I came to see you today. I just want you to explain to me how I could possibly have been infected. Please," Saul implored. "No one else has given me a satisfactory explanation. Many just dismiss me without even listening," he said. "I just want to be tested again," he added. I explained to him that once one tests positive, one remains positive for life. "If the laboratory where you tested can be trusted, it will be a waste of precious time and good money to repeat the test," I said to him. "It never changes. You don't have to go through the same exercise again if you already know the answer," I added, to make sure that he did not entertain any false hope.

"But I still have this lingering doubt in my mind. I just can't see how I could be infected. Please doctor, just do it — just for my peace of mind," Saul implored.

In the circumstances I could see no other way to remove any doubt that he was HIV positive and that he would always be HIV positive, except by re-testing him. I thought that this would help him to finally accept the reality and start living positively.

But Saul tested HIV negative!

When I gave him the laboratory report, he stared at it for a long time in meditative silence. Then a teardrop fell on the report. But he kept on staring blankly, not focussed on it.

This case of a false HIV positive had caused him so much anguish and had ruined his future with his long-term fiancée in whom he had invested so much hope and love. His future had been brutally crushed by a flawed test and an incompetent doctor who had failed to carry out a confirmatory test that would have easily exposed the error.

False positive HIV tests were not uncommon due to laboratory errors in the early 1990s; they still occasionally occur even today. I am reminded of a born-again Christian woman who was repeatedly paraded by a pastor who claimed that his prayers (after she paid a hefty fee and topped it up with a gift of a car) had cured her of HIV. Yet, in reality, it was a case of a false positive result. That is the reason why it is always recommended to do at least two tests, unless other specific indicators exist. At the JCRC we used the test called the Western Blot as a confirmatory test, but this was expensive and was also occasionally difficult to interpret. We later turned to using two kinds of HIV tests, each with different properties. This simple routine would have saved Saul and Violet so much pain. Regrettably, these mishaps still happen.

"Doctor, I know you do not give out printed HIV test results but in my case I need a report with your signature on it," he begged in a calm, composed voice.

"Are you going to sue the clinic?" I asked, thinking that if I had been in his shoes, I would consider taking such an action.

"No, I have forgiven the doctor and the clinic where this was done. It was not done on purpose," he said, his big-hearted nature and faith coming through, graciously putting aside what many would have considered unforgivable. "I need it to re-establish my innocence," Saul said. "God works in mysterious ways. Although I lost her, I will still feel better if she knew that I had not been unfaithful to her."

I agreed to his request and provided him with his laboratory results. It meant so much to him and I was not going to deny him this after all he had been through. However, as a precaution, I wrote on my phone number with a footnote that I may be contacted in case there were any questions.

"I will go to the vicar first. He had so much trust in my integrity. It was painful to see him so disappointed in me. At the time, he looked at me like I was a creepy sinner that tried to get a good girl in trouble by false pretences," Saul said. Apparently, contrary to his own sermons, the vicar had not been as good at forgiving or forgetting as he frequently urged his congregation to be. "I just want him to know that I was not the sinner he believed me to be." Saul's eyes were wet again, but this time it was tears of relief.

The nightmare had ended. Now he had to pick up the pieces, and start living all over again.

Love Killer

It started with a call that came through the main JCRC telephone exchange one Monday morning in early March 1997. "Sheraton Hotel is on the line for you," Alice Katami, our receptionist said. "John Muhaze from Burundi wants to speak with you personally." On the line was a very excited man — it was easy to tell from the exuberant tone of his voice. When I got the details, I found that his excitement was truly justified. He was getting married the following week. As I congratulated him on his engagement, I could hear his bride giggling in the background. John requested an appointment and I told him they could come in straightaway. Who would miss the chance to have a preview of the bride?

When they arrived at the JCRC later that morning, smartly dressed, it was obvious that they were in love and having a great time together.

Right there by his side was Chantal, the gorgeous bride, smiling radiantly. Their hands were all over each other. Indeed, they were a picture postcard of a happy couple. They talked excitedly about their impending wedding, and how the preparations were shaping up in Bujumbura. Invitations had been sent out to hundreds of friends and relatives, not to mention some of the country's top dignitaries.

The happy couple had flown in to enjoy a pre-wedding quiet time together, which they jokingly described as a sort of rehearsal for the honeymoon. There was no better place to stay in the city than the Sheraton — then Kampala's most luxurious hotel. And while they were in town, they could as well have an HIV test done at the famous JCRC, just to complete the premarital rituals. They were already learning to plan and do things that mattered in their new life together.

When they arrived for testing, they found that I had already made the arrangements for them to meet with our counsellor. The bride-to-be asked me whether it was really necessary to attend the session. "It is possible that one or both of you could test positive," I said to them, "in which case you need to be ready to face this news. This is also an opportunity for you to learn as much as you can about HIV/AIDS".

The jolly couple readily accepted my advice. They did not seem to be bothered by the test. Casually, the excited bride -to-be said they were so much in love that nothing would separate them. Indeed, everything seemed to be right for her, with him right there at her side and holding her hand.

Chantal tested negative but John's results came out positive. This brought the chatty conversation between them to a sudden stop. I recall Chantal looking at John as if she had suddenly bumped into him on the street. She seemed to examine his face as if a carbuncle had just materialised on his forehead. Then she took a step backwards, and the hand that previously held his now held tightly on to her handbag, as if it had suddenly become heavy. John just stared into space, stunned. Then our senior counsellor and I took them through a lengthy post-test counselling session.

I advised John to have a CD4 test to determine whether he was at a stage where antiretroviral therapy would be needed, and he agreed. Since I did not know what went on during the pre-honeymoon rehearsal before the results, I advised Chantal to undergo another test in three months time. As they left I watched the loving couple, who had embraced and kissed all the way to the clinic, leaving at arm's length. The previous night must have seemed like a long, long time ago.

The next day, sad looking, unaccompanied and casually dressed John was back for his CD4 results. He looked sick, aged and subdued as he narrated his ordeal.

"She treated me as if I was a leper." he said dejectedly. "Then she demanded to have her own room. She is gone now, and the marriage is off. Now I have the ordeal of facing the folks back home, who right now are still busy making last-minute preparations for the wedding. I don't really know how to break the news to them. They don't even know that we were crazy enough to travel abroad so close to our wedding day. But she said she will do me a favour and keep it all under wraps. You know Bujumbura is a small town, and rumours spread very fast," he added.

Talking seemed to console him a little.

"To all probing relatives and friends, we've agreed to say that we had a quarrel," he went on. "Irreconcilable differences — or something like that," he added.

John's CD4 cells were very low, indicating that he had advanced HIV disease. I explained to him that he needed to start on therapy immediately. The counselling session seemed to work well for him. The money that he had saved for the honeymoon came in handy to pay for the then very expensive ARV drugs. To make ends meet, he moved from the Sheraton to a cheaper downtown hotel, where he stayed for a week, while he got used to the drugs. The week away from home also served another purpose. The surprise and nosiness following the shattering news of the sudden cancellation of the wedding would have faded a little by the time he was back in his hometown.

John, who in the short time that I had known him, I had come to like and respect, called me from Entebbe Airport to bid me farewell as he prepared to board the plane to start on a difficult journey back home.

Deadly Desire

When I first met the courteous and well-groomed man I will call Yona Byansiko in July 1996, I mistook him for a priest who had forgotten his dog collar at home. Unlike many other people who came to my Centre without appointment, he was in good physical shape and did not appear ruffled by being in an AIDS clinic. I thought he had accompanied a patient and wanted to give me some background information. It was quite common for relatives of AIDS patients in denial or a good Samaritan to bring suspected AIDS patients to my clinic without telling them that they suspected that they were HIV positive or even that they were taking them to an AIDS clinic. In such cases, they would request to see me first and explain the situation. But Yona surprised me when he said that he had come to see me about his marriage, causing me to wonder whether that explained the missing dog collar.

Yona told me that wife had died in 1989. Two years later he had remarried, but he did not inform his 24-year-old bride that his late wife had died of AIDS. Neither did he tell her that he had tested HIV positive. Prior to their marriage the young lady had insisted that they undergo HIV testing. Yona presented her with a forged HIV test report.

After the birth of their second child, he started falling sick and feared for the worst. He worked out a devious plot to deceive his wife. He suggested to her that they undertake an HIV test, to which she readily agreed. "This is just for reassurance," he lied to her. Now he had come to see whether I could arrange to have them tested together. Yona had assumed that by this time his wife would have been infected too. This was the reason behind his scheme aimed at misleading her into thinking that he was just finding out about his HIV infection for the very first time. He asked me not to mention to his wife that he had all along known that he was HIV positive. I told him that I took strong exception to his spiteful plot. However, as a doctor, my first and foremost duty was to attend to the sick and alleviate their suffering and not to be judgemental. His wife tested HIV-negative. They were discordant.

Naturally, his wife was shaken to discover that her husband was infected and that she was living precariously. But she was the forgiving type – the legendary salt of the earth. She declared that she would stick with him regardless. In counselling sessions, I explained to them that her luck so far could not be pushed. She could get infected anytime and therefore recommended they use condoms. We talked about their good fortune of having two healthy children already, and therefore, unlike some other childless discordant couples, they did not need to take risks.

When I checked the husband's CD4, I found him so sick that I started him on combination ARV therapy straightaway. He swore that after the narrow escape of his wife he would henceforth ensure her safety by proper and consistent use of condoms. "At least my children have one healthy parent to take care of them — just in case," he said.

A year later, they were back to see me. The wife was pregnant.

"What's up?" I asked the bemused husband and his tired-looking wife.

"Please help me Doctor, he forces me to have sex without a condom, and I am at my wits' end as to what to do," she lamented as she wiped off streams of free-flowing tears.

"Why is it necessary for you to undertake this risk?" I asked the seemingly faraway husband.

"I crave "live" sex so much that I just can't help it," he replied, taking care to avoid eye contact with his wife.

"Is your urge so strong that you are willing to risk the life of the mother of your children?"

"Doctor, in matters of sex, reasoning sometimes just flies out of the window. I don't know what comes over me! I try but I keep failing. But I promise to try harder in future. I really promise," he said.

"Well it might already be too late," the wife interjected. "He must have infected me already."

"That can only be determined by another test," I said to her, "and then, depending on the results, we can discuss the next course of action," I added. But her luck was holding. She was still uninfected. I referred then to a professional marriage counsellor. They still live together, but I do not know how they are coping with their sex life.

In another case, the marriage of a couple that faced a somewhat similar situation did not survive. This was the perturbing case of a balding middle aged man I will call Samson. I first met him when his relatives dumped him at my clinic door in a semi-comatose state, and hurried home to prepare for the funeral, leaving only his 22-year old wife in attendance. I made a provisional diagnosis of cryptococcal meningitis. It was obviously an intensive-care case and I referred him to a private hospital where I was able to follow him up. Initially, his young wife was too scared to touch him, fearing that she would catch meningitis. However, when she discovered that it was all due to AIDS, fear was replaced by panic. She was counselled and advised on measures to protect herself, and she nervously stayed on to nurse her husband through the illness. Understandably she feared that she would already be HIV-infected too. Luckily she tested HIV negative.

After two months in hospital, one of which he spent in intensive care in a deep coma, Samson miraculously recovered from meningitis. However, he retained a speech impediment, and a slight limp. I started him on ARV drugs and he responded well. A few months later, with his strength recovered, he turned up with his rather fretful wife, seeking to know what they were to do about sex. "Condoms without fail," I told them.

I demonstrated to them their proper use. The couple promised to make condoms their life companion. And after such suffering and seeing the devotion of his young wife, who exhibited such maturity far beyond her tender age at the time of his greatest need, I assumed that this was the natural thing to do. A man who had suffered so much could not possibly wish such a painful fate on his worst enemy.

Only six months later the much improved Samson again accompanied by his wife was back in the clinic to see me once again. She was pregnant.

"It's quite a risk that you took," I said to the couple, for lack of something better to say in such circumstances.

"Well she just got pregnant," Samson replied rather casually, while the wife remained quiet and self-effacing. She appeared to take no pleasure in her expectant state.

"What happened to the condoms?" I probed further. "The last time we met, both of you were so keen on them. I vaguely recall that you called them your eternal companion or something like that," I added.

"He tricked me," replied the now tearful wife, "he would pretend to put it on and then instead put it aside at the very last moment and go on to do it. Now I fear I am infected. After I found out I let him do it anyway since I am a dead woman," she said in between sobs. "I had no choice." The treacherous husband just stared at the floor without any apparent remorse.

"You can't just assume that you are infected," I said. "You have to be tested and if you are confirmed infected we have to plan for treatment to protect your baby."

Contrary to her fears, she again tested negative. After the lucky escape the couple promised that from now on they would use condoms without fail. "No tricks," he promised. The wife, on her part, said she would check that "his dick was always fully fitted with the rubber" before allowing him anywhere close to her.

However, one evening, eight months after the birth of their baby boy, I found the wife in hiding behind the Clinic.

"Please help to hide me, Doctor. He wants to kill me by infecting me with AIDS. He tried all kinds of tricks in order to do it without the condom but I thwarted all his efforts." She was surprisingly composed but unmistakably determined. "Last night he tried to rape me and I fled the house," she said, while removing the cloth covering her arms to show me the bruises and scratches. She was dressed in a rather oversized dress. "I left everything there. My sister gave me this dress. Please help me to get a visa to flee the country. I have relatives abroad," she pleaded.

"You could get police protection," I said just to reassure her, though I did not really believe that the police could adequately protect anyone from this kind of domestic dilemma.

"No! That won't work. He has threatened to kill me and to bribe the police to cover it up if I don't go back to him."

"I don't know how to help you with a visa," I said to her. "No embassy will agree to give you asylum for protection from your husband. God knows they should, but I don't think they would."

I was, indeed, genuinely puzzled as to how best to handle the complicated situation. However, to do nothing seemed heartless. I suggested that she contacted FIDA, an association of Uganda women lawyers, but she declined. She was visibly disappointed that I was not of much help to her. Like a considerable number of my other patients, she had started to believe that I could fix all kinds problems. She was frustrated to find that I was powerless to help. She said she had an alternative course of action, which she did not disclose to me. I asked her to wait a little so that I could find someone – perhaps a marriage counsellor or lawyer – to advise her. She said she could not risk hanging around. She left suddenly and for a long time I heard nothing from her.

One day about two months later, Samson came in for a routine follow-up visit and fresh drugs supplies. I asked him about his wife and baby.

"You know, she was a prostitute," he replied. "She ran away and took my baby with her."

"I don't think that's fair to your wife," I said, wondering if I could squeeze some more information out of him. "If you call her a prostitute, how would you describe yourself?" I added rhetorically. "Anyway, do you happen to know where they might be?" I was anxious about their safety. I wondered if I should perhaps look up her relatives and advise them to report her as a missing person. I would not put it beyond this unrepentant bully to have harmed her.

"No, and I don't care anymore," he replied. "I have a new girlfriend, and we are happy together," he added.

I learned later that his wife had somehow made it to Europe.

Scottish Stockings

It was not always the women who were the victims of marital discord. I met a number of men who also suffered. But they were few and far between. I particularly remember one remarkable case that concerned yet another discordant couple. The man who I will call Gregory, a 47-year-old engineer, was the HIV-infected partner. He was on ARVs and doing well.

Gregory was a very conscientious man who cared for the safety of his wife. Every time I saw him in my clinic, he always mentioned how lucky he was that his wife was not HIV infected. To ensure that his wife remained free of HIV, he insisted on consistent use of condoms. Despite all his best efforts, to his utter disbelief, in early 1997, his wife - I will call her Jerulina - discovered that she was pregnant. When they came to see me, Gregory was ever so remorseful and visibly embarrassed, pleading repeatedly that it had happened despite his very careful efforts.

"When she first told me about it, I almost had a heart attack," he said, as he turned to his wife as if to get her confirmation of the events that had transpired, but she did not seem to be paying any attention. "Perhaps what saved my life was that she was so cool about it! God knows, I wouldn't have handled it if she had been as panicky as I was at the time." He laboured to explain that it was not her pregnancy that he was most concerned about. "I am haunted by the knowledge that I exposed her to HIV — that I risked her life," he elaborated.

Jerulina on the other hand appeared undaunted and unperturbed by it all. Her husband thought that an abortion would be in the best interests of his wife. "There is no justification for putting my wife's life at risk and risking having an HIV-infected baby, especially as we have four healthy children."

But his wife was against abortion and she had my wholehearted support. I explained to the husband that the chance of his wife giving birth to a healthy uninfected child was high even if she was found to be HIV infected. To my profound relief, and even greater relief of her husband, she tested HIV negative. The issue of abortion was set aside. I suspected that they did not use the condoms properly. I asked one of our most proficient counsellors to demonstrate to the couple the correct use of condoms using a dummy penis, and to explain how condoms help to reduce the risk of both HIV transmission as well as unwanted pregnancies. When I asked the counsellor how the condom training session had gone, she said that Jerulina was very good at it. "It was like she has been practicing the art of it," she said.

But just over eighteen months later, they were back. The wife was pregnant again with their sixth child.

"Doctor, I wish you would just believe me that I religiously use condoms with my wife, but— but— this has happened again" he stammered as he lamented. "Coming so quickly after the last baby, I am beginning to lose confidence in condoms. Maybe I should use two at a time. I think they don't work," he added.

"Certainly not 100%" I chipped in, just to encourage him to open up a little more, and get things off his chest. "Not many things in life, if any, work 100%," I added for emphasis

The wife was the picture of happiness, and justifiably so. She was after all still uninfected, and the gynaecologist who examined her had given her a clean bill of health.

But only four weeks later I received a rather agitated call from the husband.

"Doctor — Doctor! I am innocent," he pleaded. I was surprised. I had never directly or indirectly accused him of any wrongdoing or hinted on it in anyway during our conversations. I wondered whether I had somehow been misunderstood. My immediate reaction was to spring to the defensive.

"I'm sorry if I did not make myself clear..," I tried to explain, but he cut me short. "No, you explained everything well. It's my wife's fault," he went on to explain in agitation. "She is very silly, I am sorry to say. She is the one causing me all these problems. She is so deceiving. But last night I finally caught her red-handed!"

All of a sudden it all made sense! Several times I had thought of the possibility that the wife could be having an affair, but each time dismissed the notion. Now it seemed to be confirmed. I had been convinced that the husband was doing his best to keep his uninfected wife protected from HIV. Furthermore he always said he did not want any more children. "So, this was it," I thought to myself wondering why such an obvious explanation had not been clear to me right from the beginning or why it had surprised the husband so much.

"These things happen," I said to the husband. I could not find the right words to say, considering the sensitivity of the matter. To most husbands, it would be a very difficult situation to come to terms with. "Take your time to ponder. Don't do or think of anything rash," I counselled. "It is important for you and your wife to come in and meet with our counsellor," I said. "And I will also arrange for another special counsellor to have a word with you," I added, while trying to think of a marriage counsellor to recommend to them. Talk of jumping to conclusions — I was flat wrong!

"My wife is the one who buys the condoms," he explained. "She took on this role when she noticed that buying condoms always made me nervous. You know – it is not easy—with all the other shoppers staring at you, and everyone knowing what they are for – and that sort of stuff. She also made it her job to always put them on me, and to remove them afterwards," he explained.

"I see nothing wrong in this…" I hastened to reassure him as he was speaking anxiously. "In fact it is rather romantic, and…" But he cut me short again.

"I know you can't believe this Doctor, but my wife has been cutting off the condoms' tips with scissors and dressing me in Scottish stockings!"

Almost a year later I happened to meet Jerulina when she accompanied her husband for routine monitoring tests. She had with her a baby girl.

"Why did you put your life in unnecessary danger?" I inquired when I had a private moment with her.

"I am a traditional African woman," she replied, "and to be a full woman, I need children." She must have guessed that this answer did not address what I meant. "I was desperate for a girl. Even if I got infected in the process, I would have no regrets whatsoever. No regrets at all," she added with apparent happiness as she gently rocked her baby.

Women's Life Jacket

While some people had lucky escapes, I met many others that got infected by their spouses, though this usually happened when the infected partner was not on treatment. In fact, in Uganda, data showed that marriage was one of the risk factors for HIV infection among women. By 2010, it was estimated that over 70% of newly infected women were in monogamous marriages or long-term relationships. Most married women were generally faithful to their partners. On the contrary, many husbands were not. Yet women, especially the poor, could do little about it. The established methods of prevention, the so-called ABC (A for Abstinence, B for Be faithful, C for Condoms) mainly depended on men's cooperation if they were to succeed.

To get round this dilemma, women need some preventive methods under their own control, like vaginal gels known as vaginal microbicide that could be used as a prophylactic even without their partners' knowledge. Efforts to find an effective microbicide have been hampered partly by funding constraints. This is not an area of research in which pharmaceutical companies are interested. The vast majority of women at risk are poor, without the means to pay for the microbicides. It has generally been left to philanthropists to give this research the attention it deserves. Meanwhile, in most poor countries, including Uganda, the HIV epidemic has become increasingly feminised. As I write, young women have overtaken men as the most HIV-infected group, making the need for a preventive method under the control of women imperative. Efforts to find preventive methods under women's control have been fruitless. In fact, the first generations of vaginal microbicides that were tested tended to increase HIV transmission possibly by irritating vaginal mucosa.

But just as it seemed like no effective microbicidal gel would never be developed, a ray of hope materialised from a study coded CAPRISA 004 that involved 889 women, in both rural and urban AIDS-devastated communities in South Africa.

This landmark study was an important scientific breakthrough in the fight against HIV. When the results were first announced in KwaZulu-Natal, South Africa, in July 2010, we received the news in Sub-Saharan Africa, with excitement and a sigh of relief. At long last something that showed promise had been found. The results were also reported at the XVIII International AIDS Conference in Vienna, Austria, where it was the highlight of the meeting.

The study found that women who applied a vaginal gel containing one of the most commonly used ARV drugs called Tenofovir were 39% less likely to contract HIV than those who used a placebo. Women who used the gel for more than 80% of their sex acts had a 54% reduction in HIV infections, whereas those who used the gel in less than half of their sex acts had a 28% reduction in HIV infections.

The study also found another benefit of using the gel—it was also found to provide protection against another common genital virus, herpes, reducing the risk by 51%. The dual effect in preventing HIV and herpes had a potential synergistic advantage because genital herpes increases the chances of becoming infected with HIV.

Commenting on these findings, Dr Quarraisha Abdool Karim, one of the leaders of this landmark study, had this to say:

"Tenofovir gel could fill an important HIV prevention gap by empowering women who are unable to successfully negotiate mutual faithfulness or condom use with their male partners. This new technology has the potential to alter the course of the HIV epidemic, especially in southern Africa, where young women bear the brunt of this devastating disease."

When the data was given a more considered examination, it was clear that much more work was needed before the world could finally welcome an effective microbicidal gel. The degree of protection was still unacceptably low and the studies did not involve enough women to give an accurate picture. On a disappointing note, a subsequent study to confirm efficacy of Tenofovir gel, was a failure. However, there is no doubt at all that these findings held promise for scientists to build on in the continuing search for a solution.

Discordance Dilemma

What looked like miraculous escapes from HIV infection by HIV-uninfected wives of HIV-infected men who refused to use condoms, or the women who sabotaged condoms use because they wanted children, may not have been a result of mere luck. The situation could have been tragically different if the infected partners had not been on ARV drug treatment.

It has since emerged that in a sexually active relationship where one partner is HIV infected and the other is uninfected (a so-called discordant couple), when the infected partner uses ARVs properly, the chances of infecting the uninfected partner reduce drastically. This confirmation of the power of ARV drugs to prevent transmission of HIV came from Washington DC, on 12 May 2011, in the form of media release issued by the HIV Preventive Trials Network, which is a worldwide partnership of scientists and communities. Results of a trial coded HPTN 052, which had started in 2005 and involved 1,763 discordant couples, had evaluated whether immediate versus delayed use of ARVs by HIV-infected individuals would reduce transmission of HIV to their uninfected partners. The couples were randomised to two groups, where one group immediately started taking ARVs (immediate group), while another group only started treatment when their CD4 fell below 250 cells or if the participant developed AIDS-related complications (delayed group). There were 27 infections in the delayed group and only one in the immediate group—a breathtaking difference of 96%!

The findings were so striking that the results were released ahead of schedule. The study monitors and researchers felt that the findings were of such urgent public interest, especially to those infected or affected by HIV/AIDS, that any further delay would raise serious ethical concerns. The breaking news story was picked up by all major news media and broadcast around the world, displacing the death of Bin Laden from the headlines.

But the much-hyped study had not actually found out anything new! In reality, the power of ARVs to reduce transmission of HIV had been known for well over a decade and a half. So, what was the rush to announce the news all about? Was it actually a breakthrough?

Virtually all previous research findings with similar results were based on either epidemiological or observational studies. HPTN 052 was unique because it was the first randomised trial (a research methodology with less chance of bias) to show that an HIV-infected person can radically reduce the chance of transmitting HIV by sexual contact to an HIV-uninfected partner by starting ARV treatment early. This is important because there are many sceptics who, for various reasons not excluding politics disputed all the previous findings or minimised their significance. Here, finally, was irrefutable proof.

The secret behind the power of ARVs to reduce HIV transmission is linked to their ability to lower HIV (viral copies) in the blood. Treatment success very much depends on use of effective ARV drugs combination, adherence, and medical supervision to ensure that drugs remain effective and, if not, are changed in a timely manner. Therefore a high level of protection as found in the study may not always apply in circumstances where there is treatment failure. Thus, the study results did not spell the end of the necessity to use condoms. Condoms, together with other proven preventive measures, constitute a package of armaments in the fight against HIV.

4

The People's Medicine

Good Hope

It has since become clear that by the time AIDS was clinically described in Rakai district in southwestern Uganda in the early 1980s, scatterings of fully-blown AIDS cases had been observed within the community in the 1970s. As described in my earlier book *Genocide by Denial*, it is not known precisely when the very first cases emerged, but analysis of events in some other parts of the country will show how people coped with the very first cases in their communities. Like in Rakai, HIV had stealthily crept into villages unrecognised. Signs and symptoms of the strange disease were diverse, bizarre and puzzling. For instance, it was inexplicable that sufferers starved and wasted away even when they had enough to eat. Why were the victim's bodies rejecting nourishment?

However, not all signs and symptoms were entirely new to traditional healers and Western doctors. They could all easily recognise familiar signs and symptoms associated with common diseases for which they had effective medicines. However, to their consternation, the patients' symptoms either kept reoccurring or just did not respond to therapy.

As more and more cases cropped up, trends emerged. It appeared that traders who frequently travelled out of their towns and villages were more at risk. People speculated that the traders were being poisoned in a feud with business rivals. Curiously, I followed up this lead, trying to find out what exactly happened in my home town of Rukungiri in southwestern Uganda. One of the myths surrounding the new disease that Gershom Mugyenyi, a mechanic who lost many of his fellow mechanic friends to the scourge, told me about was that it was initially thought to be caused by a poisonous recipe. By the early 1980s rumours were rife that the suspected culprit was boiled kapa (cat meat) mixed with beef or goat meat to disguise it. I tried to find out from others in the area where this strange belief originated. The most consistent rationalisation was the widespread belief that cat's meat was both "poisonous and a curse". In fact, for a time, the strange disease was dubbed *Obutwa bwa kapa* or kapa for short, meaning cat meat poison.

Despite the many and varying presentations of the strange disease, the striking and most common aspect was gross emaciation. Some elders in southern Uganda talked of a mysterious wasting disease that was widely known as *mutigwarwanda*. I never managed to find out when the very first outbreak was, but some people, equated the most recent outbreak with the Rwanda disturbances of 1959, when refugees fleeing ethnic persecution came to Uganda. Others talked of an earlier occurrence of a wasting disease, which started around 1920s. Not much was known about this disease but stories about its devastating effects were passed on by word of mouth in southern Uganda. Nobody knew exactly how mutigwarwanda was treated, why it disappeared, and whether or not it really existed. However, the most plausible explanation with regard to the 1959 outbreak may be found within the name of the mysterious disease itself. The name mutigwarwanda, which roughly translates as "the medicine of Rwanda" refers to the treatment and not the disease. It was commonly believed that the only healers who could cure it were Rwandese traditional healers found among the refugees.

Consistently, virtually everyone who had heard of mutigwarwanda described it as a high-mortality wasting disease. It seems to have fizzled out as mysteriously as it had appeared. Subsequently, it became common to refer to any debilitating new wasting disease of unknown origin as possible mutigwarwanda reincarnated. Equating the new disease with mutigwarwanda was both reassuring and worrying. Mutigwarwanda had come and gone, therefore the hope was that the new outbreak would soon go away too.

While trying to trace the earliest cases of AIDS and how they were treated, I was told about specific cases of some people who came down with strange diseases that, in retrospect, were almost certainly cases of AIDS. One of them was a traditional healer I will call Ibrahim Kasira, who, in the mid 1970s, returned to his home village in Bushenyi, a southern district of Uganda, but no one readily recognised him, not even his own family. He also surprised them by his failure to explain what had befallen him, which added to the mystery. As a traditional healer-cum-witchdoctor, everyone expected him to know. However, he said he suspected the cause to be mutigwarwanda.

Someone who will never forget Kasira's homecoming is his nephew, a community health worker, who told me the story. "My uncle returned when he was grossly emaciated, and his mouth was white. I had never seen such a white mouth. It was as if he had sticky cassava flour around his gums. His skin had darkened and was covered in scaly patches. His hair had thinned and turned brown and he was breathing heavily," he said. "His transformation left a lasting impression on me. I could hardly believe that a strong, fat man, who had left for Ibanda and Masaka to practise his trade, would return looking so miserably thin."

A few months after Kasira's death, a trader in the nearby town of Ishaka who frequented Kampala and Masaka suffered the same fate. By that time, people in the area had heard of a few other cases in the neighbouring districts. Many thought that these cases could have been manifestations of a new epidemic of mutigwarwanda. In hindsight, many now accept that these were the earliest cases of AIDS in their areas.

In the 1970s, President Idi Amin had warned about a new incurable type of gonorrhoea. In his trademark jocular style, he called it "Good Hope" because according to him, if you got it, then your fate was sealed. All that was left was to hope for good luck. He described it as an aggressive and incurable kind of gonorrhoea that removes the hairs of its victims. Some have since speculated this to imply that Amin had seen or been told of such cases and connected them with an outbreak of a new sexually transmitted disease before it was recognised as AIDS by scientists. However, this remains speculation as there is no way to confirm it. But, almost certainly, Amin was referring to the same kinds of cases described above, which were already being seen in communities.

Later, in early 1979, a brilliant and promising young man returned to his home town of Rukungiri after successfully completing his degree course at Makerere University. Everyone was surprised to see him back in his home village, instead of staying on in the city and taking up gainful employment. He did not look well, and he behaved in a rather strange way. As his health deteriorated he looked more and more like the traders who had died of suspected kapa poisoning. People were surprised because it was thought that only traders were poisoning or bewitching each other.

I often wonder about the cases of two men whom I knew quite well. The first one was a neighbour in his late twenties, who died of tuberculosis that failed to respond to therapy, in the late 1960s. He lived what would now be considered a highly risky lifestyle for HIV. His sex life revolved around prostitutes and he admittedly overindulged. The second man whom I saw in 1975 had Kaposi's sarcoma (KS). I was sure of the diagnosis because I was a newly qualified doctor and I had trained under Prof. Sebastian Kyalwazi, whose main research interest was KS. I had seen many cases but this one was different. Unlike the middle-aged or elderly patients who usually suffered from KS, this one was a young man in his early twenties. In addition, his KS was very aggressive, unlike Kyalwazi's cases which progressed slowly. He could have suffered from HIV-associated KS, especially as he had signs suggestive of severe immune deficiency and did not live long. We now know that KS is associated with herpes virus 8, commonly known as HHV-8, first described by Doctors Yuang Chang and Patrick Moore in 1994. HHV-8 seems to take advantage of weakened immunity to cause KS.

Meanwhile, in various hospitals, especially those in the mid-southern district of Masaka and in Kampala, cases of strange diseases turned up more and more often. Doctors noticed an emerging change in disease patterns, which included body wasting and multiple infections that failed to respond to standard therapies. Mr P. Tibomanya, a Ugandan researcher, reported that in 1982 alone, 84 cases were registered in Kitovu Hospital in Masaka district. Dr Sam Tumwesigire recalls a case that, in retrospect, he realises was the first case of AIDS he ever saw in Mulago National Referral Hospital. In the early 1980s a severely wasted woman from Masaka, near Rakai, was admitted to the medical ward. She presented with a chronic skin rash and extensive oral thrush. She had been referred to Mulago because doctors in Masaka could neither diagnose the strange illness nor treat it successfully. Mulago doctors were not any wiser. They could see that the patient was starving — grossly malnourished - and that she had signs normally associated with weakened immunity but no one could find or explain the cause. They looked for internal cancer, trying to exclude it as a possible cause, but none was found. They were left with no alternative but to make a rather odd tentative diagnosis of "adult malnutrition". However, a high-energy and protein diet did not help, and her condition worsened steadily.

"I had never seen anything like it," Dr Tumwesigire recalls. "In the early 1980s; when the first cases appeared in my home town of Kabale, it was mainly the pot-bellied well-to-do who were affected. They wasted away until they looked just like the woman in Mulago."

Earlier, in the late 1970s' while carrying out postmortem examinations in Mulago Hospital, a senior pathologist, Prof John Rwomushana, noted a new trend in postmortem findings. There was an unexplainable gradual increase of deaths caused by very rare diseases. These included cases of a serious brain infection, cryptoccocal meningitis, tuberculosis outside the lungs (extra pulmonary tuberculosis) and rare types of cancers, especially KS. The pathology department was working overtime. This was a bonanza for teaching purposes but a disaster for patients.

When I met Rwomushana by chance in Cape Town, South Africa where we were both attending the International AIDS Conference in July 2009, I asked him about his experience with regard to early cases of HIV/AIDS. "One day in mid-1970s, I found a strange case of Kaposi's sarcoma of the brain. On carrying out literature search I could not find reports of similar cases," he explained. "I just had to publish my finding." Of course no HIV test was done as the disease was unknown at the time. But as we discussed this case we both wondered whether HIV could have been the underlying cause. If such a case was found today, it would be assumed to be AIDS-related until proven otherwise.

These cases provide strong circumstantial evidence that there were some cases of AIDS in Uganda as early as the 1970s. The different therapies that were first tried were targeted at presenting signs and symptoms. However, the outcome was always death.

Medicines don't Work no More

While pathologists were trying to find the cause of deaths against the background of wailing relatives, in 1986, huge crowds gathered downtown in bars and streets for grand festivities. It seemed like the celebrations would never end. Beer was being imported and even smuggled in across the porous Uganda-Kenya border – and from other neighbouring countries – as the run-down Uganda breweries could not cope with the sudden surge of thirst in the country. The air of hope and optimism for a peaceful and brighter future was almost palpable. Many long-suffering people reckoned that the turbulent times that had characterised most of post-independence Uganda were over, and that their salvation had finally come.

The reason for the impromptu festivities was the extraordinary success of the charismatic hero Yoweri Museveni. Over the previous five years, the idolised leader of the National Resistance Army (NRA) that initially started as a shadowy guerrilla force with only 25 men, had against all odds fought all the way into central Kampala. On 25 January 1986 Museveni toppled the seemingly invincible and feared army led by General Bazilio Okello. When the few brave civilians that first ventured out to test the waters confirmed that they could move freely and unmolested, word spread quickly.

Reassured, the long-besieged and hungry multitudes of city dwellers gathered courage and emerged from their hiding places that had been their uncomfortable homes for weeks as the battle for the control of the city had raged, and they poured into the streets. They were pleasantly surprised to find that the new guards on the streets, unlike the previous ones did not randomly shoot at civilians. The memory of rowdy soldiers who had looted Kampala dry amidst widespread chaos following the overthrow of the Idi Amin regime only six years earlier was still vivid. People could not believe that soldiers could be so disciplined. And in next to no time the relieved civilians were engulfed in a frenzy of spontaneous celebration to mark the end of the chaotic war. It was arguably the biggest expression of both relief and happiness Kampala had ever seen.

Earlier, between 1983 and 1986, the bad news reaching the government of President Milton Obote had not been only from the battlefront. There were also worrying reports of disgruntlement and infighting between Ugandan soldiers from the northern tribes of Acholi that dominated the army, and Obote's own Langi tribe. Trouble had been brewing amid suspicion that Obote was trying to put a Lango in command. News of people dying of a mysterious illness emanating from Rakai, in southwestern Uganda was not taken very seriously. The military campaign took priority.

While a new political chapter was starting in 1986, the spoiler that had been generally ignored was poised to strike. Scientists had earlier reported that the new disease that was killing an increasing number of people was similar to an outbreak first described among homosexuals is the USA. Therefore no one wanted to hear of it, because homosexuality is taboo in Uganda. But the death toll mounted, and the Ministry of Health was forced to respond. One prominent Ugandan medical professor was tasked to rush over to Rakai and find out the cause of the deaths. After a few weeks of "investigations" he was back with his findings.

"There is no AIDS there" he reported to the relief of health officials. "All those talking of AIDS are scaremongers. A typhoid outbreak is responsible for the deaths. All that is needed to solve the problem are Chloramphenicol capsules to treat the sick, pit latrines and good hygiene to stop the spread of the disease," he wrongly concluded.

By 1986, the HIV infection had become one of the leading causes of death in the USA. The next year, breaking news announcing the discovery of AZT, initially thought to "cure" AIDS reverberated around the world. It came with price tag of US$10,000 per patient per year; to poverty-stricken Uganda this treatment was a non-starter.

"Thank God a cure for AIDS has been found," a relative excitedly broke the news to me. "I just heard it over the radio," he said. "We may not be able to afford it today but it is reassuring to know that it exists, and that, in time, it will reach us." But it was not to be a cure. It, nevertheless, had some transitory ameliorating effects and it was better than nothing.

AIDS could not have hit Uganda at a worse social and economic time. Numerous patients with AIDS opportunistic infections flocked to government hospitals for treatment but pharmacists and dispensers just wrote "O/S" (short for "out of stock") against almost all prescribed drugs, and handed back the useless papers to patients, most of whom would have walked long distances and waited in queues for hours. They blamed and vented their anger on healthcare providers. The few health workers who bothered to turn up at their work stations when there was nothing to dispense to throngs of desperate patients, learned to brave their clients' frustration. Patients were advised to try their luck at private pharmacies but the vast majority of patients were too poor to afford the cost of even the most basic painkillers.

"They can't even provide you with an Aspirin," was not an uncommon remark. At the time all that was available to AIDS sufferers were varieties of dubious herbal concoctions, vitamin mixtures, other non-specific medicines, and so-called supportive treatment. As described in *Genocide By Denial*, many people flocked to so-called healers including an old woman who dished out tons of dirty soil to huge numbers of gullible AIDS sufferers.

In 1992, when I started looking for AIDS treatment, it was a mere six years after Museveni's force had marched into Kampala. It was the peak of the AIDS carnage. Those happy festivities seemed like they had happened a long time ago. A trail of death had spread from the initial enclave of AIDS in Rakai to the rest of the country.

New unwritten social rules had emerged. They applied to virtually anyone who returned to his home village. I was to learn about them the hard way. When I visited my home town of Rukungiri for a short holiday in 1993, I met an old primary-school mate who had not continued his education, but who lived there comfortably as a small-scale trader. As I felt about old friends, I was excited to see him and curious to learn from him how our other classmates had fared in life. This was especially the case because I was seeing very few of them around. Regardless of whom I asked about, my old friend feigned deafness. When I persisted, he snapped and retorted in broken English, "No see, no ask."

Later, when I narrated the incident to two other friends, one of them expressed surprise. "You did not know that? Man, you have been away too long," he said. "Never ask the whereabouts of anyone not right in front of you." Another friend elaborated further. "When people fall sick these days they no longer recover like they used to do." Resignedly, he threw his hands up in the air. "Medicines don't work no more," he added.

Time and again, innocent enquiries about old friends or relatives would be met with silence and faraway stares into space. Enquiring about old friends and relatives is a polite cultural norm, but the times had changed. Prudence dictated that if any such enquiry had to be made (though it was not advisable), then it was best to go about it in a roundabout way — like asking about the jobs they used to do instead. For instance, if you wanted to inquire about your old friend John who had been a church choir leader when you last saw him, you went about it somewhat like this. "Who plays the accordion in church these days?" The answer was likely to be something like, "Since John went to be with the Lord, our choir is not what it used to be."

Then you would know that if John was still playing his accordion at all, he had only a choir of angels to accompany him.

Dead Woman Walking

An attractive woman I will call Hilda in her mid-thirties, stopped at a street junction below the main city square in Kampala to ask some idle people for directions to Haji's herbal clinic. "It was like a monster had suddenly dropped in their midst," she recalled.

Hilda was among the scores of people that I interviewed trying to understand how various families of different walks of life coped with AIDS. She shared her amazing experience.

"I remember it was mid-morning in early 1991. All eyes turned and fixed on me. After a moment a number of them simultaneously pointed to the same narrow corridor between rows of shops on Luwum Street, as the rest looked on open-mouthed." She told me that the incident has remained fixed in her memory ever since.

As she made her way to the clinic, they followed her with their eyes. Hilda turned heads everywhere she went, but this time the stares were different. "They were sort of weird," she explained. As she approached the corridor everyone she met seemed to stop and stare. Then she overheard the nervous whispers.

"*Oyo affude*," (She is a dead person walking.)

"But she still looks healthy," Hilda heard another one remark. "That is very sad," he said, "because she will kill many unsuspecting people before she finally succumbs." This was an obvious reference to promiscuous sexual relationships, which were already well-known as a major risk factor for the spread of HIV.

"It's the beautiful ones that have caused us all these problems," one man responded in agreement. Hilda thought he deliberately said it loud, so that she could hear it but the way he said it was devoid of malice. Rather, it was sort of beseeching — as if he hoped it would save a life. "I increased my pace, to avoid hearing any more insults," she said.

The narrow corridor led to a spacious enclosed square that Hilda found jammed with people. The scene immediately made her understand the meaning of the bystanders' stares and remarks. No one but a fool would ask directions to Haji's clinic. People just sneaked in and out. Inside were many emaciated people.

"It was a sight to behold!" Hilda recalled. "It reminded me of pictures I saw of holocaust survivors immediately after the Second World War."

Some of them visibly too weak to stand were lying on fibre mats on the floor. As she entered, the patients, even the very weak ones straightened their frail necks to look at her. She suddenly felt nervous and out of place. It was as if they were all saying to her, "you came too early", or "you lost your way". Although she was of average weight, among this group she looked grossly overfed.

The centre of attraction in the jammed square was an obese man of medium height that they called Haji. He moved among his withered clients looking like a queen bee among starving smoke-dazed drones. Scanning the crowd, Hilda thought that it was going to be a long wait before she would get an audience with the renowned Haji. However, he had spotted her too, though not in a way that strangers usually do. To her surprise, Haji just ignored the many very sick people who had arrived earlier and beckoned her to jump the queue.

"She is rich, that's why," one woman who had apparently been waiting in the line for a long time remarked in undisguised frustration.

"No, she might be one of Haji's wives," Hilda overhead another remark, apparently trying to keep the spirits of her friend up, "I hear Haji loves pretty women."

But they were both wrong. Hilda was there on behalf of her sister Flora who, like them, was shrivelled and bedridden. Flora was kept hidden in the house away from prying eyes. When relatives or friends came to see Flora, the family lied that she was not at home.

Hilda's sick sister was not a tolerant patient. Although she was at a stage of the disease when most people would have long given up, she was still fighting to live tooth and nail. She had a little girl and that was the reason for her fight to stay alive. Her husband had abandoned them to their fate well over a year ago when he realised that they were sick —doomed. But he had not fared any better. He died first. For her daughter's sake, Flora ignored the pain and the stark odds against her, and clung on to life, hoping for a last-minute miracle cure. As time passed she became even sicker, and more and more irritable and acrimonious.

"Nobody cares for me anymore. You are all just waiting for me to die–to get rid of me," Hilda recounted how Flora repeatedly taunted the family.

"My baby! Who will look after my baby?" She cried incessantly, "Haji has a cure but none of you will go to get it for me."

When Flora's taunts became unbearable, Hilda had no alternative but to go out and find the famed Haji. Walking through that "corridor of shame" took all the courage Hilda had ever summoned up in 36 years of life. The stares, blame, hate, anger, expressions of despair – she has never forgotten. Sixteen years later, when she first told me that sad story, she was still haunted by the experience. As she talked, she was blinking, swallowing and fighting to suppress surging emotions.

After explaining to Haji her sister's state of health, he gave her a five-litre kadomola, full of a foul-smelling herbal concoction. He demanded a lot of money for it, but Hilda did not have enough with her. The whispers had been right; evidently, Haji had given her priority over the more deserving cases because they did not seem to have money. Some of them had paid all they had but had not improved. Some were back to see whether he could offer them something more effective. Haji advertised widely on the radio and was always announcing that he had discovered new and more effective AIDS drugs. Many patients kept coming back and paying more and more, until they had nothing left. They still came, regardless — in hope.

"How much do you have with you?" Haji demanded. Hilda pulled out her purse and gave him all she had. It was a big sacrifice for her to part with so much money, but she had no choice. Haji had a way of demanding payment that was not pleasant. On top of that, her sister's moaning wrath would have been unbearable if she returned empty handed. "That will do for the moment," Haji said as he pocketed the cash. "You can always bring the balance later." Hilda had hoped that Haji would discount the balance but as if he could read her mind, he added, "Otherwise this medicine will not work."

Haji knew very well that everyone so desperately wanted the medicine to work, that no one would risk not bringing the balance. He never followed up those that did not return to pay; he knew they had died. And Haji must have known that eventually all would die. Nevertheless, in the meantime, his business flourished, as others replaced those who owed him the balance.

As Hilda frantically approached her relatives to borrow money to pay for Haji's balance, she gathered that her sister had learned of Haji's "miraculous treatment" from one of his agents who went from house to house, sniffing out bedridden patients. Haji paid his agents handsome commissions.

Weeks later, the agent was back. This time, he found Hilda at home. He was bitter and upset. Apparently he had fallen out with his boss after a disagreement and quarrel over his commission. In protest the agent had quit to start his own clinic. He said that he had learned all the "tricks" that he needed to know from Haji and was ready to go it alone.

"How is it possible that Haji can cure AIDS when he has so far lost three wives of his own to the same scourge?" he asked, to Hilda's disbelief. Hilda wanted to ask why he had acted as his agent when he knew the truth about the scam. A few years later, it was not only his wives that Haji failed to cure; he, too, slowly ailed. He then started looking more and more like his patients, with similar symptoms. Finally, he died in the same way too.

The Incredible Fungus

In Ntinda, a suburb of Kampala, a closely woven reed fence enclosed a big compound where the grass had long been annihilated by heavy human traffic. Two huge saucepans were on the fireplaces in the middle of the compound boiling furiously. The slimy green contents steamed popping and bubbling for almost twelve hours a day. A huffing and perspiring shirtless man constantly stirred the contents and in between used a once-white cloth to wipe streams of sweat from his face. He kept adding more and more firewood to the fire, and baskets of mashed fresh herbs and buckets of water to the saucepans. Every fifteen or so minutes he used a jug with a long handle to draw off liquid from the saucepans to fill two-and-half litre plastic *budomola*. He placed each filled container in a line in front of a man seated on a small raised platform, who acknowledged each delivery with a gentle stylish nod.

The man on the platform was known by a single name of Okello. He was a diminutive, illiterate middle-aged man, dressed simply in a clean white collarless shirt, dark trousers and white shoes as he presided over the ritual. He wore a sagacious expression on his face. A small crowd of about a hundred people sat silently on fibre mats below him and looked up to him in awe as they patiently waited their turn to be attended to. One by one, or sometimes in pairs or groups of people entered the compound reverentially, as if the enclosure was a holy shrine. Many of those entering were very weak and were either supported or carried inside by friends or relatives. At the entrance stood a dark, slim teenage boy, the usher, who politely but unemotionally welcomed all newcomers, and led them to the back of the queue on the mats. He also directed out those who had received medicine.

A wooden cash box was placed strategically on a stool next to Okello, who occasionally tapped it as if to ensure that it was safe. But there was no cash book, and no receipts were given out. Also in close attendance was a professional-looking nurse in a white uniform complete with a red belt, similar to that worn by Ministry of Health nurses. Besides fussing over Okello and dispensing the *budomola* he prescribed to the crowd of patients, she also served as his interpreter.

Almost six weeks after her visit to Haji's clinic, Hilda was among the multitude of people in Okello's compound, once again on Flora's behalf. "Haji's medicine did not help my sister, not at all," Hilda recalled sorrowfully. "It had not been easy for her to swallow it. The main problem was the smell! Instead of making her better, her health had deteriorated rapidly. She evidently did not have long to live and had begun to accept her fate. Then suddenly another agent turned up and promised her life — once more raising her hopes." Flora's tantrums started all over again. This time her main complaint was relentless diarrhoea. The agent claimed that only Okello – of all the herbalists –had the right remedy.

As usual a full kadomola was dispensed for Hilda to take to her sister. It cost her dearly. With great difficulty the ailing sister took a cupful of the distasteful stuff. Room was made in the family fridge to keep the rest of the herbal medicine fresh. The next morning when it was time for the next dose, they found a sediment at the bottom; it was cassava flour! Up to the very end, agents came to promise Flora health. She, in her turn, never gave up trying to find a cure that worked.

At about the same time there appeared out of the blue a fast-growing "fungus" medicine that was widely used in Uganda. When mature, the fungus looked like a fluffy dog-eared mushroom. Its exact origin remains obscure. It was reported to have come from China, but some people believed it was from Russia. The more mysterious the origin of a product, the better it was thought to be. But no-one was really bothered where it came from as long as it cured the disease.

The fungus was grown in a special way. You had to fill a jug with hot water, add a lot of sugar and tea leaves. In those days, sugar and tea were in short supply, but people saved what they could to produce the "magic" fungus. Once the water had cooled, pieces of the fungus were added and it was left at room temperature for about a week to mature while floating on top of the liquid. Then the liquid was drunk and the mushroom-like fungus was divided as new seeds, to be either sold or given away to the ever-increasing numbers of people on the hunt for it.

For over two years it was the talk of the town. Vendors moved from house to house carrying kettles and jugs containing the fungus, and it was on sale at markets. Although it was advertised as a panacea, people whispered that it had wonderful effects on AIDS patients. The demand for it was such that people travelled long distances, even from neighbouring countries to buy it. For a time it was the hope AIDS patients had. Even those who were not sure whether they were infected with HIV or not, who were too scared to test for HIV, consumed it in the hope that it would protect them from coming down with the fully-blown disease. It was said to prolong life, which was exactly what AIDS patients prayed for.

Unlike *budomola* medicines which were viewed with stigma, the mushroom was used openly. People pretended to take it for the treatment of other diseases, or merely for the sake of longevity. AIDS was never mentioned. Yet it was AIDS that almost all people who used it aimed to treat or prevent. As an added attraction, the fungus extract had a rather pleasant taste. It tasted, smelt and looked a little like diluted red wine. However, as far as health benefits were concerned, it caused no demonstrable improvement. However, no-one would openly admit it was useless, as most people who used it were in a state of denial.

In time its popularity fizzled out as mysteriously as it had appeared, apparently without any discernible effect. People stopped talking about it as if it had never existed. I met very few people who admitted to ever taking it. Hilda admitted that her sister Flora tried it as her very last card. She recalled pouring away the remainder of the fungus after her sister's death. A white papery mould had grown on top, but it still smelled like stale wine.

In the absence of drugs that had been proven to be effective, claims of traditional cures were the order of the day. Healers, both local and from other parts of Africa and overseas, especially from China, repeatedly claimed to have discovered miracle cures.

All corners of the country produced strange therapies claiming to be beneficial. But as far as AIDS treatment was concerned, in the late 1980s and early 1990s, neither Western nor herbal medicine could claim superiority over the other or demonstrate any genuine breakthrough.

5

Mysteries of Ancient Cures

Healers' Secrets

In preparation for my new undertaking as the head of the Joint Clinical Research Centre, I took time off to learn as much as I could about the mesmerising world of traditional medicine. My interest in this discipline, which was new and alien to me, arose, because it had dawned on me that it would be my duty to determine whether it had a role to play in the treatment of AIDS in the era of modern medicines. I had to determine whether the medicines dispensed by the likes of Haji and Okello were of any use to the multitudes that paid a fortune in a desperate attempt to stay alive. I realised right from the start that testing of herbal preparations was a cumbersome undertaking, which was complicated by absence of modern facilities. It was of critical national importance that I did something, though my scope was limited by circumstances.

I started off by consulting traditional practitioners to gather information. I first needed to find out who was a true traditional healer, as many novice healers claiming to have cures for AIDS had jumped on the bandwagon, not because of the effectiveness of their medicines, but because of the lucrative returns. It became clear that defining a genuine traditional healer would be difficult or, at the very least contentious. They came in all forms, and appeared in all situations and places where AIDS patients would be expected.

I searched for reference books authored by people raised in a traditional African setup. I sought out those who had studied the art and practice of traditional medicine but it was not a very productive search. Finally, I came across a little-known book entitled *Medicinal Plants and Traditional Medicine in Africa* by Abayomi Sofowara, a Nigerian scholar. In it, I found a description of traditional medicine.

Total combination of knowledge and practices, whether explicable or not, used in diagnosing, preventing, or eliminating a physical, mental, or social diseases and which may rely extensively on past experience and observation handed down from generation to generation, verbally or in writing.

This was quite a mouthful but it helped me make a start at appreciating the complexity of the subject. The World Health Organisation (WHO) redefined traditional medicine at its 8th General Programme of work covering the period 1990 to 1995 as,

....comprising of therapeutic practices that have been in existence, often for hundreds of years, before the development and spread of modern scientific medicine and are still in use today.

This definition presupposes that the onset of modern scientific medicine spelt the end of the evolution of traditional medicine; and in any case, no traditional medicine for AIDS, a new disease, has existed for hundreds of years.

I opted to approach this complex subject with broader and somewhat liberal lenses. I also adopted a community perspective whereby a traditional healer would generally be defined as a person who treats ill people using herbs (plant leaves, seeds and flowers, tree bark, stem, roots, and various fungi), animal parts, minerals or earth matter. I gathered that a traditional healer could also incorporate certain special rituals as part of treatment. In effect, different kinds of stuff and rituals could constitute part of the recipe for treatment. A variety of implements and procedures, some of them secret or mysterious, were employed in the preparation of traditional therapies.

In my Bahororo community, traditional medicine is very sophisticated and defined in broader perspective. It encompasses other aspects that include special rituals and rites (*okubandwa*); mysticism, witchcraft, sorcery (*okuroga*); fetishes, spells (*engisha*); incantation (*okutongerera*); nude night dances (*okucecera*); exorcism (*okukiza-emizimu*); offerings (*okuterekyerera*); hypnotism (*okusirisya*); magic (*emigyereko*); prophesies (*okuragura*) and superstitions (*emize*); all recognised and acceptable as linked to at least some aspects of traditional "medical" practice.

I also learned of other systems for delivery of traditional medicines including voodoo, which is still practiced in West Africa. In Benin, voodoo is an ancient tradition that is mainly practised in rural areas. Its unacceptable aspect includes infanticide, used on the belief that some children are born witches. Practitioners believe that if a child identified as a witch is not killed, one or both of the parents will die. In faraway Haiti, Voodoo is a state sanctioned religion; various ailments are treated and spiritual succour is provided.

I also learned about the ethics of traditional healers' practice. Although the traditional healer usually expected some reward for their work, payment did not necessarily have to be money. The poor were never denied treatment. They were allowed to pay whatever they could afford, when they were able to. Payment usually consisted of diverse but common presents, like chickens, goats and foodstuffs. These gifts were known in my tribe as *ebyokutera ekishaka*, meaning, "presents given in recognition of efforts made to collect the medicine from the bush".

I noted that some scientists were up in arms about a liberal definition of traditional medicine. A bone of contention was the inclusion of witchdoctors, diviners and spiritualists among those they considered to be "straight" traditional healers. One other reason for their disquiet was that their peculiar practices rendered modern research on traditional medicines virtually impossible. Furthermore, if traditional medicine was to be formally recognised for treatment of AIDS, the inclusion of witchdoctors and seers complete with their traditional regalia of ostrich feathers, seashell necklaces, rattles and colourfully decorated faces standing shoulder to shoulder with doctors clad in white overcoats and with stethoscopes around their necks would be as controversial as it would be a spectacle to behold.

I found that the norms of various aspects of "traditional medicine" are seldom clear cut or uniform across cultures. For instance, some special rituals or incantations sometimes precede or follow the administration of herbal therapy, ostensibly to activate its potency. Therefore, to steer clear of such complexities and potential controversies, I confined my research on traditional medicine into observational and partial clinical testing of herbal preparations, and tried as far as possible in such difficult circumstances to adhere to modern scientific principles.

Traditional healers or herbalists, like their Western counterparts, were searching for an entirely new, groundbreaking discovery to treat a new disease. In such circumstances, it was perhaps understandable that some herbalists randomly tried out various herbal preparations, hoping for a eureka moment. Claims and counterclaims were the order of the day. Desperate patients dashed to new "healers" proclaiming miracles. On the other hand, doctors with nothing better to offer their frantic patients watched helplessly as they were deserted by their patients who headed to the supposed new beacons of hope.

Ugandans are ardent herbal medicine users with up to 80% of them reporting ever using herbs at least once in their lives for various ailments ranging from the common cold to cancer. Some herbs are known to be effective against some veterinary and human diseases. Generations have successfully used herbs for many ailments. President Museveni admitted use of herbal molluscide from the plant Phytolacca Dodecandra (*omuhoko*) on his farms to kill liver-fluke-harbouring snails that flourish in cattle-watering wells (and infect the animals). The President praises Prof William Isharaza, who developed omuhoko into an appropriate formulation for use in cattle-watering dams that has the added advantage of killing bilharzia-carrying snails. The Omuhoko has been confirmed to be highly effective and environmentally friendly molluscide. Herbs whether effective or not were all that was available to most Ugandan AIDS patients until 2003.

In the wider perspective, herbal medicine practice is not a monopoly of Africa. Virtually all communities of the world practise it in one form or another, and many have special names for it. Many books about medicinal plants have been published all over the world. Trade in herbal medicines is one of the most lucrative businesses in the world. In a number of countries, notably China, traditional medicine is a serious academic and professional discipline taught side by side with modern medicine up to university level.

Eastern Wisdom

In 1993, a humanitarian I will call Roger Bonell, who headed an NGO that specialised in traditional medicines, arranged a scholarship for me to go on a study tour of the Far East to learn from one of the ancient and well developed cultures of traditional medicinal practice. I arrived in Hanoi, Vietnam, and found a country that was struggling to recover from a protracted war with America that had lasted from November 1955 to 30 April 1975. The country was faced with such social-economic hardships, with many of their people living in abject poverty, that it was difficult for me to understand how they could have possibly inflicted such a humiliating defeat on the greatest military and most technologically advanced power on earth!

The state of Hanoi International Airport was so bad that my plane's first attempt to land had to be aborted at the very last minute. Travelling from the airport in a 40-year-old American car, I could see that both the road and the car were in a state of disrepair. Along the rough gravel road were numerous peasants carrying baskets of vegetables and fruits for sale. There were a scattering of motorcycles and many bicycles that zigzagged along the road trying to avoid the pedestrians. When the battered taxi that, for most of the journey, moved with and at the pace of the crowd, finally crawled up to the hotel, I was tired and hungry. After checking in, I went straight to the hotel restaurant but found that it had only two items on the menu: pork and rice or chicken and rice.

When I visited the main hospital the next day, the secret behind their incredible resilience was unveiled. In a sentence, it was all due to their tenacious spirit of self reliance. The hospital was like any other I had seen in many parts of the developing world, complete with medical, paediatrics and surgical wards and other specialised medical departments. However, the pharmacy was different. I was led to the backyard and shown a well-tended garden filled with a wide variety of plants. While I was being shown around the garden I recognised a number of medicinal plants that my tribesmen have also used for generations to treat various ailments. I picked up a branch of one plant, Bidens Pilosa, known as *enyabarashana* in my language, and asked my Vietnamese guide what it was used for. "It is used as an antiseptic and for dressing wounds," he replied. There were two reasons why I was surprised. First of all, I had not expected a common weed in central Africa to be found in Vietnam. Secondly, it was remarkable that it was being used in exactly the same way and for the same conditions as it was used in my home village in southwestern Uganda.

As we walked down towards a valley below the hospital, there was a cacophony that became louder and louder. We soon arrived at the source – a large pond full of frogs of all sizes — doing what frogs all over the world do best – ribbit. However, these particular ones sounded like a squad hired to blast out noise.

The hospital used the herb garden in the same way a modern hospital uses a pharmacy. The chief plastic surgeon informed me that the commonest injuries in their hospitals were burns, especially in winter. The main causes were accidental fires ignited by cheap kerosene heaters commonly used by peasants to warm their homes. Many of the burns were very serious covering high percentages of the surface of bodies of victims. But the hospital had a remarkable record of success in treating such burns some of which, in modern hospitals, would be associated with poor prognosis. This is where the farm of frogs in the pond came in. Their skins were used to dress the burns. The skins prevented fluid loss from the burns, protected against infections and promoted healing. I saw many recuperating burns patients in hospital doing very well — much better than those I had seen with similar degree of burns in some other hospitals.

"So how do the frogs' skins do it?" I asked the head of the burns unit.

"This is an ancient practice for which we have a scientific explanation now," he replied. "The skin contains a potent antibiotic that protects against infections and also has various natural chemicals that stimulate cell regeneration."

I went on a ward round with the clinicians and observed patients being diagnosed correctly as suffering from various diseases and conditions. They were all being treated with herbal preparations and various traditional recipes. That many of them were being discharged after apparent recovery suggested that the treatment worked.

During my walks around Hanoi, I saw numerous stalls and small shops selling an assortment of herbal medicines. Others advertised traditional medicine services. Modern pharmacies were very few and far in between. I was told that most of the modern pharmacies were newly established by mainly Australian entrepreneurs. Unlike the herbal clinics which were heavily patronised, I saw few customers going in or out of Western medicine pharmacies.

At a specially arranged seminar, traditional medicine specialists explained the use of herbs in the treatment of diseases in Vietnam and other areas of Asia. The delegates heard that during the long war with America all that was available for the treatment of virtually all North Vietnamese were herbal medicines.

The same fortitude and retention of what they call time-tested practices that saw them survive over the centuries are now transforming Vietnam into a vibrant, modern state.

Rebirth of Abafumu

When I returned from Vietnam, I was much more positive about traditional medicines than I had been before. I was ready to look at it with a more open mind, and try to find out how it was practised in my own country. But it was not all smooth sailing. I was initially met with a wall of silence. This was a polite reminder that secrecy is a key component of herbal medicine practice and an ancient custom of our traditional healers.

Traditional practitioners on the whole consider their knowledge sacrosanct. Only some people are permitted to become traditional healers or *abafumu* as they are called in my kihororo culture. Customarily, the abafumu hold a special revered place in society, not unlike that of a high priest in a parish. They passed on their special skills to only a select few after a long and stringent apprenticeship before declaring them eligible to practise as herbalists. This ensured high standards, quality, and in reality some sort of patent protection of their indigenous knowledge and skills.

In many parts of Africa, abafumu operate through a system of secret societies, bound by a code of conduct and their brand of professional etiquette. It was therefore quite understandable that many of them were reluctant to reveal secrets of their trade. They feared losing their monopoly, income, and their status in the community. Most herbalists, especially those who claimed to have AIDS cures, steadfastly refused to reveal the constituents of their medicines, and some of them strongly objected to any form of scientific analysis. This became a recurrent obstacle to my work, as it tended to conflict with modern scientific research methodologies.

I came across some traditional healers and authorities who vehemently defended secrecy. They argued that herbal medicines should always be tested in the form in which they are traditionally used. Their justification was that the different constituents may be individually ineffective, but may synergistically combine to become potent. Therefore, if such medicines were tested in a different form and failed to work it would not necessarily imply that the original formulation was ineffective.

Another issue that arose with regard to research on herbs concerned the uniformity of the products. The precise methods used in Western medicine preparation are not part of the usual traditional medical practice. Many herbalists insist on preparing their own product, in secret, using traditional apparatus or intuition. If you needed to study the products scientifically, batches would not necessarily be uniform, consisting of the same ingredients in similar concentrations.

Like in all professions, traditional healers and herbalists have their own quacks, and the numbers of impostors increased dramatically in the era of AIDS as need for their services increased. Many uninitiated people took up the herbal profession, for which they were not trained or suited in the traditional sense. I had to retain an open-mind and avoided the temptation to generalise that all traditional healers were quacks.

By the late 1980s, a modified version of AIDS-driven herbal medicine practice was well established and widely patronised in Uganda. It had emerged as one of the most lucrative businesses and was a money spinner. Lack of an alternative remedy forced many AIDS sufferers to pay whatever they could afford for budomola and anything that was claimed to help. The lucrative herbal medicine trade attracted a new generation of amateur herbalists who hijacked the ancient profession from its traditional owners. The assortment consisted of the strangest of bedfellows imaginable. Among their ranks were people from all walks of life, ranging from the clergy, sheiks, teachers, engineers, lawyers, peasants and street vendors down to common hooligans, conmen and layabouts. Men constituted the vast majority of these opportunists, as is usually the case when high stakes are involved. To beat the competition, some "herbalists" devised nifty plots. Some claimed to possess magical or supernatural powers that enhanced the healing properties of their herbal preparations.

The AIDS epidemic presented a serious challenge to medical doctors' dominance and monopoly of disease management. Without any effective therapy to offer, doctors found themselves in a weak position, unable to mount a robust challenge to the scores of opportunistic herbalist scammers who, to the doctors dismay, gained popularity. Since they could not beat them, a small number of doctors joined them. Amazingly, at least one AIDS stricken medical doctor was among thousands of people who lined up to receive Nanyonga's soil that she dispensed as an AIDS cure! Since they had no alternative, the doctor and throngs of other patients who flocked to Nanyonga had nothing to lose as the soil was free, except the transport cost to the place and the time they spent there.

Divine Healing

A remarkable man by the name of Joseph Mugonza had a head start over other herbalists who claimed to cure AIDS. Mugonza, the son of a peasant called Lozio Kulazikulabe and his wife Falazia Nakanwagi, was born uneventfully on 15 July 1937, in a village called Bugere, Lwangulwe, Buddu, in Central Uganda. However, his followers were told another version, which they solemnly believe.

Bhuka Bijumiro-jjumiro, whose unique name was bestowed upon him by Mugonza, is the author of his biography, entitled *Bambi Baba Redeemer of the New Age*. According to Bhuka, Mugonza was initially reluctant to be born "for a good seven days fearing contamination of illusion," whatever that means. But he was "eventually born on the eighth day of his mother's excruciatingly long labour in a moment of awe and great fear." Entunuza Beliyonda, one of Mugonza's dedicated followers, takes up the story, describing Mugonza's birth as a spectacular miracle. "His birth was witnessed by two serpents. One was positioned between the legs of the mother, while another stood aside looking on." Entunuza explains that the presence of the serpents was a source of his vast wisdom and divine healing power, leaving no room for doubt that he believed the fantastic tale.

By the time HIV/AIDS was recognised as a new disease in the early 1980s, Mugonza was already well established as a renowned herbalist, "healer of all diseases" and a "miracle worker" who solved complicated legal, social and economic problems. He claimed to be a prophet and a living saint in possession of divine powers specially conferred upon him by God. In addition to curing diseases, he claimed to have the power to raise people from the dead, to shed his human body and move in and out of heaven at will, and be in many places at the same time. Mugonza formed and led a fanatical religious sect based in a small village in Rakai, close to where AIDS first occurred in Uganda. He gave all his followers strange, tongue-twisting new names, and confiscated all their property, making them sign documents saying that it was all done with their voluntary consent. He renamed his village surrounding a "hallowed cave" that was dug in a central hill, Sseesamirembe, meaning a generator of peace.

Every evening his followers gathered in designated holy places called "discourse circles", but more commonly known in their special dialect as *enkurungo*. They took their designated places on stone seats arranged in a circular formation around a fireplace to worship Mugonza in rituals known as *kuwaaya*. Seated on an elevated platform Mugonza presided over the ceremony, preached, told tales of his heavenly escapades, cured diseases, solved social problems, arranged marriages, prophesied, rewarded devotion, punished dissent, and allocated duties and chores. Members also engaged in other rituals including stripping naked (*gerenge*), and cleansing followers of their sins by burning some of their personal belongings (*sebagengeya nkeya*). Several women alleged that they were forced into arranged marriages with older men when they were under-age. They described weird marriage rituals which they had to undergo, including mixing of their blood with that of the men chosen for them, and smearing it around their genitals.

The uneducated but otherwise highly charismatic man, who claimed to know contents of any book without reading it, attracted hundreds of followers from various parts of Uganda, neighbouring countries and as far as Tunisia, Sweden, Canada and USA.

"Mugonza has incredible psychological power over people. He is so persuasive, so convincing and so believable, that I was powerless to resist joining his sect, despite my wife being strongly against it," said Bjorn Siemensen, a Swedish industrialist who forfeited his business to the sect—voluntarily! "I really don't know what came over me," he added as he shook his head in apparent disbelief.

Mugonza's sect was known as Sserulanda Nsulo Y'obulamu, described by Bijumiro-jjumiro as "the joining of all souls to the fountain of eternal life". Membership, though dominated by peasants, comprised people from diverse walks of life including those who sought treatment for AIDS and various other ailments.

To match his status as a healer, a living saint and prophet, he conferred upon himself numerous fancy tongue-twisting, high-sounding names preceded by glorious titles. To his followers, he is officially known as: His Imperishable Glory (HIG), Redeemer of the new Age, Master of Eternal Ageless Wisdom, Sabayimira Nsibo, Sempulutusa, Lulangulankulanga, Segiringwa, Sebirindwa, Mikenkenula, Semikenkenula, Ggulingusamanhanulonkulo, Bambi Baaba Baabuwee, Doctor Joseph, Jozzewaffe, Kaggwa, Kaguwa, Kaggalanda, Mugonza.

His followers abbreviated it all by calling him Bambi Baaba which, according to his followers, are esteemed expressions, meaning "merciful, kind and humane".

In 1987, HIG Bambi Baaba was noticed by the Uganda Ministry of Health when they received news that a "man-god" based in Rakai was busy "curing" people of AIDS, using a herbal concoction that he called *Kensalata*. The Ministry of Health hurriedly dispatched a high-powered delegation led by a senior official by the name of Dr Joseph Kyabaggu, the then Director of Planning and Services, to find out whether the "saintly" man had indeed found the elusive cure for AIDS.

When the delegation arrived on the outskirts of the village, they were stopped by Bambi Baaba's zealous scouts and informed that their "unholy" official vehicles would not be allowed in the sacred village. They parked their vehicle at the nearby police station, and were transferred into an old white Mercedes Benz saloon car with all white interior upholstery, provided by Bambi Baaba. One of the Ministry of Health delegates recalled their journey to the "holy" place. "We were so mesmerized by Bambi Baaba's protocol that, as we travelled to Sseesamirembe, we were all very nervous, not knowing what to expect," she said. "Our leader was so scared that he chain-smoked all the way," she added.

When they finally arrived, they were ushered into a hostel and told to await word from the holy one. It did not take long for them to realise that they were virtual prisoners. When they requested their hosts to let them get on with their mission so that they could return to their work, they were politely informed that they would only leave at His Imperishable Glory's pleasure. Otherwise, they were treated and fed well on a purely vegetarian diet, which they described as delicious, and washed down with non-alcoholic drinks, as ordained by the sect's faith. During their longer-than-expected stay, they watched as numerous people from various parts of the country came in for treatment. They were only allowed to meet a select few, who uniformly claimed to have been cured of AIDS. However, none of them provided any proof that they had ever been infected by HIV.

By the time His Imperishable Glory was happy to let them go, they had pledged their Ministry's strong support for a health centre specially dedicated to the sect. Bambi Baaba renamed the new health centre Vumiliro. In addition, the delegation pledged government funds to run it. They also promised to support construction of a herbal medicine factory to manufacture Kensalata. Bambi Baaba promptly named the new enterprise Famacolo. He prophesied that it would soon become a monopoly supplier of AIDS medicine to the Ministry of Health. He also declared that it would expand to become a major earner of foreign exchange for Uganda from AIDS drugs export to other countries.

Over the years, the actions of the sect troubled the neighbouring communities more and more. They complained of intimidation, land grabbing and weird rituals and activities alleged to be perpetuated by the sect, and called for urgent government intervention. Eventually, an official commission of inquiry, to which I was appointed as one of the commissioners, was set up to investigate the activities of the sect. Among the terms of reference given to the commission was to determine whether Joseph Mugonza and his sect had the power to "cure incurable diseases" including AIDS. It was during the public hearings that the public learned of some gruesome allegations that a number of followers revealed in their sworn testimonies to the commission.

It emerged that Mugonza insisted on the total and unquestioning allegiance of his followers. But he did not take their loyalty for granted. From time to time, he set surprise tests to verify their continued compliance. For instance, he once asked his followers to build up their appetite by fasting overnight and most of the following day in preparation for a grand feast, when they would all eat their fill. The next afternoon, as promised, a select group of "chefs" emerged carrying big steaming pots and saucepans from a makeshift kitchen that had earlier been declared out of bounds to all other community members. They set the pots on wooden tables in front of the hungry followers who had gathered in semicircular sitting formation with their plates and spoons in front of them. "However, the aroma exuding from the pots was sort of strange," one of his followers later testified.

Bambi Baaba Baabuwee gracefully took his place of honour in a strategic position from where he would watch all his flock "enjoying" the meal. Then he invited them to serve themselves. What they found in the pots was so startling that their appetites evaporated instantly. However, no one dared decline His Imperishable Glory's specially prepared meal. Oblivious to the odd stuff, each and everyone filled their plates and returned to their places to await word from the holy one to start eating.

When they were all ready, Bambi Baaba "blessed the food", and signalled for them to start. Almost in unison, all of them dipped their spoons in the greenish murky "gravy" only to be told to stop as they were about to take the first mouthfuls. Apparently, they had all passed the test. Bambi Baaba was reassured of his followers' faith and obedience. But for one overenthusiastic follower, the signal to stop came too late. I don't know whether HIG awarded him a first class pass.

So, what did Bambi Baaba have on the menu for his faithful followers for this unforgettable feast? Hard to believe as it may be, it was a special "casserole" of cow dung and stones!

Bambi Baaba ensured that those who erred lived to regret their transgressions. One of his many centres of correction was a rectangular building known as Balora that occupied a central place in Sseesamirembe village. The feared and revered building also served as a mausoleum in which embalmed bodies were kept. Numerous followers also described Balora as a place for meditation and other secretive rituals called *okuloora*, a special privilege reserved for the initiated elite, described as those who "had passed through many stages of spiritual evolution that enabled them to see with a third eye". Balora was said to be a source of healing powers, wealth and spiritual inspiration.

One witness told the public inquiry of the time she was locked up in Balora overnight as a punishment for disobedience. "The naked bodies, including those of children were arranged in semi-standing positions leaning against the walls. "I was so scared—my heart thumped in my chest, I shivered and sweated—I thought I would die," she said. "I screamed, but the sound did not come out because I was scared that Mugonza would hear it, and give me a worse punishment. The night was long, dawn seemed to take forever to come. I am still haunted by the ghosts—especially as I knew some of them before they died."

Another follower was alleged to have been chained in the forest overnight. Evidently, whoever Bambi Baaba punished would never forget it, and others who heard of it would thereafter tread carefully lest they raised his ire.

When we visited Sseesamirembe long after Mugonza had gone to America, we were taken around by a worried and highly suspicious group of his loyal caretakers who were apparently in charge of the sect. In Balora we found only the bodies of adults, which were neatly arranged in new coffins covered with sheets of new cloth. The room was newly swept and was heavily sprayed with perfumed air fresheners, with scented sticks burning in each corner. However, we were told later by several witnesses that this was a sham show that was specially staged in preparation for our visit. Apparently, the eve of our arrival saw a burst of frenzied activity in Balora. New coffins and rolls of cloth were delivered, and old ones hurriedly removed and heaped in the store. All bodies of children were allegedly removed by a trusted group of followers who were sworn to strict silence, and hurriedly buried in a shallow mass grave a few kilometres from the site.

When we made a surprise visit to Famacolo, the supposed AIDS herbal medicine factory and Vumiliro, the sect's health centre we found both of them in very sorry state. It took a while to find the keys for the Famacolo building. While we waited, I got the impression that the delay in finding the keys was a ploy to encourage us to postpone the visit. However, if that was the intention, it failed. When we finally entered the building, it was obvious that no one had used the building in many years. There was a thick layer of dust on the floor, rats' droppings and an army of cockroaches that scattered in fright when the door creaked open. The room was covered by thick cobwebs. In one corner we found a dust-covered and pest-infested old sisal sack full of snail shells. In the opposite corner there was a tattered sack half full of dried plant roots and remains of decomposed leaves. Needless to say, if anyone was still being treated with Kensalata, it was certainly not being manufactured in this Famacolo.

As for Vumiliro we were shocked by what we found there. All I can say is that it was a misuse of words to call it a health centre. The rundown Vumiliro, had no functional steriliser. In the delivery room and what passed for a ward we found bricks being used as pillows for inpatients. We were stunned to find cotton wool, used to clean patients' wounds, disposed of in corridors, and blown all over the compound by the wind. The only pit latrine for use by the patients and staff also doubled up as a disposal for placentas. On the medicine trolley, we found a mess of used needles and gloves, mixed with medicines, dirty forceps, banana peels and pieces of decomposing oranges! It was the dirtiest and most unhygienic building masquerading as a health care centre that we had ever seen. It was appropriate that Mugonza had insisted on calling it a different name. It was apparent that instead of treating AIDS or any other disease, Vumiliro was a high-risk centre for their transmission and spread.

As the AIDS crisis was shrouded in widespread fear, stigma and mysticism, it is not surprising that frauds exploited it. It was not only amateur herbalists and the spiritualists like Mugonza that were involved. Many people of various nationalities and backgrounds at various times claimed to have discovered an AIDS cure. Sadly, many unsuspecting people believed them.

Part of my mission was to try and stop them.

6

Proof of a Cure

By God's Grace

As I started my new job at the newly established JCRC in 1992, the first hurdle was to figure out how I would tackle the monster disease. I really had no inkling how to go about it. All I was sure of was that it would be difficult. I was fresh from Mulago Hospital where for a period of over one and half years, I had witnessed AIDS carnage on almost daily basis. Outside the hospital, I had witnessed deaths of friends, colleagues, relatives and fellow citizens of all ages and walks of life. Worse still, I also knew of many other HIV-infected individuals who would inevitably follow. Every time I met them, I wondered whether that would be the last time I saw them.

I thought then that if I could not find a cure, I would, at least; find out whether the claims of various herbal cures were genuine or bogus. But, as I later found out, the sheer horror of AIDS and zeal to do something about it had blurred proper evaluation of the magnitude of challenges that lay ahead. Luckily, as it initially seemed, on my second day at work I found that my very first task was already waiting for me.

I learned of it when a bespectacled, middle-aged grim-faced man I will call Baptist Mululu – a self-declared pastor - and his associate I will name Brazier Babikoka, were introduced to me. I met this rather odd pair at the JCRC campus, in their rather dubious capacity as herbalists. As soon as introductions and pleasantries were over, Baptist, an edgy character who evidently wanted to get on with the business at hand told me right away that he had by "God's grace" discovered an AIDS cure. "JCRC is blessed to have a unique opportunity to scientifically verify my miracle treatment," he boasted.

Baptist, who preferred to be addressed as Pastor Mululu, informed me that he was a well-connected man. However, this was not entirely new information to me. I had already gathered from the grapevine that in June 1992, the twosome had met President Museveni and briefed him about their breakthrough herbal medicine that I will call Gracia. They had flamboyantly described Gracia as "predestined to save hundreds of thousands of Ugandans' lives", adding that in time, it would stop the carnage all over Africa. Mululu's newly acquired status earned him the rare privilege of hitching a ride aboard the presidential jet, comfortably ensconced in a reclining chair next to the President all the way to London, to lobby investors (though I must add, unsuccessfully), for financial input into the manufacture of his "wonder" medicine.

However, the President did not take Mululu's claims at face value. The President had insisted on scientific proof of efficacy before the "miraculous" herbal medicine could be unleashed on the impatiently waiting public. Mululu was reportedly irritated by the delay that this would cause. The reason for going straight to the top had been to fast track Gracia into mainstream medical practice. A locally based NGO headed by Malawian I will call Dan Gurudi, donated most of the funds for the research.

As the expectations were so high, Mululu had no difficulty in convincing government to donate herbal processing equipment to ensure homogeneity and standard quality for his medicine. In addition, the government released some top-up funds to help speed up the research. By September 1992, the clinical trial of Gracia — the very first formal herbal AIDS drug trial in Uganda - was under way.

At the time I did not fully understand the scope and full implications of my new job. It was already apparent that the huge task of supervising the research on the efficacy of Gracia and other claimed therapies fell squarely on my shoulders. There I was, having just taken on the job with a mission to find an AIDS cure, being presented quite early on with a prized opportunity on a silver platter. Somehow I could not shake off the lingering doubt in my mind about the competence of the two novice herbalists, who claimed to have pulled off a miracle cure that had eluded many more expert people.

My very first impression of Pastor Mululu was not favourable. Somehow, he did not exude the kind of aura expected of a pastor and discoverer of a life-saving drug. Within a short time of meeting him he talked more of what he could get out of people than what he could give in return. Far from being a fisher of men, it increasingly emerged that the pastor was, on the contrary, more like a fisher of their pockets.

However, I initially tried to keep an open mind and give him the benefit of whatever remained of my rapidly diminishing faith in him.

Meanwhile, I tried to learn as much as possible about his background. But the findings that materialised were not inspiring. I could not find anything in his past to connect him with any credible herbal practice. I was able to ascertain a genuine connection between him and an obscure religious sect that he had founded and led as a self-anointed pastor. I gathered that Mululu was not a gifted preacher. He often appeared to the congregation as a boring preacher. His finest hour was always at offertory time when, all of a sudden, he would spring to life to cajole and harangue the faithful "to give more and more to the Lord". He never forgot to tell his congregation that the good Lord had endowed him with the powers to heal the sick both spiritually and physically. "But my healing services are not free," he repeatedly reminded them, "and those who pay more will heal faster."

On the other hand, his partner, the lacklustre but gentle Babikoka, was difficult to place. He appeared rather bemused and aloof, more like a paid servant than a business partner. A little probing revealed that the almost illiterate but otherwise enigmatic Mululu needed the well-educated Babikoka to boost his credibility and help in negotiations and contracts. As far as medicines were concerned, the wily Mululu had also enlisted the services of a retired doctor to help him navigate the complex medical world characterised by cumbersome technical terms, jargon and etiquette. Evidently, and to his credit, Mululu was good at identifying and enlisting the right kind of collaborators.

Even before fully settling at the JCRC, someone I suspected to be a proxy of Pastor Mululu ensured that I got to know what was at stake. It happened one late afternoon, when a dark, muscular man with a clean shaven-head, clad in jeans, and a sleeveless dark shirt, the type of man commonly dubbed *kanyama* in Kampala jargon, came to see me in my small office. He was the kind of fellow who did not quite fit the profile of a holder of a daytime job. Initially, he appeared a little nervous and hesitant to enter. But his confidence seemed to increase as he approached. As I sized him up, something about his looks brought back fading memories of Idi Amin's dreaded henchmen of the 1970s, who used to bundle people into the boots of their cars, drive them away, never to be seen again.

"Thank you for the work that you are doing Doctor," he started off with feigned politeness, but was evidently long out of practice with good manners. "I hear you are complicating the situation for my friend," he said raising his voice by an octave or so, snubbing my gesturing invitation to take a seat.

"I am afraid I don't know what you are talking about," I uttered after a brief pause, trying to work out what the stranger was up to.

He leant his considerable bulk across my desk, a little too close for my comfort. His breath stank of a mixture of tobacco and something else unpleasant, perhaps to do with infrequent use of a toothbrush.

"I have also been told that you are a stringent researcher, but that's not what brought me here today," he said, as he pulled back and slumped in the chair. "I just came to tell you this. Nothing in the world defeats money." He paused a little, perhaps to ensure that his message was taken in. "Gracia is gold," he went on to say, taking his time on the three words. "Pastor Mululu has it all in his grasp," he added as he half-stood, leaned forward, and reinforced his message by clenching his right fist, tensing his neck and facial muscles, and gnashing his teeth as if he had practised the sequence, "and he will not take kindly to anyone trying to snatch his legitimate prize from him." With that he shot up fully, stretched his bulky frame, turned round and walked slowly towards the door, pausing only for a brief moment to offer this unsolicited advice. "Doctor, if you have any problems, the good pastor can easily sort them all out for you."

I did not know what to say to him or whether to report the incident to the police. I wondered what the police would do anyway. I was not even sure whether this would pass as a threat or innocent advice delivered by an ill-mannered messenger. I decided to forget it. But, as I later found out, it was not the end of the matter. As the work progressed, I was repeatedly reminded that the president was out there impatiently waiting for the results. "Good results," Mululu once told me, making it clear that as far as he was concerned, any other outcome was not an option. When I asked whether this had any connection with the message delivered by the mysterious man, he denied any knowledge of him.

I soon learned that there was much more to AIDS research than the familiar rigours of science. In fact, if scientific principles were all that one knew in this business, then one was doomed. As I worked on this trial, and subsequent ones, I found that courage was repeatedly required. For instance, it was unimaginable that I would have my telephone tapped, receive threatening calls, and eventually be dragged to the government ombudsman, the Inspector General of Government (IGG), because of people whom the same IGG later described in his report as "malicious". This happened because my work threatened the lucrative business of quacks, conmen and other vested interests.

My very first official involvement with the highly hyped-up Gracia research was in early October 1992. I found an impressive research team already at work. Among them was a private practitioner, the same one hired by Mululu as an advisor, who was already using Gracia for routine treatment of his AIDS patients. Meanwhile, many patients, for whom the trial seemed a lifeline, jostled to register for the study and swarmed to the JCRC.

The research manual (or protocol as it is technically known) was quite extraordinary. The introductory part stated that "two herbalists, Pastor Mululu and Babikoka, working with one of Uganda's leading physicians had discovered Gracia". It was said to be already known to cause "marked symptomatic improvement of AIDS patients". Gracia was described as "a blend of some leaves and tree bark". The document proclaimed that preliminary analysis had shown that "Gracia had astounding activity against HIV-1". Among its reported attributes was its alleged ability to destroy all opportunistic pathogens. It was also reported to be able to reverse the damage caused by HIV on the immune system. "Gracia is non-toxic, heat stable, and resistant to stomach acids." However, no evidence was provided to support all these amazing attributes of the "wonder" herbal medicine.

Clearly, in the preparatory stages of this special research project there had been some difficult questions to ponder. Prominent among them were the following: How could a herbal mixture consisting of an unspecified number of leaves and tree bark be standardised into a stable and consistent product suitable for modern scientific testing? How would homogeneity of the herbal preparation be ensured? How would suitable dosaging be determined? How does one certify that the herbalists practised good manufacturing practice (GMP) and guarantee that their products were replicable, and of consistent quality all the time?

As it was plain that virtually all herbalists intended to benefit from their products, it was understandable that many, Mululu included, were not always willing to reveal the identity of the constituents of their products or methodology of preparation. Another tricky issue to consider was the use of placebo (blank) controls – a common research method used to determine whether the treatment outcome was due to chance or placebo effect instead of the herb or drug being tested. Secondly, the Gracia study could not be double blinded (another common methodology used in clinical testing of new drugs, aimed at minimising human bias by ensuring that the researchers did not know in advance whether any particular patient was receiving the medicine to be studied or a placebo). Ideally, this testing would have required a suitable placebo identical in appearance and taste to Gracia but with no effect on AIDS.

In preparation for the Gracia study, an attempt was made to address some of these critical concerns so that this study could proceed expeditiously. A grinder to help achieve some sort of a homogenised product, and a freeze drier were donated to the herbalists. In addition, a new pickup truck to facilitate transportation of the ingredients was provided. However, the freeze drier was never used because no extraction method was involved. The herbalists were persuaded to prepare, weigh and pack the powdered herbal mixture under supervision within the JCRC premises.

In order to ensure some sort of quality control, scientists from the Royal Kew Botanical Garden, London, were contacted and they agreed to regularly carry out basic analysis of each batch of Gracia powder to ensure some sort of uniform consistency. An arrangement was made whereby the herbalists dispatched samples of each batch of their medicine to London. The results were returned directly to them.

On a highly optimistic note, the study protocol included a provision for an independent study Data and Safety Monitoring Committee (DSMC) with a mandate to oversee the project and carry out regular data review. The DMSC was also supposed to take timely action, including speedy announcement and fast tracking of any breakthrough results if the study showed "overwhelming efficacy", or quickly respond by promptly stopping the study if there was evidence of "severe untoward effects". Actually no such committee was ever set up. In retrospect it appears that this section of the protocol was just lifted from some other better planned studies.

As far as I could judge, this study had some fundamental flaws. However, as an individual just coming on board, it was too late and virtually impossible for me to radically alter the course of this project, which was already in advanced stages of execution. All that I could do short of closing Gracia down was to salvage whatever good could be harnessed out of it at that very late hour.

On Friday 16 October, 1992 I attended my very first official Gracia meeting and was formally introduced to the investigating team. My first impression was a feeling that something was out of place. Unbelievably, I found that the herbalists were members of the study team charged with what was supposed to be "unbiased monitoring and evaluation" of their own product. Yet here they were, with a vote in all aspects of the study. However, as the meeting progressed I soon found out exactly what the presence of the herbalists among scientists was all about.

Immediately after the introductions and the usual pleasantries the meeting proceeded to the day's core business which comprised five items on the agenda. All were about money! The meeting did not touch on anything to do with the welfare of the twenty patients already on the study; neither did it address clinical events like adverse or beneficial effects observed so far. In fact, no laboratory scientists who carried out the tests or doctors and nurses who were actually seeing the patients on a day-to-day basis had been invited to the meeting. There was no item on the agenda to address any possible protocol violation. Indeed, the subsequent discussion mainly concentrated on money issues, especially to do with payment to the herbalists for their product and their salaries as study investigators.

My team and I did our best to minimise the scientific flaws we could readily identify and at the same time tried to keep Mululu and Babikoka at arm's length. We ignored their vehement protests and thinly veiled threats and just carried on. Finally, thanks to my diligent JCRC technical team, the study was completed. However, the emerging data showed that Gracia had absolutely no discernible benefit to AIDS patients. Dan Gurudi, the Malawian who had provided the initial funding, would have agreed too, if he had lived to see the end of the study. I later gathered that Dan's offer to fund the research was not without strings attached. He was one of the first HIV infected clients of Pastor Mululu, who had paid dearly in a futile effort to save their lives.

To get to this stage, I had endured many problems including persistent requests by the herbalists that I send a message to the president stating that the study was "progressing well". Yet the study was clearly not demonstrating anything near the wonderful effects that the herbalists had so vividly and passionately presented to the president at their earlier meeting, in their frantic efforts to obtain funding for the research.

Following the damning results, I ordered the study closed and then stood by awaiting the inevitable consequences. At one stage, I worried that the man with the stinking breath would return. But other unpleasant repercussions followed, fast and furious. These included anonymous hateful calls—some of them too disgusting to print, as well as indirect threats, which I ignored. I understood the disappointment and fretful plight of those with vested interests, who had to come to terms with the loss of their bonanza. The study had been highly lucrative as long as it had lasted. It had expanded the market for the otherwise worthless herbs, provided a regular salary over and above other material and monetary benefits, including a free new truck. Much more had been promised. Now, all these goodies had come to a sudden end with no immediate prospects of resumption.

Long after the dust had settled, one mystery that had always lingered in my mind was solved for me by sheer coincidence. It happened when, for the very first time, I chanced to meet our former contact from the Royal Botanical Gardens, London, who had arranged for regular analysis of the ill-fated Gracia. It was at an international Traditional Medicine meeting held in Washington, USA.

"I have always hoped to meet with you, and get an explanation about Gracia," she said. "I just could not understand why you people kept sending us those hopeless samples, despite our repeated warnings that the exercise was awfully flawed. Look," she went on to elaborate, "the samples were erratic and inconsistent, and we had to stop the analysis because it was just a waste of time."

I just stared at her in disbelief. Sensing my perplexity, she added; "You never received our letters, did you?"

Almost seven years later, in February 1999, the hopeless subject of Gracia popped up once again in the form of a letter. It was from a young and apparently unsuspecting British scientist writing from south Wales, whom the pastor had apparently approached for support in a futile attempt to revive his flagging AIDS herbal medicine practice. The letter, copied to the Uganda High Commission in London, was reminiscent of the first claims that led to the start of Gracia study. In part it read, "The plant leaves' extract has a wide range of chemical classes". Now it was only a concoction made from leaves. No mention of tree bark! "I will be pleased to visit Uganda if thought useful, to ensure that all steps are taken to move things forward quickly."

However, not all was lost. The silver lining was the exposure of Gracia as a totally useless concoction. Sales plummeted as many would-be victims and those who were already using it stopped wasting their millions of shillings on the useless stuff.

Promotion to the Board

Of the many herbalists that I met, Alphonse Tulidde was the ultimate fraud. He was a trained clinical assistant, but he had abandoned that work for a more lucrative herbal trade that targeted AIDS sufferers. He lived in Luzira, a suburb of Kampala bordering the heavily fortified ten-foot wall complete with razor-sharp wire that runs around Uganda's main prison housing the country's most hardened criminals. Later, when I got to know Tulidde a little better, I had no doubt that his home address was on the wrong side of the wall.

I first met him in October 1994 when he came to the JCRC claiming that he had discovered a marvellous herbal AIDS cure. With his paramedical background, Tulidde was well versed in basic medical jargon, which he effectively exploited to con unsuspecting lay people. He widely advertised himself, as "Doctor Alphonse" as he schemed to sell his AIDS herbal medicine without the inconvenience of it being tested, to the Ugandan Army. He had targeted the military because they had a widely publicised and big budget allocation, and according to rumours reverberating around town also had a high demand for AIDS treatment.

My first impression of Tulidde was the same as I had of "Pastor" Mululu but there was a difference in character. Unlike Mululu who always looked serious, – Tulidde on the other hand, smiled constantly and infectiously. He had a sense of humour and could crack a joke or two. But I was on my guard. Therefore my immediate consideration was to throw him out. However, faced with the catastrophe of AIDS I could not entirely escape suffering such characters, though admittedly not gladly. My only consolation was that if I could prove that any fake herbal concoction claiming to be an AIDS cure was in fact useless, then this action in itself would be of benefit to AIDS patients. It would save them huge amounts of money that would otherwise be stolen under false pretences, and possibly also save them from unhygienic or toxic preparations.

Tulidde recounted bogus tales of lives that he claimed to have saved. He boasted of having successfully kept many prominent people in Uganda well and alive with his herbal medicines. "Imagine what would have befallen Uganda if it wasn't for me!" he bragged.

He blurted out many names of dignitaries that he alleged were under his care and was apparently going to mention many others when I strongly objected. I reminded him that the privacy of individual patients who came to him in his capacity as a healer needed to be respected and that I took exception to him trying to mention their names to me or any other person.

"Look! Everyone knows these guys are sick. It is no secret. I am not the one who told everyone in town that they have AIDS," he said defensively. "On the contrary, I should be given credit because if it was not for me they would all be dead. Talk doesn't do them any harm."

Even the paranoid may have real enemies, as the saying goes, for as far as rumour mongering was concerned, Tulidde was absolutely right. The gossip flying around town with regard to those infected, on their deathbeds, who infected who, and so on were just mind boggling. This was the kind of chaotic situation that Tulidde exploited. With his ears close to the ground he would sift through the chit-chat and natter in bars and various other places, picking up names of politicians or prominent people said to have AIDS. He would then claim that all of them were his clients. If anyone died he would declare that such an individual had died because he or she declined his therapy.

In my practice, many dignitaries, among others, were tested for HIV infection. I knew that many among the dignitaries widely rumoured to have AIDS by Tulidde and the grapevine were in fact HIV negative. I recall one politician duped by Tulidde saying of his opponent, who had beaten him during the previous election, that he was on standby to inherit the constituency seat since his opponent would soon die of AIDS. Unfortunately, he died, not his opponent. It was however virtually impossible to call Alphonse's bluff. He was protected by stigma that fuelled the need for secrecy. No one would dare confront an alleged AIDS victim and ask whether it was indeed true that he or she had HIV. Tulidde's innuendos, broadcast free of charge through the grapevine, elevated his stature to that of a leading herbalist to whom prominent people flocked.

To investigate his claims I was tasked to determine the efficacy of Tulidde's herbal medicine. He was a hard haggler and insisted on an inflated price which we could not refuse. With his pockets well lined he returned to his base, boasting that he had successfully had his medicine approved by the JCRC. When he delivered the first batch of his herbal concoction, I found it to be one of the worst of all herbal "medicines" that I had ever seen. It looked like it had been hurriedly prepared and was not well homogenised. I could actually see and recognise a number of leaves of some common garden plants. It was a dirty brown colour and the smell was revolting. After a few days it grew a black mould on top despite being kept in the fridge. When this was pointed out to him, Tulidde grabbed the 20-litre jerry can containing his concoctions, rushed out with it and poured the filthy contents in our compound. The next morning he turned up with a fresh supply, which was only marginally better.

It is pointless to describe the testing process and enumeration of the results. Suffice it to say, his messy so-called herbal medicine was devoid of any demonstrable modicum of benefit. We vigorously tried to disseminate this information as widely as possible so that we could save unsuspecting AIDS patients from being conned or acquiring other infections from the unhygienic concoction. We succeeded in blocking his planned business with the army and drastically reduced the numbers of prominent people going for his therapy, but failed to totally stop the activities of this determined cheat because there was no law to stop him from practising as a herbalist.

The last time I heard of Tulidde was through a newly printed glossy pamphlet that had surfaced after a lull of a few months. Apparently, he had gone back to the drawing board. In it he advertised what he described as a better, bigger and scientifically advanced team working for his "organisation". The new list of his board members was very impressive. It looked like a "who's who" directory of Uganda's top doctors and scientists. When I scrolled down the list of various dignitaries and experts, I was dumbfounded to find that the incorrigible Tulidde had "honoured" me with the membership of his board!

The Dream Cure

"I have discovered a cure for AIDS!"
This was the proclamation in a hand-written message on a page plucked from a poor quality primary school exercise book, the type commonly used in rural villages. It was hand delivered to my office on 6 July 1994. One Abdul Waaka, who also claimed in the same letter that the efficacy of his medicine was guaranteed, appended a scribbled mess which I presumed was his excuse for a signature.

"I am a living proof that it works," he explained further. "I came down with fully-blown AIDS in 1985. I was so sick — really at death's door. Then my own medicine revived me back to life," Waaka expounded. "Now I am alive and well for all to see. On top of that I have successfully used the same herbal medicine to cure numerous other people in villages across the country." He concluded his letter by requesting JCRC to test and confirm the wonderful effects of his medicine and then to recommend it for use throughout Uganda, and the world.

I gathered later that he had earlier approached his area's district council chairman, several senior district administrators and the district medical officer, who in turn had referred him to the Uganda Natural Chemotherapeutic Laboratory (UNCL) based in Kampala so that his allegedly miraculous medicines could be tested. Waaka informed me that the tests could not be completed because of a shortage of funds to buy "chemicals" for further analysis. But when I later inquired from UNCL how they had fared with Waaka's medicine they had a different version. It transpired that when he found out that there would be no payment for testing his medicine, he just melted into thin air.

Waaka was smart with the media. He had a way of getting them to be in his service. He successfully got his "amazing" story covered in the only local Luganda language newspaper at the time, *Ngabo*. In a headline feature article, he narrated the wonders of Wali Wekwesewa (WW), the name he gave to his medicine roughly translating as "Where had you concealed yourself?" He described it as "a most miraculous medicine," and went on to exalt the work going on in his mud-and-wattle home which also doubled up as a factory for it. When he later heard about the JCRC he re-named his home the Herbal Joint Research Centre.

He claimed that he had discovered WW in 1985, after ten years of intensive tests on AIDS patients, ignoring or most likely just unaware that AIDS was unknown ten years before 1985. When I met him later and challenged him with this information, he was visibly taken aback, but only for a brief moment. He recovered fast to explain that WW was "in fact a panacea".

"Besides AIDS," he expounded, "Wali Wekwesewa is highly effective against many other diseases and social conditions ranging from leprosy to poverty." I did not have to listen to any more nonsense. Such wild claims were the order of the day. They needed to be countered—strongly.

By this time I was fully aware that the majority of the people who had jumped on the herbal medicine bandwagon were after money. The tone and spirit of Waaka's letter indicated that he was no exception. Therefore I considered the matter closed. Unfortunately, things did not turn out according to my plans. Just over four months later Waaka bounced back. To my consternation, he continued to pop up every now and again, sometimes in weird circumstances, often when least expected.

On 12 December 1994, I received his second letter. It was vitriolic. Among other things he said that he was bitterly frustrated to see Ugandans dying when he had a proven cure that could have saved their lives. This time round his claim was echoed by a barrage of well orchestrated telephone calls from a number of senior government officials whom he had apparently lobbied successfully. The brazen guts of the fellow! Waaka was now almost impossible to ignore. I thought at the time that it would be prudent to invite him to the JCRC and somehow dissuade him from his unreasonable utterances. In hindsight, this was not a brilliant idea. I lived to regret it.

He promptly responded to the invitation. He turned up at my office escorted by an impressive delegation consisting of some dignitaries from the central district of Mukono, as well as a contingent of healthy looking people. They declared in unison that they were all former AIDS patients who had been cured by Waaka's magical medicine. He brought with him a sample of his herbal medicine. He explained that it consisted of a distillate from eight different barks of trees and one leaf. The clear straw-coloured liquid product was presented in an old Uganda Waragi (a local potent gin) bottle, which was a rather strange choice of utensil for a man who claimed to be a devout Muslim. The distillate smelled of eucalyptus oil and had a mild, pungent but tolerable taste. My first impression was favourable. Here was a clear fluid, unlike Tulidde's messy concoction, and it was in clear glass bottles instead of the usual opaque five-litre jerry cans. It looked like a product that could be shelved in a modern pharmacy and dispensed in measurable doses. I was forced to admit that in packaging and presentation, Waaka had won round one. Now I just had to take a closer look at him.

He was a short, medium-sized man, perhaps in his early forties. He was rather quiet and cut a figure of someone philosophical, despite the fact that he was hardly literate. The district officials who accompanied him testified to his authenticity and bore witness to the magic of his drug, explaining that they had seen the miracle of it all with their own eyes. They talked of many people in their district and beyond who had been cured of AIDS. The "former patients" who accompanied him all looked healthy without any apparent evidence of symptomatic AIDS.

Just as I was beginning to compliment him for his endeavours in coming out with a clean product, I was suddenly taken aback by what he said next. I asked him to explain how he came to discover that eight different barks of trees plus one leaf could cure AIDS. More specifically, I wanted him to explain how he was able to correctly pick those particular eight barks of trees and a leaf out of thousands of others in the bush and be so sure they would synergistically combine to treat the dreaded disease. With a sly smile and frequent lizard-like head nods, he explained that, one night as he slept, a spirit appeared to him, led him to the bushes and showed him the right plants to pick, how to mix them and out of it all he came out with Wali Wekwesewa! I had heard this kind of mumbo jumbo many times before from herbalists trying to use the mystical and the divine as a vindication of their usually randomly concocted preparations. Therefore I remained unimpressed by Waaka's claptrap and was not prepared to have anything to do with his so-called medicine.

However, and not for the first or last time, I was not to have it my way. A series of events, including intense lobbying and pressure from various quarters requesting us to confirm the efficacy of the then widely publicised Wali Wekwesewa, the tenacity of Waaka, as well as the fact an increasing number of desperate AIDs patients were using his concoction. The only way to stop the scam, was to prove that WW was ineffective. To conserve scarce resources, the study would be kept small; just a simple pilot evaluation to see whether there were any grounds to justify undertaking a wider study. It would last only twelve weeks, after which an interim assessment would be made. We planned to check whether there was any boost to the immune system as would be indicated by rise in CD4; and to check whether patients showed any clinical improvement. At that time, we had no facilities to do viral load assays, and even if we did, it would perhaps have been a waste of scarce resources to include it.

The pilot study started on 26 May 1995 and it ended on 20 December 1995. Among the patients who finished the study, some showed a slight increase in CD4, which suggested that their immune systems had remained stable, but the observed increase in CD4 was not significant and could have occurred by mere chance or by the fact that participants were being treated promptly for opportunistic infections. One of our staff who was involved in the study presented the findings to an African AIDS conference as an example of the type of research on traditional medicines that was going on in Uganda. At the time when there was no effective AIDS treatment, African AIDS conferences always had traditional or herbal medicine on the programme. In the presentation, it was emphasised that the results of the pilot study did not prove any efficacy, but Waaka understood all this to mean that his medicine was effective. However, since we could not turn down any glimmer of hope, we decided that we would study the herbs a little further. Waaka was over the moon and made sure that his entire home village got to know about it, and also ensured that some FM radio stations broadcast the news.

When I invited Waaka back to discuss the possibility of extending the study, I took care not to raise his expectations. I explained that we did not find any evidence that his medicine could cure AIDS. I clarified that we needed to carry out more tests with a bigger number of patients to see whether there was any significant palliative effect. With that, a smile materialised on Waaka's face. He had been paid a handsome sum of money for the supply of the medicine to a small number of patients. The prospect of supplying more excited him greatly. I clarified further that we could not undertake such an expensive study unless we had specific guarantees of a strictly scientific nature. It would be necessary to standardise each of the plant constituents that he used in the preparation so that the medicine he supplied for testing was uniform. I explained that we required that each batch be consistent in quality to ensure that evaluation would be meaningful. This request wiped the wide smile off Waaka's face. I told him that he could have his product tested in whatever form he liked but, in such a case, he would be better advised to have it tested by traditional medicines organisations like *Uganda N'eddagala Lyayo* instead. I patiently tried to make him understand that the JCRC only used scientific methods to determine efficacy.

The talk about scientific procedures must have sounded like mumbo jumbo to Waaka. He thought we used some sort of a crystal ball. He was apparently surprised that the process would be so exacting. He had expected an instant answer followed by publicised blessing of his medicine and a sales boom. He suspected that this was just a clever trick to rip him off. I tried to reassure him that his intellectual property, or more appropriately, claim to the medicine would be protected, and that JCRC had absolutely no interest in making money out of his product. I clarified that any benefit accruing from it would go straight to him. The mention of benefits restored a broad grin to Waaka's face, and he promptly agreed to the conditions. However, when it came to signing a routine agreement incorporating these terms, Waaka developed cold feet. He requested to take the agreement home, sleep on it and return later for further discussion. The following week, Waaka was back with a totally changed attitude. He accused us of trying to steal his herbal formulation and did not agree to any scientific testing. Swearing that he would never return, he vanished.

A few months later, news of what was described as "an amazing herbalist" who had taken the city suburbs by storm, causing much excitement among AIDS patients, reached us at the JCRC. Soon we came across leaflets being distributed proclaiming a breakthrough in AIDS therapy. The leaflets stated that the new medicine had been tested at the JCRC and found to be highly efficacious. When we inquired about the herbalist in question, we discovered that it was no other than our old friend Waaka. He had set up shop next to Mulago Hospital, Uganda's main referral hospital, where he was doing brisk business. More news about him reached us mainly from people who wanted to confirm whether it was indeed true that we had found his medicine effective. We blew the whistle on him. His shop closed down or, more correctly, relocated elsewhere. Waaka was not the kind of guy to easily give up on a lucrative enterprise without a fight. However, over time, his clientele declined as the promised cure did not seem to work. But Waaka was not to go down quietly and he decided to fight the JCRC, and me in particular.

Waaka, a formidable lobbyist, made his way to the Minister of Health in the Kingdom of Buganda and reported that the JCRC had investigated his drug, found it efficacious, stole the formulation and kicked him out of the deal. The JCRC was housed in the premises owned by Buganda Kingdom, and therefore Waaka thought that the Kingdom's officials should somehow compel the JCRC to endorse his medicine. "As a loyal Muganda who loves the Kabaka (official title for His Majesty the King of Buganda) with all my heart, I seek the Kingdom's intervention," Waaka pleaded.

He also managed to hoodwink some journalists from the leading newspapers to take an interest in his "sad" story. The latest version of his ever-changing story was that the government had allocated a huge amount of money to be used on the research of his medicine, and that he was entitled to a big chunk of it, but the JCRC had left him out in the cold. Furthermore, he alleged that JCRC stole his herbal medicine and used it to make AIDS drugs to treat patients at the Centre. Fortunately, both the principled Buganda Minister of Health and a newspaper journalist contacted me and I explained our side of the story. However, while the minister was satisfied with the explanation, the journalist sniffed a scoop in Waaka's fantastic story, and was not about to drop such an opportunity. Nonetheless, the overwhelming evidence showed that Waaka was very economical with the truth. The journalists admitted in the interviews with us that there was no merit in Waaka's version of the story, but one paper still went ahead to publish his allegations, albeit an evasive and watered-down version.

When the heavens failed to fall as Waaka had expected, he retreated back to his village, but like the legendary bad coin, he bounced back. Meek and apologetic, he turned up unannounced at my office, referring to all that had transpired as an unfortunate misunderstanding. Now he was all ready and very anxious to have his medicine tested according to scientific requirements, and this time he was happy to have the constituents of his concoction standardised, provided he was well paid. However, the snag was that he had "forgotten whether the tree barks were five or six and whether the leaves were three or four". But he told me not to worry too much about that because the dream would come back to clear up all the uncertainties. "Just pay up and I will be back with the information." I did what Ian Robinson, our old headmaster at Kings College Budo used to do to a recalcitrant student, which was to show him the door and ask him to use it.

Unfortunately for Waaka, we had moved on. Advances in AIDS research had surpassed the initial makeshift stage following the discovery of ARVs. Our efforts were now focussed on the new challenge of trying to find ways of reducing the cost of the exorbitantly priced ARV drugs so that our patients could have access to them. However, we realised that even in the best of circumstances, getting the cost of ARVs reduced to a level at which it would be universally accessible was still a long way off. Therefore we continued the search for and tested other preparations that appeared more promising than Waaka's random concoction of herbs. As the bitter and disappointed Waaka left my office with his shoulders drooping, I thought that it would be the last time I would see him. And for many years he seemed to have faded in oblivion but, as I was to be rudely reminded, this was not his style.

Eleven years after Waaka last walked out of the JCRC, he turned up again on 21 September 2005, as a special guest on a Kampala's FM station's prime chat show. Waaka and the sensational presenter captivated the listeners with an embellished story of his miraculous discovery of "an AIDS cure that could have saved so many lives" if only it had not been thwarted by Dr Mugyenyi at the JCRC. Waaka was out for my blood. In response, some outraged listeners flooded the station's switchboard calling for action against me. Some other callers described in vivid terms the wonder of Waaka's medicine and described how they were miraculously cured of AIDS in the same way, even using the same words as Waaka had used to describe his own cure. As the competition for audiences was stiff, many stations searched out anyone with a hot story to boost their ratings. This situation was very opportune for Waaka, who had promised the radio presenter a highly sensational story. It gave him a unique opportunity to vent his venom and relieve the frustration emanating from his decade-old rancour.

When even this did not seem to help, Waaka resorted to his old friends, the press. Understandably, newspapers all over the world love miraculous medical stories because they captivate readers and increase sales. By any standards, Waaka's story was too far-fetched to take seriously, but unbelievably an editor of a daily newspaper was so taken up with Waaka's story that he appointed a senior journalist to write an exclusive on it. "This will be the biggest story of the year," he reportedly said to him. But when the journalist reported that there was no merit in Waaka's allegations, the editor was enraged and ordered him to go back and find something. "This guy discovered an AIDS cure, and JCRC sabotaged it," he said. "We can't allow them to get away with it," he added. The journalist contacted us once again and we explained the whole saga again.

At the time the JCRC was using the highly effective ARVs and involved in research to test a newer generation of drugs. Happily, the previously rampant death rate due to AIDS was declining rapidly, corresponding with increased accessibility to ARVs. Waaka's concoctions clearly belonged to the dustbins of history. But this was not the case in the eyes of the editor who went ahead to publish Waaka's incredible "AIDS cure story". The editor followed it up with publication of a special letter to the editor in which I was castigated for giving Waaka a raw deal, and an editorial appealing for Waaka's "dream" medicine to be recognised as a promising AIDS cure.

Nobody took up the request.

Cheat-A

A seven-foot, hefty stranger with a stern expression unexpectedly burst into my office one morning in November 1993. He quickly closed the door behind him as I stared at him in perplexity. He approached my desk and signalled for silence with his finger across his lips, though no words had been exchanged. I was gripped with a mixture of curiosity and anxiety, wondering what the rather weird intruder was up to.

"Sh! Sh! FINISHED! FINISHED!" He boomed, and then seemingly realising he was talking too loudly, lowered his voice to a whisper as I remained transfixed in my chair speechless. After a short while, he pronounced his first full sentence.

"Do you understand what I am saying?" he asked as he stared at me, perhaps trying to assess the effect his dramatic entrance. "I said, fi-ni-shed!" he added, after a rather long pause, pronouncing each syllable with emphasis. Continuing with his erratic actions, he briskly moved to the window and scanned the areas outside, apparently to make sure that no one was eavesdropping. Seemingly reassured, the towering figure returned to the desk where I was still immobile in my seat, not sure what would come next. He seated himself in the adjacent visitor's chair. Meanwhile, I was in a state of trepidation, trying to figure out whether the fellow was deranged, or since I had never set eyes on him, just a simple case of mistaken identity. The scenario did not look good. Suddenly I saw a trace of a smile on his face. I assumed that he flashed it on to reassure me as my concern and puzzlement must have been apparent.

"It's AIDS!" he said.

"What about AIDS?" I asked.

"I HAVE FINISHED IT!" he thundered once again.

Then, in a much softer voice fading to a whisper, "I found the cure," he said, as he leaned back in the chair, this time with a broader smile. His mood kept changing. In a flash, he was serious again. I wondered whether he suffered from a psychiatric condition. "You know, my formula may be stolen," he said in a muted tone, "Many people are after my discovery. Walls - they have ears. Windows - they have eyes. Nobody must hear us discuss this subject. Keep your voice low!" he said, as he took an odd look around the office.

It seemed like I had a crazy guy with a wild imagination, or perhaps some sort of a conman, the kind I had become so familiar with, trying to grab a quick buck, in my office. My immediate thought was to throw him out, but he thwarted this by quickly introducing himself. He was Dr Richard Changa (not his real name), a medical doctor, born in Gatundu, Kiambu, central Kenya. He was a medical graduate of the University of Nairobi. Following his internship, he had held a series of jobs, including that of medical officer in infectious diseases, malaria research assistant, assistant lecturer in anatomy, and private practitioner. Among his professed work experience, before he entered medical school, was a stint working in a herbarium identifying and classifying plants. He produced a certificate of full registration with the Uganda Medical Practitioners and Dental Surgeons Council. It was genuine. Thus, being a bona fide fellow doctor, I thought that, at the very least, he deserved a courteous hearing. Changa presented me with a research protocol outline, and a list of requirements that he explained were absolutely essential for demonstration of the marvels of his "curative" drug that I call Cheat-A.

His bizarre behaviour aside, Changa was otherwise quite organised. He had prepared a methodical study protocol for testing his medicine. He planned to treat a small number of patients with his medicine for only a fortnight, followed by a period of four weeks of observations. During this period, he said, he would demonstrate unmistakable improvement in all his patients as evidenced by a steady rise in CD4. He promised that previously confirmed HIV positive patients would turn HIV negative.

"All these results," Changa declared, "would be self evident within three months."

He had with him several written reports of seemingly impressive treatment outcomes for eight patients whom he claimed to have cured using his Cheat-A therapy. To facilitate his work, he requested to use a special laboratory capable of carrying out HIV culture. At the time, this was virtually impossible to provide in Uganda, and even in many other parts of the world. He also demanded accommodation for up to six months, transport to and from the airport whenever needed, two or three patients on whom to demonstrate and a two-room office.

Interestingly, Changa did not initially mention money or anything to do with reimbursement for his work. He said that all he wanted was to demonstrate the effectiveness of a drug that would save mankind. He claimed that one of his Ugandan patients had already attained impressive improvement in CD4. He offered to let me observe his patients' progress while he administered his treatment. I saw this as an opportunity to call Changa's bluff, by scientifically demonstrating the senselessness of it all, and to save patients from what I suspected to be bogus therapy. However, I insisted that he had to get research ethical clearance, which he agreed to, but I found out later that he had not complied with all the requirements.

A week later Changa sent me a message explaining that the Cheat-A, which I had hitherto thought to be a herbal concoction, was in fact a synthetic drug. In a surprise move he now demanded payment of £480 for the drug and a per diem. "I already consider myself a member of the JCRC," he said to my bemusement. I declined his request and barred him from JCRC. After a brief period loitering in and around Kampala, Changa vanished, and I hoped this was for good, but I was to find out that he was more tenacious than I first thought.

I continued hearing from him from time to time. The first time was only three months later, when I received a telephone call from the Kenyan police. Apparently, the long arm of the law had caught up with him and he was safely behind bars for malpractice. The police wanted to know whether JCRC had indeed tested Changa's drug and found it efficacious. I was relieved that he was out of circulation, but only six months later, I gathered that he was once more at large, out of his shackles and back in private practice in Nairobi. He did not seem to have benefited from his stay in correctional centre. I wondered whether 'kitu kidogo' (a Kenyan euphemism for bribery) could have fixed it for him because he was back to his old mischief. By then, his operations had extended to the internet. He sent me an email drawing my attention to his website. There he was once again announcing his "AIDS Cure in only 28 days." I noted that he had doubled the cure time from the fourteen days that he had started with.

Guess where the alleged data that brought him to that conclusion came from? According to him, he claimed that his "100 percent guaranteed cure was validated by the WHO Centre for Research and Training in Nairobi and the Joint Clinical Research Centre in Kampala."

Old Black Magic

When a middle-aged stranger, of pleasant disposition and carrying a fairly bulky black plastic bag was ushered into my office one morning in 1995, I guessed immediately that he was not Ugandan, which was soon confirmed by his accent, which sounded South African, as he politely acknowledged my welcome.

He was accompanied by an officious-looking man clad in a smart black suit and a matching tie, who was clearly in a hurry to finish his assignment and scram. This man remained standing, not even trying to disguise his impatience, while the stranger accepted a seat. The man pompously introduced himself as the personal assistant to the vice president of Uganda, Dr Samson Kisseka. He then handed me a letter, explaining that he had strict instructions to hand it to no other but me and to deliver it personally. He then excused himself, explaining that he had to rush back to attend to other important state duties. The letter, typed on official headed paper of the Office of the Vice President was brief and to the point. It was an introduction of the stranger, Mr Thabo Motsamai, described as a South African *sangoma*. The letter requested me to avail to the sangoma all the necessary facilities for him to demonstrate the effectiveness of his "wonderful AIDS medicine" and, secondly, to make expeditious arrangements for him to start saving lives of Ugandans who were dying in droves.

I already knew the meaning of the word sangoma which I had learned of during my exile days in Lesotho in the late 1970s. It was a Zulu name for a traditional healer-cum-witchdoctor, who held a special place of respect in his or her community. I saw a number of them in Lesotho, a country that officially recognised them as part of the broader healthcare providers to the community. Traditional healers known as *ngaka* in Lesotho were taken so seriously that they had a Minister of State in charge of their affairs. However, there was a nagging feeling at the back of my mind that there was something not quite right about this particular sangoma.

Then all of a sudden it clicked! It was the attire – or more correctly lack of it. Unlike typical sangomas that I had seen in Lesotho, Motsamai did not wear a leopard skin, had no ostrich feather in his cap, no coloured ash paint on his cheeks, no crocodile tooth necklace, no gourd rattles or other traditional implements that give the sangoma his special identity. When properly attired, a sangoma was always unmistakable. Wherever and whenever you met the sangoma, a feeling of awe would strike you. On the streets of Kampala, Motsamai could have passed for a kiosk trader, or any other low-income struggler. No one would have given him a second glance.

Motsamai waited patiently, stealing occasional glances at me as I read the letter. When he sensed that I had finished, he suddenly sprang up, taking me unawares. He burst out in a melodramatic chant in an incomprehensible language, interspersed with some parts recited in English for my benefit, I presumed.

"I see death all around! I see bad air, contamination – evil spirits," he chanted.

The sangoma's expression had suddenly changed, transformed into a stare, his hands were raised above his head while his body shook all over. Then, in a broken, tremulous musical voice, he continued with his ritual in unintelligible language. After a while he again switched to broken English.

"The devils – yes – devils, were conjured into the black man by the white man. Yes – I see white ghosts – a white cloud – hovering over the dead—the lifeless African children—I see mothers crying, who will save us? Blood! Desolation – everywhere. Who will save us now? Oh! Oh! Oh!" He uttered a few more, similar phrases.

Meanwhile, his eyes appeared to protrude, rolling like globes. Shivers started at his head and increased rhythmically downwards, until his whole body was shaking vigorously. Then he fell down hard. The shaking subsided, and he finally collapsed on the floor almost lifeless, remaining in a trance-like state for a while. Slowly, his fingers twitched, followed by limb movements, and then he sat upright, his eyes darting from side to side as if he was trying to work out his whereabouts. Coming back to life, he lifted himself back into the chair, taking up an upright sitting posture. Whatever Motsamai may have missed in regalia, he more than made up for in his spellbinding sangoma act. After a short break, he appeared to be preparing for a second round of his rituals, but I would have none of it. What I had seen was enough. "Stop it!" I shouted, as I simultaneously banged the table to command his attention.

This effectively brought Motsamai to a jerky stop. Apparently, he was not used to rude interruptions in the course of his ritualistic performance. It was indeed ill-mannered and insolent of me to interrupt a sangoma in the midst of ceremonial chanting. It is almost unheard of. Few people would dare risk his wrath by being so recklessly rude. Traditionalists believe that if a witchdoctor is upset, he could react by unleashing *mayembe* (evil spirits) and all kinds of unpleasant consequences that go with it. But in the midst of the AIDS crisis, trying to cope with so many demand on my time by patients, and my frantic efforts to find a remedy, patience with people I considered time-wasters was not my strong attribute. With an apparent expression of surprise and disbelief, the sangoma paused his rituals for an explanation. The stern look left no doubt that no ordinary explanation would be entertained.

"I am not impressed by your theatrics," I had the impudence to say to him. "And I really do not have time for more of it," I added. As he just stared at me without uttering a word. I elaborated. "Here we practise a different kind of medicine, and this kind of mantra is not part of it," I explained rather impatiently but in a toned-down voice. This did not seem to go down well with him. "Look, you brought me a letter from the vice president. In it he asked me to evaluate the effectiveness of your medicine and report back to him as quickly as possible," I said, trying to cool his apparently rising rage. "I apologise for the interruption, but I need to get on with the work." This seemed to have the desired effect. Once again, he was all ears. He must have feared that I had scrapped the whole thing. "Can you show me your medicine please?" I asked eyeing his bag, which I expected to contain the usual kind of budomola or improvised bottles containing the varieties of herbal concoctions that I had become familiar with.

"Yes, of course," he said as he unzipped the big black bag. What followed was a total surprise!

He plunged his hands inside, and in a fraction of a second, scooped out the contents, which he threw high up in the air. He then swiftly knelt down to observe and note the positions where the various items settled. He resumed the chants as he described the meaning of the ground formation of the strange items.

"The bone went west," he started off, never mind that the bone had actually rolled in a southern direction. "Oh that's a bad omen, look the feather is spinning, it's spinning upside down – oh no!" I could see no spinning feather, but a very light woolly feather floated for a brief moment. "This can't be happening! Oh! Oh!"

I was lost for words as I observed the contents of his bag. It included a dried chicken head, what appeared to be human hand bones, colourful feathers of various birds, multicoloured beads, shells of different sizes and shapes, and various other strange items and artefacts I could not immediately place. There was also a sealed transparent polythene bag that contained a bloody fluid. This perhaps explained a peculiar odour, almost like decomposing foliage, that floated over the room the very moment he opened his bag. I worried that the fragile-looking fluid bag could burst and add to the mess which the sangoma had already made in my office. Up to the time the bag was flung open, I had taken it for granted that Motsamai's medicine was some sort of herbal preparation, and that the hypnotic chants were just a ritualistic prelude.

I was getting increasingly edgy as this man was wasting time that I could ill-afford to waste on that busy morning. I was gearing up to say something rude while kicking him out of my office, but curiosity got the better of me.

"Mister Motsamai," I called out, controlling my impatience and annoyance. "That's enough. Quickly get your things back in your bag." For the second time, he came to a jerky stop, as he stared at me in unconcealed anger. "I have just one more question for you, before you go," I said as he began to gather his ungodly stuff in disappointment. "Did you actually put up a similar show for the vice president?"

"Yes, of course I did," the sangoma retorted angrily. "How else would I have convinced him to refer me to you?" Obviously not expecting an answer, he continued to gather and throw his stuff back into his bag.

I couldn't help wondering what the vice president had thought of this show, if it was even true that Motsamai had staged it for him too. What exactly did the vice president expect from me? Become a sangoma initiate? I could understand that AIDS was driving people to desperate measures but this was just too much.

As the obviously disappointed and crestfallen sangoma prepared to leave, I irritably reflected on the depths to which I had to stoop in order to find a relief for the AIDS scourge. Did I really have to suffer this nonsense? Was it actually nonsense? Obviously, the sangoma and I lived worlds apart. Perhaps he just had a different concept and approach to disease and treatment. Were the sangomas of this world entitled to their beliefs, or was it their livelihood? I pondered. Should our differences make us so infuriated with each other? I felt guilty for inflaming his ire. Certainly there was food for thought here.

The sangoma as the protector of the community from evil spirits has a special place in traditional African culture. What other spirit could be worse than AIDS, which had hit the community, wreaked havoc, and had even defeated modern medical practitioners? This mysterious and relentless killer disease had rejuvenated and galvanised an ailing ancient practice. Without any Western medical alternative the sangomas and traditional healers (sometimes difficult to separate), were all that the community had to believe in, during the desperate times. At least in this situation there were no credible rivals. It was therefore not surprising that the sangoma had strayed so far from South Africa and had trekked all those thousands of kilometres north to Uganda, despite the fact that Uganda had its own sangomas, known in western parts of the country as abafumu. Just as there was an explosion of AIDS-driven Western NGOs fanning out in Africa, and especially Uganda, the sangomas or abafumu, though with much less pomp and publicity were, like their Western counterparts responding to the AIDS crisis and the side booming business AIDS created. At the time, in terms of what they could do about AIDS, and in terms of what they had to offer, none could claim superiority over the other.

As far as South Africa was concerned, the same scenario happened in reverse later. Many Ugandan abafumu moved to South Africa in the mid-1990s in response to the surge in AIDS cases there and became sangomas. When the Ugandans arrived in South Africa they found some sectors of society very superstitious and the demand for sangoma services very high. Some South Africans revered sangomas and considered them holy; they believed that sangomas had supernatural powers to bring good luck, to chase away evil sprits, make the poor rich, immobilise business rivals, restore soured love affairs, and predict the future, among other things. At the time when AIDS was killing an increasing number of people, the community looked to sangomas to provide a cure. The vast majority of Ugandans who flocked to South Africa and ended up working as sangomas were quacks. They turned the ancient profession into a scam. They advertised widely, under fancy names like Doctor Ndugu Shaba Shaba, and kept changing names to appear like they were new in town.

Sangomas from distant places can be very appealing as they are shrouded in mystery; yet they had a relatively easier job, because they did not have to chant in strange tongues. Their own tribal languages, which could not be understood by distant tribes, would do just as well, even if they just sang children's lullabies. Not surprisingly, in such lucrative circumstances many quack sangomas, mainly illegal immigrants, exploited peoples' desperation.

As the Sangoma, prepared to leave my office, which I must say he cleaned painstakingly, I felt a sudden change of heart. The short time that I spent watching him carefully putting back all his tools in his bag one by one, paying particular attention to each, and the care that he took to ensure that my office was as clean as he had found it, must have done the trick. There and then, I realised that I had been unnecessarily harsh, even though I did not believe in the sangoma's practice. At least he deserved some traditional African respect in keeping with his profession. This gentle mannered man had done nothing wrong. Surely, he was no different from all the others - of all walks of life, from all parts of the world that I had met, either trying to do something about AIDS or trying to get something out of AIDS. This was the only remedy to a strange disease that he knew. Although sangoma practice was linked to voodoo, juju, witchcraft or whatever it may be called, it was in reality comparable to some of the peddlers of various concoctions in the early days of AIDS, who blindly tried out various therapies randomly. The numerous quacks that knowingly dished out or mixed totally useless medicine and profited from it were perhaps no better, and in some cases that I got to know of, much worse. Certainly the likes of Don Blockbuster, an incredibly sophisticated American high-tech quack I describe later, could not have possibly stood on a higher moral ground than a sangoma. The pharmaceutical companies that in some cases did not participate in the discovery of ARVs but refused to make it available to the millions who perished, just to protect their profits, have no moral authority to pass judgement on the sangoma.

At least the sangomas did something for poor Africans. They comforted them when death hovered all around them, and gave them hope at the time when their hearts were broken, and something to believe in when their faith was all but gone. They lifted their sagging spirits out of despair and encouraged them to hold on to life, even if it was just for a little while. Surely, the sangomas' rituals, though useless, could not possibly kill anyone, but denial of effective drugs did. I recounted the details of the carnage in my book, *Genocide by Denial, How profiteering from HIV/AIDS Killed Millions.* Such callous treatment of the poor would shock this humble and cultured sangoma to his bones.

As the sangoma stood up to leave, I certainly had a better understanding of him than I had had at first, when I felt like pouncing on him for no other reason than that he had messed up my office. Remorsefully, I unreservedly apologised to him for my uncalled for inconsiderate treatment. I expressed my regret that our different kinds of professional etiquette prevented us from sharing a common ground in our approaches to life, diseases, including AIDS, death and matters of the spirits and beliefs. I wished him well, and suggested that he considered the option of joining hands with the Ugandan abafumu, who would perhaps share their experiences with him and advise him on more appropriate clientele for his speciality. I also explained that due to my profession, I belonged to a different world of medical practice based on scientific evidence, where patience and understanding of traditional health practices were not our strongest attributes. The return of a faint smile on the sangoma's face signalled a move towards forgiveness. Or so, I hoped.

After a warm handshake and exchange of pleasantries, the rather surprised but forgiving sangoma and I parted ways to our different worlds, to continue the same struggles against the same monstrous HIV/AIDS scourge on which none of us was making much progress at the time.

7

A Cure at Large

Pills and Chopsticks

The message from the permanent secretary was brief and authoritative. "You have to leave for Beijing immediately," he said. "This can't be true," I thought to myself. It was Christmas and I had accepted an invitation to and paid my contribution for a grand party to usher in the New Year at the Kampala Club.

I found out much later that it was a message from the Ugandan Embassy in Beijing, which had triggered the frantic events that ruined my family's plans for the festive season. The letter, classified Very Urgent – Restricted, had arrived by diplomatic bag on 19 November 1992. In those pre-Internet times, the diplomatic dispatch to announce the Chinese discovery of "an AIDS cure" was the fastest means the embassy had at its disposal to send bulky documents that included cuttings from Chinese English-language newspapers and brochures from the manufacturers of the claimed breakthrough drugs.

At the time, the Chinese media were awash with claims of discoveries of cures for AIDS. One of the articles, headlined "China claims herbal treatment for AIDS virus" that was faxed from Beijing talked of a pharmaceutical factory in northern China that had signed a contract with a Danish firm to export US$260 million worth of anti-AIDS herbal medicine each year. The mention of a technologically advanced Western country seemingly giving its seal of approval to the newly discovered drug lent credence to the validity of the claims. The pamphlets that accompanied the message from Beijing explained that the wonder medicine had been discovered by a "Western-Chinese Medicine Combination Research Group". It described the medicine as "safe, effective and used to cure HIV infection". It claimed that the results of their studies were confirmed by the specialists of the Chinese Academy of Medical Sciences certified by Board of Health of Datong on 22 January 1990. Everything looked impressive and authentic.

Accordingly, an urgent appointment for a Ugandan delegation to meet the Chinese scientists in Beijing, and negotiate terms under which Uganda could acquire the drugs was fixed for 28 December 1992. I was appointed to lead the delegation.

Within the short period before our departure, news of the Chinese breakthrough spread. People whispered that I was about to go and fetch home the cure for AIDS. One patient who learned of the news shed tears of joy. "Hurry, hurry, before we all perish," the terminally ill patient said. "The Chinese have come up with a great kung fu leap to karate-kick out the AIDS virus for us," he managed to quip, "yet here you are, not responding fast enough," he added, joking in an unsuccessful effort to mask his anxiety. He was, of course, wrong to accuse me of lack of enthusiasm. I was certainly fired up to find anything that could alleviate the suffering and carnage. But there was a visa to be arranged.

Notwithstanding the bad timing, I had always longed to visit the famous Great Wall of China and travel beyond Beijing to see for myself the changes taking place in a previously poor country renowned for "barefoot doctors", now beginning to drive to their practices in Lexus luxury cars. I wanted to see for myself the social-economic transformation that was taking place in China. While Africa's development was being undermined by the AIDS epidemic, China, on the other hand, had become one of the fastest-developing countries in the world. However, the weather and the tight schedule of our mission conspired to deny me the chance to do any sightseeing.

The other members of my delegation were Drs Nathan Odoma and Francis Murungi (both not their real names), and a Chinese woman by the name of Ji Ai Hua who had been co-opted as our official translator. We arrived in a freezing and snow-covered Beijing early on the morning of 28 December 1992, and there to meet us was Prince Simbwa, a long-serving Ugandan diplomat. Remarkably knowledgeable about China, the Prince who was a member of the royal family of Buganda Kingdom, briefed us about the country as he whisked us to our hotel. "I like the Chinese people. They are welcoming, hard working and progressive. However, be aware that the Chinese eat many varieties of foods, like snake and dog meat which most Ugandans find revolting," he said, immediately making me decide to avoid being too adventurous with exotic foods.

On arrival at the hotel, he allowed us a few hours to freshen up before returning to take us to our first appointment with the Chinese AIDS drug pharmaceutical company representatives. When we assembled in the lobby to await the arrival of the prince, I was taken by surprise when Odoma suddenly pounced on me. Heatedly, he challenged my leadership of the delegation. "Who appointed you a leader of this delegation? I do not recognise your leadership. You are self-appointed," he fumed. "No sensible person can ignore me — the real AIDS expert — and appoint you instead." He looked around as if to see whether Murungi and our interpreter who did not seem to understand what he was talking about, were in support of his mini revolt. But he did not seem to like what he saw. Undeterred, he pressed on, "Mugyenyi, what do you know about AIDS?" the irate doctor charged once more. "Nothing, nothing at all," he added, answering his own question. I replied that it did not really matter who led the delegation, since we were volunteer colleagues working together for the same cause.

"It is because of your renowned expertise that you were selected to be on the delegation," I commented trying to be as cordial as possible. "We fully acknowledge and respect your expertise, which we need on this mission and we will be guided by it," I added.

However, as I found out a little later, my reconciliatory remarks cut no ice with him. Fortunately, the timely entrance of Prince Simbwa temporarily ended the unease that was beginning to build up, and I thought that would be the end of it. To my discomfort, it resurfaced as soon as we reached the embassy when I came under attack once more. In a loud voice, Odoma claimed that he was the true leader of the delegation. This time round, I did not say anything. I just produced my appointment letter and presented it to the ambassador as Odoma stared at it in apparent surprise. Although Odoma had been officially informed before we left Kampala, in my presence that I would lead the delegation, he had not been present when I was given the official letter of appointment. In faraway China, out of reach of the authorities, he must have thought he had a better chance of bluffing his way to the leadership. I had accepted the appointment as a mere formality to facilitate communication and decision making, especially as it did not carry any personal benefits. It never occurred to me that leading a delegation of three for a very brief period would in anyway be contentious. I had not even planned to present the letter but it seemed to unravel a sticky situation, as he seemed to accept the reality with a mixture of impotent resentment and embarrassment. To my relief, this restored some tranquillity to the mission. Luckily there was Murungi, a perfect gentleman, who had no leadership ambitions or any sort of axe to grind, on the delegation. Cautiously and patiently Murungi and I worked to achieve a fair working atmosphere for the duration of the mission. I remained courteous towards Odoma and allowed him as much leeway as possible in all the discussions, and only intervened tactfully when he went astray.

The Chinese delegation from the Datong Pharmaceutical Company based in Chengdu City, Sichuan Province, in the hinterland of China consisted of two smartly dressed men and a woman. They arrived complete with their briefcases containing samples of the drug, and copies of business proposals ready for signature. To our surprise, none of them was either a doctor or even a scientist with credible experience in AIDS treatment or any kind of medical research. Apparently, their sole mission was to sell us their AIDS drug, imaginatively named, China Formula One. They appeared to have no other interest or mandate other than haggling out the best possible price, exchange some token gifts and thereafter head straight back to central China to pack the merchandise and ship it to Uganda. They were visibly surprised when we did not immediately address the cost issue.

I insisted that we needed to talk to a doctor or a scientist able to explain the medical aspects of the medicine, including the results of their clinical trials, the dosages, and its status in the Chinese pharmacopoeia. Here we drew a blank, as this group was clearly out of their depth regarding these matters. Exercising my reclaimed authority, I told the Chinese that either they find us a competent scientist to answer our questions or the deal was off. The Chinese left the room for private consultation in the corridor and to make a secure telephone call to their company. On returning, they announced that a scientist was on his way and would attend a follow-up meeting the next day.

When the meeting reconvened early the next morning, the promised scientist- a young man in his late twenties or early thirties - joined the Chinese delegation. However it became apparent that their "expert" would not be helpful. His knowledge of scientific research methodologies for drugs development and testing was rudimentary, though we were able to gather some useful hints and information that made it possible for us to decide on the way forward. He explained that China Formula One was made from a soil fungus and that it had only been tested on a small number of patients, as there were very few Chinese infected with HIV. The few research subjects they could find came from Shanghai, which had the highest numbers of AIDS cases in China. When we asked him about the results of their research, he described the treatment outcome as "very good" though he could not say exactly what the indicators were. When pressed further to explain how they came to this conclusion he just said that "all treated patients were cured". Further scientific enquiries raised more questions than answers. I was surprised that despite all these flaws, Odoma put up a spirited defence of the Chinese standpoint and urged us to accept China Formula One. We gave him a polite hearing, as he explained his point of view. "I studied medicine in China and I know the Chinese make wonderful medicines," he said. "In any case, I am in the best position to take a decision on Chinese medicines." However, I remained unconvinced and insisted that we needed to carry out our own scientific study to determine the efficacy of China Formula One.

The Datong team, on the other hand, remained adamant that their medicine needed no more testing. "We guarantee 100% that our medicine cures AIDS," their leader insisted. They swiftly dismissed my suggestion that their company fund a clinical trial in Uganda, and declined my invitation to them to participate in any role in such a study. In this, they had Odoma as an ally, arguing that it would be a waste of time and resources to retest the drug in Uganda. Nevertheless, at the risk of provoking his ire, I stood my ground because I could not discern any evidence that any credible scientific research had ever been carried out to prove the drug's effectiveness. Murungi concurred.

Faced with the impasse, the genial ambassador, Major General Fred Okecho, a skilful diplomat, set to find a solution. He sent an urgent message home — a sort of SOS - to inquire whether the Ugandan government would be willing to foot the bill for the study. To my profound relief the response was positive. However, considering the frantic demand for therapy and the desperation of AIDS patients in Uganda, I felt that I had no alternative but to agree to the request that the study was conducted simultaneously with a compassionate treatment programme. This compromise thrilled Odoma, but not as much as the Datong delegation. At long last they had achieved the very first item on their agenda, namely the cost and amount of the drugs to supply. They could not hide their excitement.

I left this part of the transaction to the Ugandan embassy and I turned my attention to another Chinese, Professor Lu Weibo, who seemed to promise a better scientific approach to AIDS treatment than the officials of Datong Pharmaceutical Company. He was a man of many titles and a remarkable background, having first qualified as a doctor in modern medicine before undergoing traditional Chinese medical training. He rose through the ranks to the chair at the Beijing Chinese Traditional Medical University.

Since the days of President Nyerere's Ujamaa (socialism), China had had a longstanding collaboration with Tanzania. Lu Weibo was involved in a joint study with the Tanzanians, testing a Chinese candidate AIDS drug named Glyke at Muhimbiri Hospital in Dar-es-Salaam. I had heard of his work earlier and had sent my deputy to Tanzania to touch base with him and to invite him to work with us. When the opportunity to travel to China arose, I sent him a message requesting to meet and visit his place of work to learn and see how the research on Glyke was proceeding.

Lu Weibo was a very pleasant man. He hosted a truly memorable dinner in the famous Peking Restaurant and also took us on a tour of his university campus and laboratories. We found the research laboratory well equipped with modern research and diagnostic equipment, including the then relatively new Polymerase Chain Reaction (PCR) system for measuring HIV viral copies in the blood. It was evident that the University was involved in serious work on a mix of ancient Chinese and modern medicine. I asked Lu Weibo if he could extend the partnership to us in Uganda to speed up tests on Glyke and other Chinese medicines. He promptly agreed to do all he could to help, but apologised that he had no funds to support a study at another site outside Tanzania. However, he agreed to ask the Glyke manufacturing company to sell us the drugs at subsidised prices for our own tests and to give us some technical support.

The New Year found us still in Beijing waiting for flights back home. I had the rare opportunity to be invited to the African Ambassadors' diplomatic party, which was held to welcome 1993. As expected, the diplomatic party was orderly; more like a Christian brethrens' get-together, without noisy fanfare and fireworks characteristic of end-of-year celebrations, like the one that I had missed at Kampala Club.

Freezing Beijing was most inhospitable for a tropical being like me, and it was getting even colder. It became so bad that we remained confined to the hotel for most of the time. Being snowed in provided an opportunity for me to have a long chat with Murungi, who was particularly fearful of the cold. Besides, he was ill and rarely left the comfort and warmth of the hotel, not even for a stroll to the nearby shops. He disclosed that he feared for his life because, like hundreds of thousands of fellow Ugandans he also suffered from AIDS in its advanced stage. He feared that exposure to cold weather could easily result in life-threatening pneumonia. Naturally, he had a personal interest in getting a cure for AIDS, and a valiant determination to survive. Accordingly, he obtained some samples of both Glyke and China Formula One, which he started using straight away. He joked that he was the first guinea pig. "If these drugs are effective, then I will not only survive but will also be an educated witness," he said jocularly.

Three weeks after returning home we received a big consignment of China Formula One drugs and a few weeks later a much smaller consignment of Glyke, the latter parked in neat, professional pharmaceutical containers. In contrast, China Formula One's cherry-red capsules were sealed in polythene envelopes inserted into thousands of plastic school lunch boxes - each one accompanied by a pair of decorated chopsticks.

The study to test the drugs together with a compassionate treatment programme started as soon as it was approved by the AIDS Ethical Research Committee. The study was planned to run for six months. However, there was to be an interim analysis at three months to capture any early response to inform prompt decisions like widening access to other AIDS patients. As the study got underway, the Datong Pharmaceutical company sent me a message, requesting an invitation to Uganda to see how patients using their drugs were doing. I was delighted that despite their refusal to fund a study of their own drugs, they were at least showing some interest in the study progress. On 14 April 1993 I sent them a letter of invitation through the Ugandan Embassy in Beijing to visit the JCRC. Meanwhile we prepared a research progress report to present to them and we looked forward to their technical input.

I was disappointed to find that the delegation consisted of the same laymen whom we had met in China and their two elegant female companions. I soon found out that they had come with a different agenda. They showed no interest at all in the work going on at the JCRC, which was in the midst of testing their product. They did not even bother to inquire about the research progress or study findings. Instead, they spread out in Kampala, apparently on a sales promotion exercise. They held dinner parties for doctors in private practice, pharmacists, and drug importers, and struck lucrative deals with some downtown businessmen. They sold all the stock of China Formula One which they had brought with them. For their long-term business interest, they appointed a local Chinese businessman as their representative and main distributor. Then they were off to the airport to continue the same mission in other AIDS-affected African countries, starting in Tanzania.

The study findings of China Formula One treatment were very disappointing. Patients on neither the study nor compassionate showed any signs of improvement. Their CD4 cells continued to decline, indicating that the drug had no effect on the immune system. A small number of patients voted with their feet and abandoned the therapy. But the majority plodded on simply because they had no alternative. Some hoped against hope that the drug could be a slow miracle worker and that the benefits would somehow manifest later. Sadly, no such optimistic wishes materialised. The final analysis of the study results was damning. There was absolutely nothing in China Formula One treatment to indicate any modicum of effectiveness against HIV/ AIDS. Yet our stores were full to the brim with the useless fungus stuff, in a heap of cartons containing lunch boxes and chopsticks that our country had paid for dearly.

Murungi was not physically present to witness the hopelessness of China Formula One. Despite taking the Chinese drugs, he had by then succumbed to AIDS. The bright doctor had known he did not have long to live and I had forged a closer relationship with this pleasant and resourceful man. I highly appreciated his kindness, concern for patients and value as a scientist. He was an example of the bright people the country could ill afford to lose, and yet who were daily victims of the scourge.

With regard to the other Chinese drug, Glyke, there was slight evidence of transient benefit to AIDS patients. This was mainly in the quality of life and some minor improvement in the symptoms. The immune system also seemed to stabilise for a while but this did not appear to be sustained. A further study would have been desirable, perhaps using a higher dosage, or in combination with other drugs, but failure to demonstrate convincing evidence of potential benefit was a constraint to acquisition of funds to carry on. Fortunately we had a fall-back position. Prof. Lu Weibo was involved in another study on the same product in Tanzania and China. I thought that if there were any significant findings we would hear about it from him. We never did.

The promised China Formula One cure, which had once been colourfully described by one of my expectant patients who has since died, as "the great kung fu leap against AIDS", turned out, as the Chinese would say in Chairman Mao era jargon, to be "a leap of a paper tiger on the strings of the Datong Pharmaceutical Company." Regrettably, the demonstrable uselessness of the two drugs did not entirely stop other conmen peddling a flood of other bogus AIDS cures descending on battered sub-Saharan Africa to reap from the desperate and the dying. I still felt a great deal of satisfaction for putting the Datong Pharmaceutical Company out of business in Uganda. The sales of other bogus Chinese drugs plummeted as the news of the uselessness of the Chinese AIDS drugs spread widely.

However, this left me in the same situation as where I had started. There were now many more desperate patients and their relatives whose hopes had been raised. They were crying out for something, anything, to save their lives. Therefore I had to set aside our disappointment, pick up the pieces once again and continue the search.

French Connection

By mid-1993, the numbers of AIDS patients besieging the JCRC was rapidly building up. Whispers about promising Chinese drugs being tested at the Centre had spread far and wide. This fuelled rumours that JCRC had discovered a cure for AIDS but that it was being kept quiet.

As soon as a new wave of rumours proclaiming a new AIDS drug trial passed, overwhelming numbers of people would arrive, each one hoping to be the first. My phone kept ringing as frantic patients and their relatives attempted to jump the queue. Some even managed to locate my residence and waylay me on my way home. We tried to inform patients that we were only at the time testing various drugs without any guarantee that they would work, but we could neither dampen the determination of those who wanted to participate or convince them that we had not found a drug that worked. "How come people you treat improve?" I was frequently challenged.

It was, indeed, true that many of our patients improved but this was because we treated their opportunistic infections. These improvements were usually temporary. We tried to address this issue by producing pamphlets that we distributed to patients who came to seek treatment and those who volunteered to participate in our trials. We explained that AIDS had no known cure. We made it clear that none of the drugs that we had tested so far had been found to be effective. But few people believed us. On the contrary, gossip about "a secret cure" having been discovered at JCRC spread beyond Kampala to the rural areas and as far away as neighbouring countries.

I remember one ailing mother of three who kept turning up, week after week, to seek treatment. She was always accompanied by her eldest child, a seven-year-old girl who carried a bottle of water and supported her mother. I once asked her why she kept coming when we had nothing to offer to her. "I come just in case…" she replied. When she finally stopped coming, I was sad, though not surprised.

In the middle of this gloom and feeling the heat, I turned once more to a 67-year-old retired pharmaceutical chemist who lived in the hinterland of France, for help. My French connection had started way back in 1990, just before I joined Mulago Hospital as a consultant paediatrician. I was introduced to a pleasant French businessman called Pierre Lys. Pierre was the president of the Paris-based Ugandan-French Association, which aimed to promote friendship and business between the two countries. He was concerned about the AIDS catastrophe in Uganda and interested in doing something about it. He introduced me to a French scientist by the name of Maurice Rouchy, who was working on the development of AIDS drugs. I learned that Mr Rouchy had developed an anti-HIV medicine which was already being used on trial basis to treat patients in France. I gathered that some prominent international personalities and celebrities were beneficiaries. Pierre had described their response to treatment as "impressive outcomes". With awe, Pierre had described Mr Rouchy as "a brilliant pharmaceutical chemist, a sort of recluse but a very compassionate man."

Rouchy was a credible scientist. His impressive CV included discovery and successful patenting of various drugs, most of which were for veterinary practice. I later saw his patent documents, of which a number had expired after the stipulated twenty years. Among his discoveries were drugs reportedly active against animal retrovirus diseases. As the HIV is related to the retrovirus family, it was reasonable to expect drugs that act on retroviruses to have a fair chance of success against HIV as well.

"His innovative drugs are cheaper, safer, and more effective than AZT," Pierre explained. This news was welcome at that trying time in 1990. I felt like dashing out to meet this redeemer.

I set off for my first rendezvous with Rouchy in late November 1990. Pierre met me at Charles de Gaulle Airport, and hosted me for the night at his spacious bungalow. However, I was not to enjoy a full night's sleep. I was woken up at 2.00 a.m by Mrs Lys who offered me a cup of strong coffee. Pierre drove me for a distance of about 300 kilometres out of Paris to meet with the awesome Mr. Rouchy. I had heard so much about him that I felt rather apprehensive, not least because the rather eccentric scientist had scheduled the meeting for 6.00 a.m sharp. True to his word, he was right there when we arrived, clad in a dark-blue striped suit, standing in front of a big castle. Rouchy had a wide grin on his face, seemingly oblivious to the bitter weather.

Pierre informed me that our host, the owner of the ancient castle, was a senior French high court-judge who was Rouchy's close friend. I was later informed that the secretive Rouchy did not trust people sniffing around his laboratory and thus chose this exotic venue a couple of miles away for our meeting. Pierre had further explained that Rouchy's paranoia was not entirely unfounded. It stemmed from a prolonged court battle he had had with a pharmaceutical company that had violated one of his patents. I saw little of the judge except at lunchtime, when he served us with a generous rare steak, which he had prepared with expertise of a master chef. There was another memorable event in the castle. For the first time in my relatively sheltered life, I saw Champagne being served as part of early morning breakfast, the same way some people serve orange juice.

Right from the moment I met Mr Rouchy, it was clear that communicating with him would be cumbersome because he did not speak English and I didn't speak French. Initially, we just exchanged bemused smiles, and uttered some pleasantries – he in French and me in English, while Pierre fumbled as interpreter. Rouchy believed that his drugs were superior to Zidovudine, then the only approved ARV drug, but which was failing. He insisted that I had to learn as much as possible about his drug so that I could use it properly. A crash course in pharmaceutical chemistry related to his drugs followed, which Rouchy unleashed on me in French, of course, as Pierre, a layman, struggled to translate the technical terms. Fortunately, many scientific words and terms are of Latin origin and therefore common to both English and French, so I was able to follow the discussion and to understand the chemical formulations and permutations of Rouchy's new drugs. The drilling lasted the whole of the first day and most of the second one except for brief breaks for coffee and snacks.

Rouchy explained to me at length how his medicine worked (mode of action) and the expected outcome. He was very concerned about the poor nutritional state of African patients and believed that treatment without nutritional supplements would, at the very best, be less than optimum. He therefore recommended including Oligomines, a thick dark brown, pungent liquid mixture consisting of essential minerals, trace elements and multivitamins as a critical supplement to the treatment. The slimy fluid exuded a foul smell bordering on nauseating. On pointing this out to Rouchy, he just responded by pouring out a cupful of the dark fluid and gulping it in a second. Licking his lips gleefully, he declared the product palatable.

Rouchy was also concerned about opportunistic infections that are normally associated with advanced AIDS. He emphasised that the infections needed to be vigorously treated, or better still, prevented, in order for his anti-AIDS drug to have maximum effect. He therefore recommended inclusion of an antibiotic, Doxycycline, as part of the treatment regimen. He explained that it would act as prophylaxis against many common opportunistic infections. "In addition," he observed in his characteristically firm but rather jocular voice, as Pierre translated patiently, "it has the added advantage of being synergistic with the anti-AIDS drugs."

I couldn't help but like what I saw of Mr Rouchy. He was indeed a very curious man, well read in his speciality and up to date with AIDS research. His explanations made sense, and his adherence to scientific principles as well as his background in pharmaceutical research convinced me that he was a worthy partner to work with in the race to find a cure. I was further reassured when I found out that, unlike many others I had come across, he was not putting money above science. Indeed, he offered to relinquish all his rights to the AIDS drugs to us if we found them efficacious. This was a powerful humanitarian gesture. However, I remained with one major concern: I was uncomfortable with his belief that his drug could cure AIDS in just one month. No one, at the time, knew half of what we later learned about the treacherous bug.

The remarkable Rouchy had not always been a chemist. He had studied economics as an undergraduate and boasted of having had President Valéry Giscard d'Estaing as a classmate. His transformation from an economist to a scientist was precipitated by a family tragedy. His father to whom he was very close, died of cancer that could not be treated. The final stages of his father's illness were very painful and tormenting to young Maurice, who watched helplessly as his father fought a losing battle. From that moment he wanted to find medicines that could stop death and alleviate suffering. He enrolled to study chemistry and paramedical sciences and specialised in pharmaceutical chemistry, which later became his main career.

The multitalented Rouchy had some odd hobbies. He had a small chicken farm as a side business, and his eggs sold like hot cakes. The secret behind his success in chicken farming was the special but secret diet of his chickens which caused them to lay eggs readily flavoured with spices. In fact, Pierre bought some to take back to Paris with him. Rouchy also loved nature, and treated plants with respect, tenderness and admiration. I once saw him walk to a plant, gently holding a leaf to his nose without plucking it off its stem, and then lifting up his head with apparent pleasure at savouring the scent. If Rouchy had been Ugandan, I bet he would have made a good herbalist and probably a witchdoctor as well. In fact he asked me how African traditional healers practised their trade, and whether they had effective medicines for conditions such as high blood pressure.

Rouchy hosted a farewell dinner on the eve of our departure. For the first time I encountered a type of cheese that was said to be a delicacy in France, and a favourite of Rouchy that, to me, smelt worse than Oligomines – a possible explanation for Rouchy's tolerance of odd smells. I also remember that dinner for another, more personal, reason. Seafood is my preferred dish whenever I travel to Europe or America. That night, as I made the order from the set menu, Rouchy strongly advised me against it.

"Before you order fish, you must always ask if the sea is within a hundred kilometre radius," he advised. "If the answer is no, order something else."

I paid heavily for my failure to heed Rouchy's advice. The next morning as we travelled back to Paris, the full effects of food poisoning hit me hard. Yvelyn, Pierre's companion who was travelling with us had a look at me as I lay in the back seat suffering cramps of pain.

"Poor Peter," she said to Pierre, who kept interpreting French for me. "There is no way I can possibly tell how seriously sick he is," she lamented. "He can neither blush nor flush and if he did, no one would notice."

Cat's Lives

On 3 November 2004 a peasant woman I had known for 13 years and who I shall call Evelyn Oleto strolled into my office. She looked healthy, and confirmed that she felt fine. Anyone seeing her then would have needed some convincing to believe that over a decade earlier her relatives had given her up for dead. She was an example of what later became known as Lazarus syndrome — rising from the dead.

Evelyn had just been to our AIDS outpatient clinic for a routine checkup where she was found to be doing very well. She had been provided with three months' supply of ARV drugs. She was ready to start on her 150 km journey back to her rural home in a small town in northeastern Uganda. She explained that she had peeped in to say hello and to enquire about the health of Maurice Rouchy, whom she had never met. She also wanted to say farewell to me as she would in future be getting her medications from a clinic that we had opened closer to her home. Over the years Evelyn had become almost like family.

Back in early 1991 when she was seriously ill, there was no effective AIDS treatment. She became the first patient that I tried on the new AIDS medicine codenamed KS3 that I had obtained from Rouchy. This was the reason why she was concerned about the man she called her saviour. But Evelyn almost did not get the drug. I recall telling her that I would not start her on the new drug because I was not sure of its efficacy.

"This one may or may not work, and I can't just prescribe it for you," I said.

"You wouldn't deny treatment to a dying patient, would you doctor?" she asked.

"What if there was a possibility that the drug was toxic?" I probed.

"But Doctor, I trust you. I know you wouldn't give me a poisonous drug," she replied.

This was precisely the dilemma. Doctors are not supposed to prescribe to patients drugs of dubious efficacy, and I had no way of knowing.

"AIDS is going to kill me anyway," she pleaded. "It is better to die trying to find a cure, than to die too scared to try." Evelyn's philosophical remarks made sense, but did not make the situation any easier for me. Indeed, no bona fide doctor would contemplate giving a patient a questionable drug except under research conditions.

I had met Evelyn following my very first trip to France to meet Mr Rouchy. Her cousin, Ruth, was a nurse on Ward 1C, Mulago Hospital, where I was also working as a paediatrician. Ruth had taken particular interest in my quest for AIDS treatment, and was keen to learn more about my trip to France. One morning during our coffee break I heard the reason for her interest though I should have guessed. She had a cousin who was dying of AIDS.

"Could you please try her on the new medicine?" she pleaded. "The poor woman is married to an alcoholic, and she is the family's breadwinner. If she dies, I shudder to contemplate the fate of her five children."

In 1991 only Zidovudine (AZT/ZDV) was available, which, besides being unaffordable, was toxic because of the high dosage used at the time. It was already clear that on its own, it had no survival benefit. Without any therapy Evelyn was doomed to die, within a year or so. If the KS3 proved to be even partly effective, she could get relief and even live a little longer. Even if the drug had no effect, presumably no harm would have been done provided, of course, there was no serious toxicity. Absence of toxicity need not have been absolute. Some approved cancer medicines have the potential of causing terrible side-effects that could be life-threatening. Such drugs would be totally unacceptable if it was not for the fact that cancer like AIDS, without treatment, was always fatal.

Before the outbreak of AIDS, recent medical history of infectious diseases had not encountered or described a challenge of such magnitude. In this case it seemed to me that the only person who could decide whether to risk an untested medicine was Evelyn herself. My job was to give her all the information I had so that she could make as much of an informed decision as was possible. After a full explanation, Evelyn still begged to be started on therapy immediately.

I had to be realistic, and avoid giving her any false hope and as she was not in immediate danger, I asked her to come back a week later. I needed to buy some more time to think over the matter and consult colleagues. The doctors I consulted were unanimous in their verdict. "Go ahead and treat her," I was advised. Some went further to state that delaying or denying her a chance to try out the only possible treatment available would be unethical. I felt isolated.

I decided to go ahead and to start Evelyn on the drug, but this was on stern condition that she would strictly adhere to Rouchy's recommendations. I had to check her for reaction daily for at least the first month. She did not merely agree, she jumped up in excitement. I wondered whether I had raised her hope to unrealistic levels. There was still the issue of the cost of her monitoring laboratory tests. I had no alternative but to pay it myself. I alerted Rouchy that I was about to start my first patient on KS3. I requested him to remain on standby to provide advice in case I ran into complications.

The following month of treating Evelyn was difficult for both of us. At the time, Rouchy believed that KS3 would cure AIDS within a month, but to achieve this, the patient had to adhere strictly and take the medication every four hours, even through the night. Evelyn thought this was a minor sacrifice to make, considering the alternative. "If I don't stay awake to take my medicine, the disease will put me to sleep forever," she quipped. I could see that Evelyn still had a joke or two left in her. My role was anything but a joke. I had to see her at least twice a day, check all her vital signs, record all her laboratory tests, and keep Rouchy informed.

Over the first few days everything seemed to go well but, on the fourth day Evelyn and I got a scare. Despite feeling generally well, she reported that her urine had suddenly turned bright yellow, which I confirmed when she provided me with a sample.

"This is deep jaundice!" I thought. I worried that the drug had knocked out her liver. I promptly took a blood sample to be tested for signs of liver failure. I also sent an SOS fax to Rouchy to inform him of the unwelcome developments and to seek his urgent advice.

In the laboratory I hovered over the technologist as he performed liver function tests that seemed to take forever. I insisted on a repeat when the tests finally came out normal. I just could not accept that Evelyn's liver was perfectly normal, as the repeat results confirmed, because the yellow colour of bilirubin, normally associated with jaundice, was a red flag for liver problems. I was about to demand a third retest when a messenger brought a fax from Rouchy. It contained a couple of sentences in French. I rushed out to find a translator. Huffing and puffing I found a Rwandese woman who could read French. The surprised woman first looked at the message and then stared at me in disbelief – wondering what the huffing and puffing was all about.

"The message just says, this is good news. It means she is taking the drugs in adequate dosages. The urine colour is only the natural pigment of the drug."

The only other major drawback Evelyn had to endure was the bitter taste of the drug. It initially made her feel nauseous the whole day long. It had a pungent, garlicky odour that smelt in her breath, her urine, and her stool. "I can even smell it in my sweat," she complained. After a week, she started getting used to it, and by the end of the third week she had learned to live with it though she always kept a piece of lemon handy, to suck when unexpected nausea hit her.

After a month, that felt more like a year, I sat down to review her results and to reflect on the treatment outcome. I found that there were some positive blood changes, that could be construed as improvement. Other parameters including liver and kidney tests, remained normal, which suggested that the drug was not toxic. However, without CD4 it was difficult to be sure of any immunological improvement, though Evelyn claimed she had not felt better and stronger in a long time. I could not take this as indicative of improvement. Her feeling of well-being could have been a placebo effect due to the euphoria resulting from the knowledge that something was being done. Initially, I did not discern much change though there was no sign of deterioration. Later I noticed some subtle signs of improvement: Evelyn's skin rash improved and her oral thrush – an opportunistic fungal infection and a sign of advanced AIDS – became less troublesome, though it was not completely gone.

Rouchy, though pleased with the progress, was rather disappointed that I had not found the more dramatic response he had expected. In view of the fact that the patient was doing well and quite comfortable on therapy, he advised that I extend it indefinitely and, to my delight, with much less intensive monitoring than before. I changed to weekly reviews and asked Rouchy to tone down his incessant demand for progress reports.

Six months later it was apparent that Evelyn was doing well. Rouchy advised that therapy should be stopped and that I should merely continue with observations. Evelyn remained reasonably well for over a year, but slowly symptoms started creeping back. In 1992 when I took up the new job at the better equipped JCRC, I started preparing for a formal drugs trial of KS3 and its newer analogue drug, which I renamed Jocecylon and Joceclovir respectively. I restarted Evelyn on Joceclovir, and she seemed to respond well.

However, by 1994, her symptoms returned and it became clear that she was no longer benefiting from the treatment. I then switched her to the then newly introduced antiretroviral bi-therapy consisting of Zidovudine and DDI, which was an improvement on Zidovidine monotherapy. However, its effect was also temporary.

In hindsight it is tempting to deduce that Rouchy's medicine did the trick for Evelyn, or that it helped in some way to keep her going for almost four crucial years, until better treatment became available. But it would be scientifically flawed to conclude that Rouchy's medicine was effective based on Evelyn's case alone. Her apparent improvement and survival could have been due to some other factors, not excluding placebo effect. The fact that she was closely monitored and treated promptly for opportunistic infections, and the concurrent use of Doxycycline prophylaxis could, in combination, have helped to keep her going for so long.

However, when new ARVs became available, her new problem was the high cost of the drugs, which was well beyond her means. I felt obliged to help her out the best I could, as indeed she had been some sort of a research subject. Her pioneer use of KS3 also opened the gates to trying other patients on the same experimental therapy.

In 2006, fifteen years after Evelyn was first treated with KS3, she visited my office and reported that she was doing well on ARVs, which she was getting from a new AIDS clinic close to her rural home. Her children were grown up. Fortunately, none of them was HIV infected. However, like many other Ugandans she had sad stories to tell. Her husband, her cousin Ruth – the nurse who first introduced her to me – were among many extended family members who had perished.

"The irony," she recalls with humble disbelief, "is that I was the sickest, and was expected to die before all of them."

It must be said that fate favoured Evelyn. Just as she was running out of money to sustain her family and pay the cost of drugs on her limited income she earned from her small-scale trade, free AIDS drugs became available under President Bush's Emergency Fund for AIDS relief (PEPFAR).

Evelyn seemed to have nine lives!

Victim of the Same Scourge

The death of 29-year-old widow I shall call Peace Guliwano was announced in early August of 1991. But several months later, she (or her ghost as her stunned workmates initially thought) turned up at her workplace smartly dressed and ready for the day's work.

Peace, a well-educated woman, worked with Greenland Bank. I first met her in late July1991 under heart-rending circumstances. The meeting resulted from a request by the medical superintendent of Mulago Hospital, at the time my boss, Dr Kihumulo Apuuli. He asked me to see a patient who was reportedly in urgent need of medical attention. I later gathered that Peace's alarmed uncle, whom I call Kasozi, had rushed to Mulago Hospital to seek emergency medical help. As a paediatrician, I found it odd that I was being asked to attend to an adult but I guessed that the whispers about the AIDS work that I had embarked on was behind the request.

Kasozi led me to a house in Kansanga, a suburb of Kampala. There I found an emaciated and almost lifeless female patient. She was so ill that the very act of lifting her eyelids seemed to cause her pain. Her lips were dry and cracked at both corners. Her hair was thin and scanty. Clinging on to her frail body was a sickly and agitated toddler of about three and a half years. Hovering over the bundle of pain was a graceful middle-aged woman I shall call Gloria, who reassured Peace, "My child, we are all praying for you. God will heal you. Everything will be alright." By her worried expression, I could sense that she did not believe her own words. I later gathered that Gloria was Peace's auntie.

Gloria tried to drag the clinging baby from her mother so that I could examine her. The child screamed uncontrollably, determined to resist attempts to pull her off her mother. "I want my mummy. Don't hurt my mummy," she screamed in an ear-piercing tone as she tightened her grip. She eventually lost the battle as a no-nonsense woman who had been called in to help unceremoniously yanked her off, ignoring her kicks and screams and my appeals to let the child remain, and carried her out.

The scantily furnished and poorly-lit room smelled foul. Looking around, I focussed on a plastic pail by the patient's bed — actually a mattress on the floor - half-full of some mucky fluid. This partly explained the source of the smell. Gloria wore a bewildered expression, as if expecting something awful to happen, and it did. Peace suddenly burst into a spasm of coughing, jolting Gloria into action. Squatting besides Peace she propped her up, and started patting her gently on her back. This seemed to trigger an explosion of projectile vomiting, and a torrent of profuse diarrhoea that resulted in almost unbearable stench. I helped to lift Peace out of the soaked bed onto a clean and dry spare mattress, then I stealthily retreated to the window to catch a whiff of fresh air while the auntie tidied up.

Hardly had a minute passed when Peace suddenly screamed in pain. Gloria dropped the towel and took a step back, shrieking in fear. I hurried back and found Gloria staring at a large red linear wound on the right side of Peace's groin. "They must have burned her with hot liquid," she shouted. I diagnosed it immediately as a severe ulcerative stage of shingles known in Uganda as *kisipi*. I thought I could allay Gloria's fears by telling her what it was, but it was not to be. Gloria bolted out of the room in utter terror. After covering Peace with a clean sheet and patting her reassuringly, I scrambled after her auntie. I caught up with her at the entrance to the bathroom. She had with her a packet of soap powder and a brush.

"There is nothing to be scared of," I attempted to reassure her. "Kisipi is not contagious."

"But kisipi means AIDS, doesn't it Doctor?"

"Not always," I mumbled hesitantly, wondering how to communicate to her truthfully without making her panicky state worse.

"Doctor, I am so frightened and I have already exposed myself extensively. I fear I am already infected."

"No, you are okay," I interjected.

"She must go away but I don't know where to take her," she snapped.

It took me a while to set her mind at rest, and a little longer to convince her to resume cleaning up for Peace.

"But that raw wound, I can't touch it, Doctor."

"You don't need to worry about that," I said, encouragingly. "That bit is my job. I will take care of it for you."

An hour or so after I had got a drip of saline and glucose going, and Peace's condition had stabilised, I then sat down with Gloria, who had calmed down considerably, to take the history. The distraught and visibly tired woman narrated a dreadful story of the events of the previous evening. "Right now she is much better," Gloria said, even though those seeing Peace for the first time would have found it difficult to believe that she could have possibly been any worse. "Last night I did not think she would make it to this morning."

Gloria had returned from work at about 6.30 pm. Her house was locked up because it was her domestic help's day off. Just as she was about to open her front door, she heard faint whimpering sounds. She beheld the sorry sight of a starving child and a dying woman beside her door. She initially mistook them for vagabonds who had come onto her porch. On closer scrutiny she realised that it was her own niece and her child. Hungry, worn out, and dressed in a dirty nightdress and soaked in urine, the child had collapsed on top of her mother, who was too weak to help. There was a roughly folded note beside them, which she picked up. It contained one brief scribbled sentence.

"Here are your corpses," it said.

"When I touched the sweaty forehead of my niece, I found she was running such a high fever, that my hand was instantly hot and wet. I fetched some water in the bucket and started sponging her, to cool her down—she was on fire," Gloria explained. "Then I hurried to a nearby clinic and found a nurse in one of the clinics who resuscitated Peace while I fed her starving child."

One would be excused for thinking that the most urgent action to take in such circumstances would be to rush the patient to hospital. But at the time, few people had hope that a hospital could provide assistance. More often than not, there would be no doctors on duty, drugs would be out of stock, virtually all space would be crammed full of critically ill patients and, not infrequently the bodies of those who had not received attention would still be lying there. Any nurse found on duty in a government hospital would be overwhelmed by the desperate calls of dying patients' relatives. Occasionally the nurses would be assaulted by irate relatives and some of them would in turn react with less than professional patience. Hospitals were not pleasant places to be, especially if one was very sick!

Knowing that the hospital was unlikely to offer a cure or effective palliative care, many families did what they could for their sick relatives at home. The small minority that could afford it took their sick to the numerous private clinics and nursing homes that had sprung up as the AIDS situation deteriorated, where some of the doctors and nurses, missing from their duty stations at government hospitals would be found moonlighting. Other medical practitioners had fled the country altogether in search of greener pastures. For a big proportion of patients, especially in rural areas, all they could afford were the services of herbalists and traditional healers. When the situation deteriorated, they called in priests or pastors of which there was no shortage. Numerous sects had sprung up to pray for or prey on the escalating numbers of AIDS patients.

It took a whole week for Peace to recover sufficiently and regain her composure to properly recount the details of her ordeal. I still recall her perturbed expression as she recounted the events of that fateful morning. She was at home on extended sick leave and had just crawled out of bed to reach for some milk, which a kind neighbour had warmed up for her child, when she saw a taxi mini-cab arrive. It was followed by a dilapidated old Toyota car which she recognised as belonging to her brother-in-law. The two brothers and the sister of her deceased husband had arrived. The very sight of her brothers-in-law was enough to send a chill down her spine as the two brothers never got on with her husband.

"As the only family member who had made it to university, and later got a good job, a wife and house of his own, they were intensely jealous of their brother's success," Peace explained. "Initially, they made unreasonable demands — that he should share his salary with them. When he refused, they ostracised him."

Her late husband tried to appease them by setting up a family business where he hoped they could all work together. Instead, the brothers ran it down. One of the brothers used the business capital to marry a second wife. When her husband got tired of funding a futile venture and withdrew from the business, it collapsed and his brothers blamed him. From the grapevine, Peace and her husband heard of undisguised threats against them. When her husband died, they did not attend his funeral. Now, here they were, suddenly arriving at her house, where they found her weak and defenceless with only her orphan child. She had always prayed that if ever she had to confront her in-laws, they would find her well and ready to defend her family's property, just as she had promised her husband before he died. Their visit could not have happened at a worse time.

Peace thought that the only line of defence was politeness, even if it was pretence. Accordingly, she summoned her remaining strength went down on her knees to greet and welcome her in-laws according to her kiganda custom but she was not allowed the honour. Unceremoniously, the two men shoved her aside and burst into her house. They told her that they had come to reclaim their late brother's property and that she and her child had to leave immediately. Menacingly, they accused her of having killed their late brother by infecting him with the HIV.

"We won't allow you to pass on our late brother's property to your relatives," her sister-in-law said. "You and your AIDS-infested child, you are both doomed. And I hope you suffer and die horribly for killing our brother."

Roughly, they bundled her into the taxi with her screaming child, without even a change of clothing and drove them across the city to Kansanga, where they dumped them on the veranda of her auntie's house. She recalled that one of them scribbled something on a piece of paper and threw it beside her. Gloria had not told her the contents of the note.

We later learnt that soon after this incident, the brothers-in-law had gone to the bank where Peace worked, and informed her employer that she had died and had already been buried in her ancestral village. Peace's workmates had obviously observed her progressive loss of weight. She knew that they were whispering behind her back that she had AIDS. They had worried when they saw her hair lose its lustre, and had noticed that she tired easily. And when she developed a skin rash that, over a period of months, spread to her arms and legs, forcing her to wear long-sleeved blouses and trousers all the time, they knew the end was near.

One of Peace's workmates later painted a picture of what went on in the bank while Peace ailed. Her workmates had maintained a façade, trying to make it look like nothing was wrong. They pretended not to notice Peace's ailments, but they always came up with a variety of excuses to avoid working too closely with her. They never mentioned the word AIDS within earshot of her. When she finally failed to turn up for work they took it with a mixture of relief and grief. They did not expect to ever see her alive again.

When I first examined Peace, I found that the immediate problems we had to address urgently were pneumonia and dehydration. Accordingly, I treated her with intravenous fluids and antibiotics. I also attended to her wound. Her condition gradually improved. However, as it was apparent that she was already in advanced stages of AIDS, I started her on KS3. As I had already started using it on a few other patients without any evident toxicity, I was confident that it would at the very least not harm Peace, though I was still unconvinced with regard to its effect on HIV/AIDS. Under the daily care of Gloria and a local nurse, Peace made steady progress and, to our delight, she started regaining her weight and strength.

Just over two months later the rejuvenated woman showed up in the bank lobby dressed in a sleeveless blouse and a skirt, looking healthier than ever before. Some of her workmates later confessed that they thought she was a ghost. Although her job had been given to someone else she was reinstated on account of her previous good work record.

Later I was told that this courageous woman also surprised her brothers-in-law when she suddenly turned up at her house. She was accompanied by her lawyer carrying a court eviction order. One of her brothers-in-law was already well settled in and had started redecorating the house to suit what was described to me as "his demonstrably bad taste". Peace tossed him out.

Unlike many widows who had their properties grabbed, Peace was one of the very few lucky ones who got a second lease of life.

Unfortunately she died of breast cancer about four years later. In order to avoid the house being seized by her in-laws, she had sold it and bought a smaller property elsewhere. She then invested the rest of the money for the future education and maintenance of her daughter who, to my delight, I had earlier found to be free of HIV.

Certainly, the care Peace received from her caring auntie and the nurse at Kansanga, and the treatment of opportunistic infections, all helped to prolong her life. But I still wondered whether Rouchy's AIDS medicine had not also helped in some way.

Rouchy's Medicine

It seemed like Mr Rouchy had, indeed, found the elusive palliative to HIV/AIDS. He had developed two anti-AIDS drugs at the time when AZT was the only US approved ARV drug. AZT, then used in high dosages was already known to be associated with some serious side effects. Its benefit was mild and also transient. According to Rouchy, his own drugs were safer and certain to work better than AZT. Rouchy codenamed the first compound KS3 and the second one KS3-TH, but for purposes of easy reference, I took the liberty of renaming the first compound Jocecylon and the latter Joceclovir. Rouchy believed that Joceclovir would be more effective.

Rouchy had explained that the mode of action of the drugs was through "blockade of the last stages of HIV maturation". If I had not recorded this back in 1991, one would be excused for deducing that Rouchy was referring to the more modern AIDS drugs of the class of protease inhibitors (PIs), which act on the HIV virus at almost the same stage of viral maturation. The confirmation of the efficacy of the PIs later in 1995, especially when combined with other drugs, was to become a turning point in AIDS treatment. However, I cannot confirm whether his drugs were PIs.

During the discussions, Rouchy raised a pertinent economic issue. His economics background had apparently not gone to waste. He explained that manufacturing the drugs in France would be too expensive. He did not want his products ending up like AZT, which the poor could not afford. He explained that it would be much cheaper to manufacture only the powder form of the drug in France, to ensure purity. The encapsulation could then be left to be done more cost effectively in Uganda. He offered to train me to make the capsules.

He suggested that, on returning home, I could either continue to do it myself or train someone else to do it. Without much ado, he sat me down in his class of one and I immediately started on my very first lesson in drugs manufacture or, more specifically, making capsules. He treated me like a student who had to be readied for a fast approaching final examinations. The standards were stringent, and he emphasised that this was essential. Frequently peeping over my shoulder, he kept checking that everything was progressing well. It would have been tough to have Mr Rouchy as your primary school teacher!

"There must be no contamination, and each capsule must weigh 300 mg plus or minus 10 mg," Rouchy commanded through the translator as I tried to master the new skill.

The tools for the job were basic. They included a scientific weighing scale, sterile dressings, an encapsulating mould — plus lots of patience. The mould allowed for manufacture of up to ten capsules per round. It was essential that the gelatine capsules were filled uniformly. Then every 100 capsules were weighed and a random sample of ten would be reweighed, to make sure that the whole batch was uniform. He drilled me until he was satisfied that I was doing it right.

As I prepared to return home, Pierre turned up with a special bag with multiple pockets of varying sizes, much like those used by drug smugglers. Rouchy and I systematically filled the pockets with empty gelatine capsules, KS3 powder, 2 litres of concentrated Oligomines, Doxycycline capsules and the encapsulating mould — each one in its own chamber. I headed for Charles de Gaulle Airport wondering whether I would be mistakenly arrested for peddling illegal drugs, or whether this would happen on arrival back home in Uganda. With my bag and contents I looked like I was "in the big time". However, the trip passed off uneventfully. I declared the contents as experimental AIDS drugs at Entebbe Airport and they were cleared. However, I still recall the brief encounter with one of the customs officers. "I hope they work," he remarked as his colleague examined the multi-pocketed bag, "otherwise we shall all be dead." Then, as I was leaving he suddenly seemed to remember something. "Excuse me Doctor," he hurriedly said as he drew me aside. "Can I send my sick sister to volunteer for the tests? My other two sisters and the only brother I had are already dead. Only two of us are left. Otherwise, by the look of things, I will soon be left alone. That is, if I am safe," he added. I wished I had something comforting to say to him.

One would be forgiven for assuming that, as soon as I arrived home where numerous AIDS patients awaited me, I started using the medicine immediately. "Suppose the drug harmed my patients?" the question kept reverberating in my mind. However, in time, Rouchy's reassurances, especially the numbers that he reportedly treated without any serious complications, the deteriorating state of Evelyn's health, the desperate pleas of her relatives, and the encouragement of my fellow doctors, gave me courage to start using the drugs. Evelyn's lack of any apparent side effects that could be attributed to the KS3, reassured me and I extended it to a few more patients.

Demand for the drugs shot up as news spread that some AIDS patients were on trial drugs. But I could not raise the funds to order new supplies from France, even though Mr Rouchy charitably charged only for the materials and transport costs. By that time my own small savings were used up, and there seemed to be no other way to proceed. Then one of my colleagues brought in a well-to-do patient nicknamed Tycoon, who offered to pay all the costs involved for me to travel to France and bring in the experimental drug for him. I explained to him that, I was not sure that the drug had any effect on HIV, and that I had many other patients with similar need but too poor to have the drugs sent to them from France. I told him that as a public sector doctor, it would be unethical to ignore the needs of so many and go on to attend to an individual who had a way out. I suggested to him that since he could afford it, it would be better for him to travel to France and be treated by Rouchy himself.

"I agree with you, Doctor," he surprised me with his prompt understanding of an intricate dilemma that also affected his own life. "I am not alone," he went on to explain. "I have a few friends who are also sick and we would like to be of assistance to you. We have joined hands to help you get enough medicine for some other patients as well." This was a pleasant surprise. "But you know Doctor, virtually everyone in Uganda is sick. Surely, we can't be expected to provide therapy for everyone. We shall offer what we can afford," he said. "Beyond that, you will need to find some other ways to help others —and may God help you."

Twenty years later, Tycoon is still alive, because he could afford ARVs as soon as they became available and, as I write, he remains in good health. His business has flourished. His kindness to others in need continues and he helped me to develop a programme of cost-sharing whereby patients who were too poor to pay even the consultation fee had their expenses subsidised by the wealthy volunteers, a strategy that saved many lives.

When I joined the JCRC in 1992 – then a marginally better facilitated research unit than Mulago Hospital – I got the opportunity to formally test Rouchy's drugs. Based on what I had seen so far, I had grounds to believe that they had a good chance of success. I planned to scientifically study the drugs to ascertain their efficacy. However, this brought in some special challenges. To begin with, I needed to ensure uninterrupted drugs supplies to participants in the trial. Secondly, I needed a second opinion.

I made an appointment to meet Mr Rouchy in Brussels in June 1993 on my way back from the Berlin International AIDS conference. I asked two senior Ugandan doctors who had attended the same conference to join me. Mr Rouchy came, accompanied by Pierre to interpret for us. After listening to him and considering the evidence that he provided, the three of us were unanimous in our verdict that Rouchy's drugs had scientific merit and deserved to be studied further. We were gratified when he promised to provide free technical support.

A few months later I returned to France to follow up on the details. Once more Mr Rouchy subjected me to the same rigorous training and made sure that my understanding of the work was up to scratch. This time round, I received a very rare praise from him in form of what he described as "your quick grasp of a new and difficult subject". He again saw me off, loaded with enough drugs to start the trial, and assured me of subsequent supplies. On this occasion I found that Mr Rouchy no longer believed that AIDS could be cured in a month. "I now know a little more about this virus than I did last time you were here," he explained as Pierre interpreted, "but I am still confident that it can be successfully treated." He was now talking merely about suppressing the virus. He promptly agreed to my proposal to extend the clinical trial period to at least three months.

Rouchy's firm belief in his products' effectiveness encouraged me to go on with the study. I never quite believed that his treatment or any other that existed at the time would provide a cure for AIDS. But based on what I had learned, I was cautiously optimistic that it would at least be the beginning of a long process to finding an effective medicine to prolong life. I also hoped that if it worked it would offer relief to other African countries that I knew were equally tormented by the scourge. Nevertheless, I deliberately remained neutral to avoid raising expectations, as the fiasco of Gracia-1 was still a recent memory.

The preparation period took us much longer than initially anticipated, mainly because we had to check every detail. As HIV science had advanced, I insisted that we had to use the most up-to-date tests including CD4, then the state-of-the-art test. However, we desperately needed funds and I appealed to everyone I knew for help, but nothing was forthcoming until several months later when Dr Ben Mbonye, who was then the secretary for defence, succeeded in getting us the necessary funds to go ahead.

In preparation for the study, we constituted a team of investigators comprising clinicians, laboratory technicians, nurses, counsellors, a health visitor and a biostatistician. We included in the study only patients who were in advanced stages of AIDS equivalent to category 3 and 4 of WHO staging based on the severity of the disease, whereby stage 4 is the most advanced. The funding enabled us to include the CD4 test to accurately measure the level of immunological improvement among participating patients. The first trial patient was enrolled on 23 January, 1994 and there was a rush by many others to join. Many more volunteers than we needed came forward. At the end of the first phase of the trial which was completed on schedule on 28 June 1994 we faced a dilemma. Many patients who had felt well on the drugs had no follow-up therapy.

As the study progressed, the indications were that for the first time, we had a drug that showed genuine promise. Most patients on trial treatment reported a sense of well-being that they had not felt in a long time. A good number of those who had been experiencing general body weakness and drowsiness excitedly reported that they felt much stronger, more alert and had a better concentration span. A number also reported improvements in appetite, fewer episodes of diarrhoea, decreased malaise, evening fevers, skin eruptions and body aches. However, on average, there was mild weight loss among the study group, and the course of some of the opportunistic infections remained generally unchanged. But considering the short period of therapy this was not entirely unexpected. Overall, most patients praised the treatment and felt that it had helped them a great deal.

Detailed analysis of study findings revealed interesting results. The scientific indicators for body immune function seemed to support the patients' reports. The CD4 of those in the group that received Jocecylon, increased by 20% from baseline after six weeks. At the time there were very few AIDS drugs on clinical trial that could effect this change. Those in the group that received Joceclovir maintained a stable CD4 count through the three months of treatment and observation. A small number among them experienced a modest rise in CD4, but unlike Jocecylon, this was not statistically significant. There were too few side effects to warrant any terminations.

While I celebrated the results Rouchy, on the other hand, was rather taken aback by the findings. He had expected Joceclovir, his newer discovery, to do much better than Jocecylon. But the study results suggested the opposite. Of course, there could have been some other explanation, including the short period of therapy, the dosage or timing of doses since the pharmacokinetics of the drug was not known. Since patients being treated did not deteriorate, Joceclovir also deserved a second chance to be studied further on a larger number of patients, using different dosages, before coming to a reasonable conclusion. I was convinced that the two drugs deserved a more intensive scrutiny to further define their effects. This necessitated a larger and more expensive study.

But no funding source was immediately available. If our pilot study had been carried out in a rich Western country and the same results obtained at the time, Jocecylon would have been on the fast track with a view to developing it into an anti-AIDS drug. It would have attracted lots of investors, and pharmaceutical companies would have been interested and eager to fund it. Considering the non-deserving drugs that made it to the media at the time, this one should have hit the headlines too. There were several possible reasons why this was not to be. First, pharmaceutical companies had sensed that AIDS drugs would turn out to be highly lucrative business. But due to the high price they could reap in rich countries where they would also be on demand, poverty-ridden Africa was left out in the cold, because it did not constitute a profitable market. Secondly, Mr Rouchy was averse to the idea of big pharmaceutical companies getting hold of his products unless they guaranteed that the poor would have access to it.

The only way we could see forward was to lobby for private funding. Judging by how difficult it had been to secure funding for the initial small pilot project, the prospects of finding funding for a greatly expanded study did not look good. Nevertheless, I started on a fundraising mission while at the same time trying to put together a team of local and foreign partners to work with us on this project.

However, some serious issues needed to be ironed out first. Even if the funding became available, how would we fare with the unwieldy task of developing the drug to the standards required for quality pharmaceutical products? How would we set up a manufacturing process, and let alone obtain the necessary regulatory licences? To address these challenges, I again turned to Mr Rouchy to tap into his wide knowledge of the pharmaceutical industry. In his usual philosophical way he urged patience until a pharmaceutical plant in Uganda capable of undertaking local production of the drugs was set up. "Only then," Rouchy said, "would you ensure that the medicine would be accessible to your people." He promised to provide the necessary technical help in getting the process going. Jokingly, he added as Pierre interpreted, "If the sharks get hold of it…" He did not complete the sentence but made a brisk cut-throat sign.

When I informed a senior government official about Mr Rouchy's offer of help, he enthusiastically promised to facilitate the project. A few weeks later, he informed me that a decision had been taken to invite Mr Rouchy to Uganda. I was thrilled by this development, and pleased when I was assigned the pleasant job of passing on the invitation to him. With a spring in my step, I boarded the plane for France. I looked forward to the moment I could pass on what I thought would be Mr Rouchy's most exciting news since his retirement. I knew that he longed for a time when his drug would be accessible to the poor. The critical constraints to this happening seemed to have been overcome. The pharmaceutical company that would manufacture his drug had been identified. It seemed like the pieces were falling in place: the elusive medicine to alleviate the agony of AIDS would finally be available, right here in Uganda.

However, when I arrived in Paris things did not go according to plan. As usual, Rouchy welcomed me warmly and immediately asked how patients, especially those who were taking his medicines, were doing. However, his mood changed when I told him about the invitation. It was a cruel anticlimax! I was astonished and puzzled by his response. Although I was used to his rather unconventional character, and had learned to expect the unexpected responses, this one, was to say the least, a little over the top. To add to my confusion, Mr Rouchy did not explain his baffling reaction. However, by his uncharacteristic shilly-shallying, it was plain that some sort of battle of thoughts was going on in his mind. Piecemeal, and over time, the real reason emerged in a roundabout way. He first inquired whether there were passenger ships from France to East Africa. Then finally he owned up. My hero, the great Rouchy, was scared of flying. So overpoweringly scared that at his advanced age, he had never been in an airplane! And he made it clear that he had no intention of doing so, then or ever.

I had relied on Rouchy's acceptance of the invitation, and I had no plan B ready. But I returned home to work on it. My initial idea was to persuade the pharmaceutical company that had been identified for the task to send their technical staff to France for training. Unfortunately, my ideas did not fit in with their immediate priorities. At the same time, reports of other AIDS drugs, from up and running Western countries' pharmaceutical companies, were coming in.

I remained in touch with Mr Rouchy. Over the years he has become a good friend. Even at his advanced age, he zealously keeps in touch with the developments in AIDS treatment research. He regrets that his drugs never made it. As the saying goes, for the lack of a shoe, the kingdom was lost!

Cure Enterprise

They arrived in a spectacular fashion, but without appointment.

Impressed, Santrina, my long serving secretary, ushered them into my office, explaining that they were on what they had described to her as "a very important and urgent mission". Dr James Okot, a jovial Ugandan-born scientist working in Britain, led the delegation which consisted of a good-humoured, English businessman, Gregg Billinghurst who was holding on tightly to a leather briefcase as if his life depended on it. Then there was Sarah Reed his secretary, and their aid de camp, George Kapere, a local recruit (all not real names).

Dr Okot, reminded me that we were contemporaries at Makerere University Medical School, explaining that he was two or three years behind me. I could hazily recall a diminutive scholarly young man now evidently transformed into a well-groomed gentleman. He introduced his companions after which he left it to Gregg to explain the purpose of their mission. In an apparently well-rehearsed drill, Gregg winked to the secretary as he handed her the hitherto closely guarded briefcase. On cue, she sprang into a patently practised routine. With a slight touch, the brief case flew open and she removed neatly arranged documents and an expensive pen.

"Before we can say anything to you, you must first sign these documents" Gregg said with an inviting smile as he took the papers from Sarah. "Secondly, anyone in this institution who will directly or indirectly have anything to do with this project must also sign similar documents," he added in a measured businesslike tone, as he politely handed me the pen and papers pointing to a dotted line.

"I just can't sign documents blindly," I pleaded, but still impressed by the smooth flow of their act "at least I need to know what it is all about."

"Fair enough," Gregg shrugged courteously. In matters of etiquette it was difficult to fault him. "It's all about protection of privileged information," he said as he gestured in an apparent invitation for me to go ahead and scan the document.

The professionally written document was faultless. It meticulously explained the discovery of a new AIDS medicine by Dr James Okot. Okot was described as a cancer researcher working in the UK. Apparently he had, in the course of his work, discovered a group of molecules that boosted the immune system of cancer-afflicted mice so much so that the tumours just melted away. The question as to whether these molecules would do the same for AIDS patients then arose. Very preliminary tests indicated that the substances, indeed, had some immune modulating effects in humans. This attribute would, if its effectiveness was confirmed, come in handy to repair the damage HIV causes to the body. Dr Okot was optimistic that his discovery could in future form part of an AIDS treatment regimen. First of all he needed to demonstrate the proof of the concept. The next logical step was, of course, to go out and test the drug on AIDS patients. But this required money – and a lot of it too – which Okot did not have.

Although all the details were never fully revealed to me, I gathered that Okot had started looking around for a sponsor. He eventually found a benefactor in the form of a young, upcoming businessman, Gregg Billinghurst. Gregg, a meticulous man in his business endeavours, was initially sceptical. At first he found it hard to believe that an unpretentious young African was on the verge of making one of the century's greatest scientific breakthroughs, one that had eluded so many other well facilitated and high-profile European scientists. When Gregg made inquiries about Okot's credentials from the university research unit where he worked, he was awestruck by the high esteem in which Okot was held by his peers. Having established that Okot's work was bona fide, Gregg explored the business potential of AIDS drugs on stock exchanges. Any remaining doubts were dispelled and he realised that huge amounts of money could be made out of Okot's discovery. But he understood that this was only possible if it made it to the highly lucrative pharmaceutical market without middlemen.

Gregg, a shrewd businessman, came up with a road map for a successful enterprise. He was not only going to find funds for the clinical trial but would find partners to float a pharmaceutical manufacturing company that would have monopoly rights and patent protection to make and market the new drug worldwide. The company I call Goodway was registered in a tax haven offshore island of the UK. Okot became one of the directors. It was agreed that Gregg would take care of the business side of the project while Okot concentrated on the science. This marked the beginning of a partnership that seemed destined for great medical and commercial glory.

As the drug's efficacy results were needed fast, Uganda, then the epicentre of the AIDS epidemic, was the natural choice for the study. Gregg had it all planned in such minute detail that even the day and time for the media conference to announce the "breakthrough" news after the successful drug trial, and launch of the drug were all fixed. Enthusiastically, he showed me a diagram with my designated seat at the momentous media conference at which he would break the news to the world. He had timed the event for 7.00 pm — the UK's peak TV viewing time – leaving enough time for the next day's papers to prepare the headline story in their late editions. Nothing was being left to chance.

Preparation for the trial of the pioneer Goodway Pharmaceutical product, which I will call Aidsvir, proceeded swiftly. The scientific and ethical review boards readily approved the well and professionally written study protocol, thus paving the way for it to proceed. Preliminary results were ready in just over 28 weeks.

However, to Gregg's profound disappointment, the results failed to demonstrate the clear efficacy that he had so eagerly anticipated. In contrast, Dr Okot was able to discern what he described as "some highly optimistic trends". First he observed that the patients on therapy did not deteriorate as would have been expected if the treatment was totally ineffective. In addition, there was, on average, a fair rise in CD4 cells, suggesting some beneficial immunological benefit. However, these findings were not good enough to reach statistical significance necessary to put the issue of efficacy beyond reasonable doubt. Quite clearly, the trial findings did not point to an outright failure, but cried out for more research. It was back to the drawing board. Fortunately, Okot had plan B in form of other promising related molecules, ready for testing. However the success of Aidsvir had been taken for granted. Now, all of a sudden, more funds were needed to carry out a new study. In the interest of speed, Okot requested the JCRC to advance some seed money to get the drug trial under way quickly, promising to refund the money later. As the integrity of Okot was beyond reproach, I readily agreed to his request. However, with our limited resources we could (with belt-tightening) afford only a meagre amount, which was just sufficient to get an expanded study started.

The welcome news of a possible funding breakthrough reached me while I was in Yokohama, Japan, attending an international conference on AIDS.

"I have very good news with regard to our study in Uganda," Gregg said by phone. "However I need your help to seal the deal. And I need it most urgently. Would it be possible for you to fly to London immediately? Goodway will take care of logistics."

At Heathrow Airport, I was met by a uniformed chauffeur, who drove me straight to my hotel for a much needed rest. The next morning Okot and Gregg met me in the lobby and briefed me on the day's programme. We were scheduled to meet high-ranking officials of a big investment company.

"Your role is to make an impact on them as a serious scientist — someone who could be trusted with such an important study," Gregg explained.

The meeting took place in a big office block located in the West End of London. Dr Okot was introduced to the meeting as "one of the most brilliant scientists in Britain today". This was followed by the reading out of his short-version but still impressive CV and retracing his past and present research work that had ultimately led to the discovery of the candidate AIDS drugs of unprecedented promise. As a fellow Ugandan, I felt buoyant and very proud of him. In my turn, I was just introduced as the "Ugandan scientist who carried out the initial tests on the drugs". The meeting was informed that we had successfully tested the first of a series of related drugs that showed promising results, though not sufficiently significant to be defined as efficacious. This was yet another reason why I liked and respected Okot. He always insisted on the truth. That is the main reason that I stuck with him even when the going got tough.

When the time came, the clinical research expert advisor to the investment company called upon me to give details of our research findings. I presented our results which, as Okot had already explained, did not establish clear efficacy. I explained that the results could not be construed as outright failure because the data demonstrated some unmistakable positive trends. "Quite clearly, the findings call for further studies using different dosages of Aidvir as well as testing of other drugs in the same class of compounds to see whether a better outcome could be achieved," I concluded my submission.

The scientific advisor had also independently studied the data and had come to the same conclusion. He concurred with my explanation, and agreed that more research was justified. Okot briefed the meeting about other possible clinical applications of the drug including potential use as a supplement to cancer therapy as a possible immune booster. At the end of it all, the company was won over. However, it soon became apparent that they were powerless to take a final decision on their own. They needed the blessing of their company headquarters in the USA before any deal could be sealed.

Early the next morning of 23 May 1995, Gregg and I, boarded Continental Airline flight, destination Dallas Texas. Dr Okot was scheduled to follow on a later flight. There to meet us at Dallas Fort

Worth Airport was Jose Martinez, a senior official of Goodway USA Inc. Jose briefed us on the programme for the next few days, which was to start that very afternoon.

The first meeting turned out to be a courtesy call on Gregg's US counterpart, the director of Goodway USA Inc, whom I call Secretary George McMahon. The reason why he was called secretary instead of director was clearly displayed on the wall behind his desk. It was in form of a framed letter signed by the late US President Johnson appointing him secretary of a government department in the 1960s. As is customary in the US, the title remained his for life.

The main meeting was scheduled to take place two days later but there was a pre-meeting rehearsal planned for the next day. I had never witnessed the like and my first reaction was to object to the whole exercise. Indeed, I had to be convinced that this was really necessary. I considered my role as scientist in this whole venture to be merely that of presenting the scientific data accurately and truthfully. Therefore, I did not see any need for a dummy run.

"It's not just the facts that matter. You need to be cool, man. Folks here need to form a favourable first impression of you, to keep this in mind as they ponder the decision," Jose explained enthusiastically. "Investment companies don't give a shit for scientific complexities. They wanna see a smart guy before dishing out the bucks, man."

"I agree to this on one condition," I said as Jose appeared to get increasingly edgy. "I will strictly stick to the facts."

"Sure! We're all for the facts, man," Jose retorted.

The rehearsal was more involved than I had anticipated. A devil's advocate was on board to ask the hard questions that the investors would be expected to pose. I was asked to go over the scientific results of the study again and again. Each time I covered the findings in much the same way as I had in London. At the end of the session, the devil's advocate cut in. "At this juncture I will come in to ask you a vital question," he said. "What is your gut feeling about the potential of these drugs?" He then paused to critique my answer.

"Well, my answer would be the same as I said in my conclusion; that the results so far, called for more tests because the first study was inconclusive," I replied.

"Well that is the best way to lose us the funding," the devil's advocate replied.

"I have to speak the truth," I pleaded.

"There are many ways of presenting the truth," he snapped. "What would be wrong with you also informing them that if the drug trial findings turned out to be positive there would be millions of AIDS patients in Africa ready to use the drugs?" he asked.

"Well, that statement would be true only if the drugs were affordable and accessible," I replied.

"Goodway would guarantee that," he clarified.

"In that case, I could live with it," I replied.

"Great!" Gregg cut in. "Now we are making some progress."

The next day I was asked to come smartly dressed in a business suit and a matching tie. As we headed downtown, Gregg inspected my attire and declared my tie compliant with American standards. "It's what they call a power tie here in America," he commented approvingly. "Now we are all set."

Thanks to the intense preparations, the meeting proceeded flawlessly and according to plan. Whatever questions the investors did not ask were brought up in the discussion by our side, followed by the well practised and smooth, flowing answers. It was an impressive presentation and a resounding success. Yet, to my surprise we were not home and dry yet. I was to learn that serious investment companies do not just dish out money — not even to smart guys. They sent us on a three and half hour flight north to New York to meet their counterparts for more discussions and consideration.

The New York meeting took place in a Manhattan hotel, and lasted for about two and a half hours. We met more officials of the investments company who mercifully did not put us through the same rigorous interview process as their London and Texas counterparts had done. They were more interested in financial management issues, which I mainly left to Gregg to address. I only responded to questions about research standards and conditions in Uganda, which I answered to their satisfaction. And that was it. Mission over, I was driven to JFK Airport to catch the evening British Airways flight to London connecting on to Entebbe via Nairobi.

Jet-lagged, I arrived back home, ending a journey in search of an AIDS drug that had taken me through four continents in just over a week. There was a fax waiting for me on arrival. The funds for the next part of the drugs trial had been obtained and I was asked to make the necessary arrangements to get it going as soon as possible. That was the last I ever heard of funds from the investment company. As far as Goodway was concerned, I had played my part to help secure the necessary funds and with that my role was over. My job now was only to concentrate on the science and deliver on the research aspect of the project, and that's exactly what I set out to do.

This part of the clinical trials involved new drug formulations and we planned to carry it out in two phases. The first phase proceeded well, but preliminary results, though much better than the first, still fell short of a conclusive outcome. But we had not designed this phase of study as an efficacy trial, therefore there was a need for a follow-on study.

Preparations for the new drug trial were well under way when heads started rolling in Goodway. I do not know exactly what triggered the debacle, but Gregg, Sarah, Kapere, Jose and other officials I had met in London, Texas and New York were all axed. Legally worded letters with lengthy microscopic text footnote, flooded in, warning us that any further dealing with the fired officials would be at our own risk. This was followed in quick succession with yet more messages informing me that Goodway UK and Goodway USA Inc had all been dissolved and had already closed shop.

That was the end of another promising lead towards an AIDS cure. But we still remained with unfinished business with the dissolved Goodway companies. They owed us money. We were informed that the companies had gone into receivership, but they were quick to reassure us that the company receiver would settle their debt with us. They never did!

Jewish Saviour

In early September 1996, a new ray of hope was kindled.

It came in the form of a highly promising message concerning "an effective and affordable AIDS cure made in Israel". It was reported to have been developed with the help of renowned and time-tested German expertise. The bearer of the news was a genial man I shall call Eugene Ndagije, a Burundi-born engineer who had taken German citizenship. He was the kind of man who would always make his presence felt anywhere he went, not only by his bulky frame but also his gentle and engaging personality. Eugene was apparently doing well professionally, as the head of the African branch of a big engineering firm that specialised in road construction. A senior government official who introduced him to me asked me to act on this matter with utmost urgency, explaining that it was "a chance to rescue our country from the scourge of AIDS."

I took a liking to Eugene the moment I met him. He was a pleasant, soft-spoken man with whom I established immediate rapport. He informed me that a German private practitioner working with Israeli scientists had developed a highly efficacious AIDS drug. "This drug will put a stop to the carnage of AIDS in Uganda," he said. He told me that the doctor, whom he apparently knew very well and regarded in high esteem, was willing to share her research results with us. Furthermore she was willing to help develop the promising AIDS cure into an affordable therapy for Uganda and other poor African countries in the region.

"Although I am not a medical doctor, I have been assured that this drug is not like any that you know of," Eugene elaborated. "It has special attributes that make it particularly appealing to poor countries." He added that when he got to know about it he took the initiative on humanitarian grounds to try and help alleviate the suffering of AIDS patients in Africa. "Has it been tested?" I asked him, wondering whether this one would be any different from many other claims that I had chased after before.

"Absolutely," he replied promptly. "I have been assured that this seemingly unconquerable bug has been tamed by a mere herbal extract from a plant growing wild in Israel."

The next day I found out that Eugene had already taken the initiative of talking to senior officials of the ministries of health of the neighbouring countries of Rwanda and his native Burundi.

"I am happy to inform you that both countries have expressed their readiness to contribute to the drugs' production costs, which would make it that more affordable for all," he said. "Please hurry to Bonn and meet this doctor, so that you can start saving lives immediately," Eugene urged me.

However, I remained doubtful, notwithstanding his enthusiastic announcements.

Although my instinctive reaction was to dismiss this latest claim outright, I soon found out that I would be departing for Germany sooner rather than later. The senior government official whom he had contacted had already made travel arrangements. He said that many AIDS patients were demanding the drug. "I hope you will return with the wonder medicine that I have heard so much about," he wrote in a memo to me.

As I prepared to depart I was approached by a diligent Rwandese physician I will call Tom Karenzi. Dr Karenzi, who later became a cabinet minister in his country, offered to work with me on the acquisition of the so-called wonder drug. However, he too had some concerns. "We need to make sure that we are not being taken for a ride," he warned. "I detect commercialism in the whole exercise." I later found out that he had been contacted earlier by Eugene and had already been to Germany to meet with the scientist concerned. It was unfortunate that he did not disclose this important piece of information to me. It would have cushioned me from a few surprises.

I arrived at Cologne Airport on a chilly morning on 15 September, 1996. I took a taxi to my hotel in Bonn and immediately contacted Eugene. He had scheduled my appointment with the doctor whom I shall call Kristin Reiter, one of the developers of the drug, for the following afternoon. I had a day of rest to freshen up and recover from the long journey but my afternoon siesta was interrupted as usual, by the phone. It was Eugene on the line. He explained that he had a VIP with him whom he wanted to introduce. The VIP turned out to be a Canadian businessman I will call Steven Campers. "He is a very nice man to know. In fact he might come in handy as a partner to help with drugs' procurement," was Eugene's liberal recommendation.

As soon as Eugene put the telephone down, Steve's call came through. With a jovial but rather boastful voice, he introduced himself, insisting that I call him by his first name. He claimed to be very familiar with Uganda, and well known personally to President Museveni and the former Canadian prime minister, Pierre Elliot Trudeau. He boasted about his high-level connections and his "booming businesses in Africa, Europe and the Americas", and promised to assist Uganda to develop the new AIDS medicine. "It's a matter of a telephone call to the Canadian prime minister and his counterpart President Museveni and all will be fixed," he bragged. He promised to meet me at Eugene's residence where we were both invited for a welcome dinner that evening. However, when it came to dinner time, Steve was nowhere to be seen.

The next day my meeting with Dr Kristin Reiter was delayed for an hour as she finished seeing the last couple of patients on her day's list of appointments. When she was through with her clinic, the doctor received me warmly. Over a cup of coffee, she told me about the anti-AIDS drug. She showed me photographs of wild plants with bright yellow flowers reportedly taken in Israel, from which, the claimed drug was extracted. She had some dried flower samples in her office, which she gave me to examine.

"These plants thrive in tropical climate, and can therefore be grown in Uganda, and be processed locally," she said. "This would save your country huge amounts of foreign exchange and make the product both affordable and sustainable," she added, making good sense as far as cost-effectiveness was concerned.

"What about the research data proving the drug's efficacy?" I asked rather impatiently. I was beginning to feel uneasy, as she seemed to be concentrating more on pleasantries instead of addressing scientific issues regarding the drug that had brought me all the way from Africa to the hinterland of Europe.

"Don't worry about that!" she brushed aside my curiosity. "Research carried out in Israel and Germany has established that it is a highly efficacious and non-toxic agent against AIDS."

"Would it be possible for me to see some samples of the drug?" I asked. After all if what she just said to me was true, she held the lives of millions of AIDS patients in her hands. "No. That's not really possible because it does not exist," she replied, taking me by surprise.

I thought of the great expectations and the optimistic note from the VIP back home.

"It would cost money, you know," she said. "And the whole venture needs a donor."

"So what is the way forward?" I asked hardly able to conceal my disappointment.

"Perhaps you should talk to Steve," Kristin said.

"I am surprised you know Steve too". I remarked as I pondered what the triad of Eugene, Steve and Kristin were up to.

"I think Steve will get us the exact connections to ensure that this project works out well for all of us," Kristin said in a matter of fact way.

It was becoming clear to me that something strange was going on between the gang of three. I could also see that, at the very least, they had some undeclared interest on their agenda that was not of a purely humanitarian nature. The question was now, whether it would be possible to work out an arrangement with them if, indeed, they had a promising AIDS drug. I also wondered whether they had just cooked up the whole story and I had been sent on a wild goose chase, or whether they were using me as a pawn or bait in some sort of scheme to fleece an unsuspecting donor.

I could not form an opinion about the hitherto unseen Steve, but it was evident that both Kristin and Eugene were respectable, bona fide professionals. I had seen Kristin at work in her obviously successful medical practice. Eugene was a senior civil engineer trusted with the headship of a big road construction project. It was therefore inevitable for me to conclude that perhaps it was Steve, somewhere in the background, like a barracuda that lies low to spring a surprise on other fish, who was pulling the strings. Yet I knew nothing about the mysterious man. But since he was highly regarded by people of such demonstrable professional integrity, it was only fair that he be given the benefit of the doubt.

To try and blunt the edge of my mounting anxiety and curiosity, I decided to do a little background research on Steve. The only place I thought of, to start, was the Ugandan Embassy in Bonn. As it turned out I was spot on. Steve was, indeed, very well known to Ambassador Samson Bigombe and other embassy officials. When I asked a senior diplomat to explain to me who exactly Steve was, he responded rather light-heartedly, describing him as, "a man whose promises are not always compatible with his actions."

The immediate natural reaction was to warn Kristin. I called her up straight away, using the embassy phone. "Dr Reiter, I just found out that Steve may not be such a trustworthy partner."

"Oh! Is that so?" She sounded surprised but the tone of her reply was cool.

I wondered whether she had known all along that Steve was a dubious character, or if she was just an unfortunate victim of circumstance just like me. However, she seemed to recover quickly, promising that she would follow up the matter.

"Never mind," she said. "Steve had only offered to help, but he is not involved in the development of the drug. I will take up the matter directly with the Israeli scientists and get one of them to come to Uganda as soon as possible to work directly with you on the development of this drug," she reassured me.

Perhaps she thought that this was something positive to tell the senior government official, and the people anxiously waiting back home – the good news of the Jewish saviour who would soon come to Uganda to save them from the killer scourge.

It has been a long wait, but waiting for a Jewish saviour, needs faith and a lot of patience.

Norwegian Cure

The fame and fortune to be made from developing a promising AIDS drug brought together two peculiar individuals — two of a kind. Without AIDS, it would have been virtually impossible to imagine that their paths and mine would ever have crossed.

One of them was a man I will call Brian Saunders, a down-to-earth middle-aged British businessman. His working-class Yorkshire accent betrayed his modest educational background. Saunders, an old fashioned, strict schoolmaster type, took life and himself seriously. He spent most of his time focussed on his business ventures and had hardly a minute for recreation. In sharp contrast, his partner a highly educated Norwegian scientist I will call Hansen Van Grouch, was young, easy-going and had an active social life outside work. Both had their eyes fixed on the prize of a lifetime but with different roadmaps towards its achievement. They were prepared to put aside their differences and work together as they travelled on the long road to their mutual goal.

The two men were first introduced to me by a Ugandan politician-cum-businessman whom they had met in London. They had informed him of what Saunders was later to describe as "a veiled gold mine, in the form of a highly promising new AIDS drug, which only needed to undergo a final efficacy test". They asked the awestruck politician to identify a competent Ugandan research institution that would be interested in testing their new drug.

At our first meeting at the JCRC, I was spellbound as Dr Van Grouch narrated how he had discovered the new drug. He made it all sound very easy, as if the discovery was almost by accident. Apparently he had been testing various candidate drugs for possible effect on HIV in his research laboratory in Oslo. At first he had ignored one candidate drug because it was thought to be least likely to have any effect on HIV. For this reason, it was just included to serve as a control, but it provided surprising results. He found that it inhibited HIV much more effectively than the trial drugs. He repeated the experiment many times but always came up with the same results. He also established that it was able to do this at a very low concentration and without damage to cells.

With mounting anticipation, he requested a few of his colleagues to repeat the experiment independently but without revealing the identity of the drug to them. The results were the same. Van Grouch knew that if this drug could safely do in humans what he had observed it do in his laboratory tissue cultures, then he was on the verge of discovering the elusive AIDS cure. He kept the findings close to his chest as he sought a trustworthy sponsor and a site to test it on real AIDS patients.

Van Grouch had thought that it would be easy to find a pharmaceutical company to sponsor a clinical trial of such a promising drug, with the potential to earn billions in profits. But all the major pharmaceutical companies that he approached for sponsorship of the clinical trial of his "breakthrough" AIDS drug declined to have anything to do with it. I gathered that one pharmaceutical research scientist was brutally honest with him, and told him the reason for the repetitive rebuffs. "It's just too good to be true."

Virtually all pharmaceutical companies must have experienced many candidate drugs that promised them gold turn to dust — just as I had also found out the hard way.

After a long, frustrating search, Van Grouch chanced to meet Brian Saunders, a businessman of modest means who was captivated by the discovery and especially the business part of it. Saunders was a smart entrepreneur. He knew that AIDS drugs were money spinners. He saw this proposal as the ultimate investment opportunity that comes once in a lifetime. He knew very well that success depends on striking while the iron is hot. This looked like a viable business opportunity, and the prize – if the drug proved to work well – would be enormous.

As the sole financial backer of the project, he anticipated having the exclusive rights to exploit the new discovery. However, he could not have imagined the long tortuous road and pitfalls that are almost always part of new drugs development. In fact, out of thousands of candidate drugs tested, only a handful ever makes it to pharmacy shelves. And in this case the drug involved was very special, with a rather curious twist to it.

When I first scrutinised the details of Van Grouch's new "wonder" drug which I codenamed Vitoviral, I could hardly believe my eyes. I was astonished to find that it was not exactly what one would call a high-tech invention. In reality, there was no "discovery" to talk about. I wondered whether poor Saunders, who had committed all his savings, had been conned. Did he know that the so called wonder drug was not new at all? However much I stretched my imagination, I still could not see him laughing all the way to the bank unless there was some hidden twist that I had not figured out.

Vitoviral was in fact an old, common, low-cost, over-the-counter drug. It was available in many village shops in Uganda and readily available in virtually all other developing countries. It had no patent protection, and was being freely manufactured locally by most pharmaceutical companies as a cheap painkiller and an anti-inflammatory. My immediate reaction was to steal a glance at the calendar to reassure myself that it was not April Fool's Day. However, I could not see the highly professional Van Grouch trying to con anyone. Van Grouch was confident that he was on the right track, and that Vitoviral would ultimately rank among other great scientific discoveries.

I wondered whether this odd couple really knew what AIDS was. AIDS had killed millions, bamboozled the very best brains in the world and kept thousands of scientists busy looking for the elusive cure. Was it possible that the answer to the century's most devastating epidemic was a simple non-prescription drug? If this turned out to be the breakthrough, what would the scientists who had been toiling so hard chasing red herrings think of themselves? That aside, if indeed Vitoviral was proven to be the answer, as Dr Van Grouch claimed vehemently, how would Mr Saunders make his billions out of it? Any patient could access it from any drug shop without paying royalties. Any country in desperate need would just expand its manufacturing capacity to cope with the rising demand. It would be virtually impossible to patent a cheap, common drug already in widespread use for ordinary ailments.

However, Van Grouch had ready answers to all these concerns. As far as he was concerned, he had come up with a discovery that created a new use for an existing drug—an application that was hitherto unknown to modern science. Millions of people in Europe have sat under apple trees (just as millions of Africans sat under mango trees) and saw millions of fruits fall down, and yet did not know (or if they figured it out, did not document it) that it was gravity causing the fruit to fall. Isaac Newton, on the other hand, is world famous because he did not merely do what everyone had done for centuries before him namely to pick up the fruit, eat and have a siesta.

With regard to AIDS drugs there was a precedent. Zidovudine, a drug that had been discovered long before we knew about AIDS, was initially developed for treatment of cancer but it had flopped in clinical trials. It was then shelved as an orphan drug but was later rediscovered as an AIDS drug. Likewise, Dr Van Grouch had rediscovered Vitoviral as a powerful inhibitor of the HIV virus in the laboratory though it was in use for another purpose. He planned to take it one step forward and test it on humans to see if it could treat AIDS. If it succeeded, Van Grouch would claim credit for the new knowledge about its use as an AIDS cure. This would earn him all the honours and recognition that go with it. As the saying goes, it doesn't matter if the cat is black or white as long as it catches mice. Likewise, if a common painkiller and anti-inflammatory cured AIDS, who would complain?

Still, the million-dollar question remained unanswered. If the trial proved that Vitoviral was indeed efficacious, how were they going to keep our mouths shut? Surely no one could possibly expect us to keep secret information about a widely available and affordable drug if it proved to be effective while our people continued to be decimated by AIDS. Apparently, Van Grouch and Saunders had considered this too, and had come up with some safeguards. These included a confidentiality pact that emphasised non-disclosure of the drug's identity and results without clearance from the sponsors. Of course, we could not agree to this condition without taking care of our own interests. I insisted that if the drug proved to be effective, all poor patients would have immediate and unrestricted access to it.

The professionally written Vitoviral study sailed through peer and ethical reviews and had no problem getting clearance to go ahead for testing. After all, the drug's safety profile was well known. The initial study was to recruit only sixty patients and run it for 24 weeks. If the preliminary results seemed promising, then the study would be expanded immediately to include many more patients.

The recruitment of volunteers was brisk. As expected, AIDS patients, in the absence of an alternative therapy, queued up at JCRC in large numbers to join any drug trials. This was the only way poor patients could access any kind of AIDS care and treatment. The study proceeded according to plan, and was completed on time. Most patients reported that they felt better and indeed looked so. To our disappointment, though not entirely unexpectedly because of the small numbers involved, the study results were inconclusive. However, there was, undeniably, evidence of some clinical and immunological improvement among the participating patients, but these findings were not robust enough to be considered significant. Yet, quite clearly, the results could not be described as indicative of outright failure either. Like in the case of Aidvir this situation also called for an expanded follow-up study.

The new study was set to start when all hell broke loose. Mr Saunders and Dr Van Grouch had a disagreement. The bone of contention was – as is usually the case in such partnerships – money. Both sought to strengthen their position in the joint venture. In a relationship that was at the best of times on edge, it was not surprising that disagreements would occur. However, I could not work out what the trigger of the acrimonious split was. As far as I could discern, Van Grouch talked to another possible investor in an effort to procure more funding for a much larger study so as to get the final and definitive results earlier. This appeared to me to be a reasonable plan. The large numbers of participants involved would inevitably make the follow-up study very expensive to conduct. Mr Saunders may not have been aware that unless a large study was conducted, the final results would not be readily acceptable internationally. Yet Saunders' funding was far short of the required amount. As he was new to the sophisticated industry of clinical trials and mistrustful of his partner's motives, he must have become suspicious.

Letters started flying in from London and Oslo fast and furious. Each one requested that we totally ignore the other, and each also contained unflattering descriptions of the other. I had no alternative but to hold back and watch the unsavoury events as they evolved. Basically, the two men tore each other to pieces. I waited impatiently for a lull in the brawl so that I could throw in a word of mediation, but it was all to no avail.

Just as I was beginning to think that calm and tranquillity had finally been restored, I received a telephone call from London. It was Saunders. He was obviously a troubled man, judging by the tone of his voice. He told me that his partner was impossible to work with. I asked him to explain how he had come to that rather strange conclusion. He replied that he heard rumours that Van Grouch "goes to the nightclubs and dances with young ladies". A week later I received disconcerting news from London. Saunders had suffered a massive heart attack. He underwent emergency bypass surgery and fortunately pulled through. I am not sure whether he decided to take it easy, as is the usual recommendation after such a life-threatening episode, whether he lost interest, or if he had no fight left in him, but I never heard from him again. My get-well messages and subsequent inquiries about his health did not attract any response. I don't even know if he received my messages.

Despite his shortcomings, the otherwise amiable Saunders appeared to have been the engine behind the whole initiative. In his absence, Van Grouch could not keep the fire burning, and eventually the whole project stalled. The last time I heard of him several months later, he had apparently taken a break from his absorbing scientific work. He was back in Uganda with his girlfriend on their way to a safari park holiday, and possibly a tango or two to go with it.

However, we did not just let the matter drop. The first phase of the trial had accumulated a lot of data that we studied carefully. We all agreed that it was not worth pursuing Vitoviral since it seemed to offer only mild symptomatic relief.

Yankee Drug

When I first ran into a tall middle-aged white man on the streets of Kampala in May 1996, I thought it was a coincidence. But I was to learn later that our meeting was part of an elaborate plan. The serene-looking man introduced himself as Don Blockbuster, a doctor of medicine from Texas USA, and then asked me who I was. When I introduced myself, he became very excited.

"You must be the guy I have all along tried to reach, to deliver great news to!" He said as he squeezed my hand shaking it rather too vigorously. He did not beat about the bush. "I have a cure for AIDS right here in my bag. I have only come to give you the privilege of sharing in the glory of being associated with the world's most miraculous discovery," he whispered to me with a broad grin.

Don had flown in from Abidjan, Ivory Coast where, according to his business card, he was the head of the Institute of Virology which specialised in AIDS treatment and research. He explained that he had discovered an effective AIDS drug which contained Interferon. The mention of Interferon immediately rang a bell. Alarm bells! There was a notorious case of a Kenyan doctor who announced the discovery of an AIDS drug in the early 1990s. The much-hyped medicine called Kemron was also an interferon-based drug. At the time, it was the talk of the town—the great hope for wealthy AIDS patients. But very few among those treated remained rich. Just one month's supply of Kemron cost more than the annual income of the majority of Ugandan senior government officials. And, as explained earlier, a 1991-2 study showed it was useless for treating AIDS.

When I told Don the story, he sprang to the defensive. "No! This is nothing of the sort," he said, bringing out a glossy pamphlet. "Our product is high tech. Besides Interferon, it also contains other sophisticated ingredients including germanium and hydroxybenzene derivatives. This is no voodoo medicine. It is from America."

Don explained that, unlike Kemron, his drug which I will call Virucide, had already been proven to be highly effective against HIV-2, the milder but more difficult to treat type of HIV found in West Africa. "Unfortunately," Don lamented "I could not find sufficient numbers of patients with HIV-1, to enable me to prove conclusively the efficacy of my drug," he elaborated. "I am confident that within a year I will have introduced a life-saving drug to the world." He complained that West Africans moved too slowly for his very fast schedule of work, and that this was one of the reasons for his relocation to Uganda. "I left them crying over there," he said. "I don't have time to waste with snails. This work must run fast, because there is a lot at stake." I later confirmed that, indeed, some people in West Africa had been left crying by Don's departure, but their tears were for a different reason.

"I know Uganda will do it fine. I know your president has done great work on AIDS. Now Uganda is going to be even greater. Imagine an AIDS cure being discovered right here, under your very nose," he said as he pointed his index finger at my nose, forcing me to duck. "And as for you Dr Mugyenyi, I will elevate your ass in the scientific world and beam it in neon lights, up there in the skies," he pointed up, staring momentarily in the air as if my ass was already floating up there. "As for your little Joint Clinical Research Centre, I will make it a great big research institute, just like mine in West Africa," he boasted as he stretched out his hands to symbolise vastness. "I even heard that you have no proper library. To begin with I will donate to your institution the most up-to-date medical textbooks." I thanked him profusely for his generosity. Later, however, I regretted accepting his offer.

That was the start of a turbulent relationship with Don. Initially Don could hardly be faulted. He was all smiles and sweetness itself. He requested that I immediately started preparations for "the greatest AIDS drug trial in Africa". In the meantime, he needed to go and wind up his business in West Africa before returning to concentrate all his efforts on the new drug in "a more promising country," as he put it. Don must have sensed my lingering doubt, because he tried to reassure me with news of the wonderful effects of his drug.

Don was a jet setter. During the one month he was away, I received faxes typed in all capital letters, sent from various cities in Europe, the US and West Africa. I also found from the addresses that, besides the Institute of Virology in West Africa, he was also head of a number of other institutes based in Europe and USA. It looked as if Don ran an international network of virology institutes. However, on his return I was surprised by his latest business card. It had an address of a brand new Institute of Virology right here in the city of Kampala! In addition, his plans and scope of projects had multiplied and diversified. He talked big. Well, nothing wrong with that, after all, he was from Texas, the renowned home of big things.

His new plans included a huge pharmaceutical manufacturing plant to manufacture Virucide and many other drugs. "I will soon be the sole supplier of drugs to the entire Ugandan Ministry of Health," he boasted. He also planned to start another factory to make condoms, gloves and syringes, and also build a vast housing estate on a hill overlooking the city. He never bothered to find out whether the hill was for sale or not. He just behaved like his money could buy anything he fancied. Then, to crown it all, he announced that he had another surprise drug. He said that it was a special cancer drug that he planned to launch in Uganda. He never explained what type of cancer his drug would treat.

I started thinking Don was more of an opportunistic businessman than a scientist. It was increasingly clear that, at the very best, he had many eggs in his basket. To allay my increasing unease, I needed some answers to some tough questions — fast. There was no better place to start than his CV. His excuse for a CV typed in capital letters, raised more questions than answers. It was distinguished by paucity of details and contradictory data. Don's CV inexplicably stated that he had studied medicine at the American College of Medicine in Beirut. Unlike other doctors, Don had not done an internship. Instead, he had made his way to Bangkok, where he became involved in unspecified work. After that he got an "important" job as personal physician to an unnamed wealthy Arab ruler. Don then held two consecutive positions as an airline executive in Europe and America. I could not help but wonder how his medical training could have prepared him for this post. Moving on to Mexico, he changed career again and became a "university instructor". He did not specify what sort of instructor. Between various other odd jobs in Laos and Cyprus, there was an unaccounted-for gap, when the maverick Don seemed to disappear from the surface of the earth. When I pressed him to explain this gap, he said with a finger across his lips, that it was "hush-hush".

Later Don acted as a business representative for a number of American and European companies. But most amazing of all, he also became a consultant for Kenya, Uganda, Tanzania, Ghana, Burundi, Rwanda, Gabon and Cote d'Ivoire on HIV/AIDS research! How was he doing it? Did he look up the countries in an atlas? How could so many countries that did not have coordinated AIDS programmes have zeroed in on him? His CV showed no past HIV experience or any credible AIDS related scientific attribute that could have made such an overwhelming impression on divergent countries to simultaneously appoint him to similar positions. In any case, how was Don managing with such huge responsibility? At least as far as Uganda was concerned it was easy to confirm that his claims were bogus. Who exactly was Don? What was he up to? One had to wonder how he had made the transformation from a personal physician and all these other divergent jobs to the discoverer of an AIDS drug. But the wily Don just brushed all these queries aside. To put it mildly, this guy's background was suspicious.

Unfortunately this kind of "expatriate" is not uncommon in Africa. Sometimes Africa's would-be benefactors ignore the well qualified local experts, opting for the likes of Don, notwithstanding their miserable CVs. This is partly the reason why some potentially good projects in Africa fail. Don must have known that, more often than not, African vetting systems were weak, and that the AIDS crisis had made the bad situation worse, creating favourable conditions for the likes of him to operate. Such a situation is well known in Uganda as *kulira mu kavuyo* translating roughly as "gain from chaos". Don seemed, like many other opportunists hovering over our AIDS-battered city with various food supplements, exotic antioxidants, vitamin pills, derivatives of various plants or extracts of this or that rare potato, beetroot or herbs from all parts of the world, intent on fleecing the soon-to-die AIDS patients. No wonder relatives of AIDS patients found many varieties of pills and herbs, when they cleaned up after their relatives' deaths.

In the midst of AIDS chaos, Don did not expect anyone to take time to scrutinise his CV, especially not if he promised an AIDS cure and some dollars to go with it. His CV was, by any standards, grossly deficient. It was so haphazardly put together that even the incorrigible Don felt obliged to apologise and promised to improve it, but failed. Even so, ignoring the likes of Don is a gross mistake, as it would not mean they would go away. On the contrary, they would either go underground or transform into the likes of Gasket and become even more treacherous. The desperation of many AIDS patients was such that they were ready to starve, take their children out of schools, wear tattered clothes and sell their assets to pay for anything to anyone who promised to save their lives. In such a desperate situation it was better to keep such characters under close observation and give them enough rope to destroy themselves, and to expose their spurious claims of AIDS cures under safe and transparent research conditions.

The only ray of hope I saw in this quagmire came when Don claimed to be working in partnership with qualified scientists. He said they included a university professor from Houston, USA, and some doctors from East Germany, who would form the core of his research team to work with us. This was a welcome development, though I kept wondering how their CVs would look.

Don requested me to sign a memorandum of understanding, so that business between him and the JCRC could commence immediately. I refused. Surely, I could not possibly sign an agreement on the "strength" of his CV. But he was back a few days later, pleading that he needed to ship in sophisticated research equipment from his previous laboratory in West Africa in preparation for the arrival of his colleagues to start on the work. He explained that he urgently needed a letter of support from the JCRC confirming that he was known to us, so that he could use it to apply for an import licence for his AIDS trial drug. That sounded like a reasonable request which I could accept since there were strong safe guards in place. The equipment and trial drugs would all come to JCRC, the proposed study could not proceed unless it had been reviewed and cleared by institutional and national ethical and scientific committees which would also vet the scientists he promised to bring on board to ensure they were competent. After consultations with regulatory authorities, I provided him with a letter of introduction, making it very clear that it was for the sole purpose of supporting his application for importation of trial drugs and research equipment, but subsequent developments caused me to regret this decision.

I asked Don and his partners to present their research proposal to the Institutional Review Board (IRB) and National Ethics Committee for their approval. I informed him that no research could be undertaken by the JCRC unless it was first cleared by the regulatory and ethics committees. This surprised Don. He had apparently not expected such stringent requirements. I told him that he needed to provide all the details related to the drug quality including good manufacturing certification, results of animal tests, and a scientific report of its safety profile. A few days later he handed me a grossly substandard protocol which I rejected. He hired a scientist to write it up for him, claiming that he was very busy with other more important work. By 24 July 1996 the revised protocol had been improved significantly but still did not meet our minimum standards, and he went back to work on it.

Meanwhile, Don's plans became even more grandiose. He bragged that he planned to fly in his own personal security team from the US to protect him and his big investments. Don's showy lifestyle exuded wealth. He had taken up an exclusive suite in the Sheraton Hotel in Kampala, and got the hotel to assign a personal chef and waitress for his use.

A series of disconcerting events finally compelled me to throw Don out. The letter of support I wrote to enable shipment of his AIDS drugs, research and scientific equipment from West Africa clearly stated that all imported materials would come to the JCRC. We expected about ten cartons of supplies, but received a copy of a letter faxed from West Africa stating that Don planned to ship in 89 cartons containing foodstuffs, patient supplies and what he declared as apartment utilities, to be followed by other cartons containing computers and heavy equipment. Customs officers at Entebbe Airport were astonished to find a commercial cargo plane offloading a big consignment of goods without any import licence. Contrary to what Don had told us, the consignment was from Texas, and not from West Africa.

Justifiably, the customs officers had cause for concern and wanted the items checked. Suspicion was raised further when they found documents that described the cargo as giant Sony television sets. Certainly, the packages conformed to the shapes of TV sets. However, Don vehemently insisted that the boxes contained dried food for patients. He pleaded that this was merely a typographical error by some sleepy officer. He put up a ferocious fight, which was later likened to that of "a lioness trying to protect its cubs". In the heat of it all, I received a call from a bewildered customs official requesting that I confirm that the consignment belonged to the JCRC. I explained that we knew of Don's plans to import some medical supplies only. The customs officials agreed to release the goods on the strict understanding that the consignment would be delivered, stored and used only at and by the JCRC. Don readily agreed but never delivered anything to the JCRC. Instead this clearance opened a floodgate, which he exploited to bring in more of his goods. I became very concerned and immediately sent a warning and a disclaimer to airport customs and security.

Another event compelled us to intensify our investigations of Don's affairs. It was during the JCRC annual staff party to which we had also invited a number of Americans from various organisations in Uganda when Don was introduced among the guests. One of the American guests recognised him instantly.

"That guy over there - do you know him?" she asked, sounding very concerned.

"Yes, he claims to have discovered an AIDS drug,"

"He does get around, doesn't he? Many people are looking for him," she said wearily. "I will be back to you about him tomorrow," she said.

The next day she sent us a copy of a letter from a US law enforcement agency. Apparently, Don was a wanted man and was possibly on the run. The most remarkable aspects of the letter were the very detailed descriptions of his peculiar characteristics, some of which I had also witnessed. Those people, whoever they were, knew their man well. They described what he was likely to wear, his arrogant manner, his fleeting and grandiose ideas, the kind of things he would be interested in, including his craving for green chillies. They also mentioned the kind of places he would frequent, and what he would do there. The letter explained that while he was in West Africa he had set up shop in a hotel and had people flying in and out from all over to see him, allegedly to get AIDS treatment. His conduct and behaviour was said to have "embarrassed the expatriate community".

I inquired about his Institute of Virology in West Africa. "Nothing of the sort exists," was the answer. What about the address on his business card? "Oh yes that did exist. It was a hotel room!" What about his Texas branch of the institute? "None known round here, thank you," was the reply. What about his medical training? Who exactly was this man? Did he have a genuine AIDS drug to test or was he on a different mission? I decided to end our association with him, and hoped that the evidence we had gathered would be enough to have him interdicted. I had a letter informing him of my decision hand delivered to his hotel suite. Then all hell broke loose.

If Don had been like a lioness protecting its cubs while he cleared his cargo from customs, in trying to force me to reverse my decision he was more like a charging rhinoceros. He first tried persuasion and flattery, making all sorts of promises, and saying how great the JCRC was. He then talked of the incentives that would accrue from the trial if it went ahead. When this did not achieve the desired results, he resorted to thinly veiled threats and indirect hints of unpleasant things that could happen if I didn't reverse my decision. When this failed, it was gloves off. Don telephoned to say that he would get me "fixed", whatever that meant. "In just a week you will get to understand who Don really is," he threatened. "You will be thrown out of your miserable office and I will have you begging me for mercy," he concluded before he banged down the phone.

What followed was very close to what he had threatened – a week of hell. Indeed, Don knew how to play dirty. To begin with, he accused me of stealing his medical books (which were in our library) and demanded that I pay for them. These were books that he had "generously" donated without being asked!

"The lives of Ugandans are at stake because of an unpatriotic young doctor at JCRC," Don charged. He went on to issue an ultimatum to my boss. "The country has a choice to make, either you get rid of this scoundrel or lose the benefit of an effective drug and a big funding opportunity to go with it. It is the only chance to put a stop to the carnage of AIDS in Uganda," he fumed.

These were no idle threats which could be dismissed offhand. Don had done his homework well. Indeed, I was amazed at his lobbying skills. He had succeeded in infiltrating upper levels of the Ugandan hierarchy, targeting influential people, especially those who were my direct superiors who could have easily fired me from my job. As they did not know the whole background and the scientific issues at stake, they believed that he was a compassionate man and a discoverer of an effective drug, capable of stopping AIDS carnage in Uganda. Don could be persuasive!

Unfortunately for him, a few influential authorities did not believe his accusations. A meeting was organised and arbitrators appointed to resolve the matter. Don had not anticipated that it would come to this. He could sense that these people were not in a hurry to dismiss me. He had lobbied very hard for my dismissal, so that he could have a free reign to work with a new head of JCRC. Don, the master tactician, had already approached someone he thought could take over from me, and made some tentative arrangements to work things out with him.

Now the schemer, changed tactics. As I walked towards the reserved table in a restaurant where the dinner with the arbitrators had been arranged, he called out in a friendly, jocular voice. "Here he comes" he said as he offered me a seat with a friendly pat on the shoulder. "Welcome to the fold old boy," he said as he scanned his distinguished company, perhaps to demonstrate to me that he was highly connected.

Suddenly, Don did something that amazed me. He apologised for all the false accusations that he had made against me. He was meek and remorseful as he enumerated the lies that he had told. I was shocked at the extent to which he had stooped in order to hurt me. If this had happened back in the days of bad old Ugandan governments, such accusations would have been enough to cost me my life. After a full confession, Don and the arbitrators expected that fences would be mended, and all would be forgiven. However, they were surprised at what they described as "my intransigency". Unsuccessful attempts were made to compel me to change my decision to dissociate JCRC from Don and his activities, but I refused. An attempt was made to reassure Don that an alternative venue would be found for him to carry out the study in Uganda. He protested that unless the study was done at the JCRC it would not get the necessary international recognition. It was then proposed that a private talk with me would smooth out the matter and Don left the room.

With Don out of the way, I laid out the evidence I had against him on the table and produced the damming documents implicating him in an international scam. To my surprise this did not impress the arbitrators. "What concern is it of ours if the guy is a crook?" one of them asked, to my consternation. "What if he is wanted for criminal offences in his own country? That is none of your business," he added. "Here you have a unique chance to carry out a historic project and you want to throw it all away?" he asked with an expression of disbelief. "Even if the trial turns out to be rubbish, as you say, at least some Ugandans would have benefited from the money. What do you have to lose? Wizen up," he concluded.

Hearing this from a notable person I had long respected was a sad moment for me. We agreed to disagree and parted. I did not know what they later told Don but the next day he was at my door, a changed man once more with civil manners. This visit turned out to be his last to my office, and also the most revealing. Apparently he wanted to make a personal apology and come clean as far as the allegations that he had levelled against me were concerned. He had brought with him a letter of apology typed in his trademark capital letters. To make up he also had a present for me. It was a plastic key holder in the shape of a human skull, like the type on pirate flags in old films. However, his visit did not go according to plan. He must have suffered goose bumps when he ran into someone from his past he would rather have preferred never to see again — at least not at that crucial moment — wearing his new hat of a physician and research scientist.

It started to unfold as Don was waiting in my secretary's office. Another visitor entered, recognised Don instantly and addressed him as Ben. Don was visibly startled. The guest was Samuel Matsiko, a former general manager of Hotel Diplomate, in Muyenga, a suburb of Kampala. The two had a rather curious dialogue that went something like this:

"It's good to see you Ben," Samuel said.

"I am not Ben," Don retorted, "and who are you?"

"You forgot? I am Sam. Remember Hotel Diplomate — where you stayed in early 1987 or thereabouts?" Samuel said

"No, you've got me mistaken for someone else. I do not know any Hotel Diplomate. I am new to Uganda and I have never set eyes on you."

Don closed the topic as he prepared to enter my office. So, when he saw me he was a little thrown off balance. However, he proceeded to tender his apologies and appeared to be genuine about it. He went on to surprise me with something totally out of the blue. Don, or Ben, in the dark about my reasons for terminating his work with us, inadvertently disclosed other scandals about himself that I had not even been aware of. Apparently, he had left West Africa in disgrace. He was accused of gross unethical conduct with regard to a group of drugs trial patients whom he was alleged to have abandoned without help. Believing that I had heard of it, he pleaded that these were blatant lies and should not have led me to cancel his trial. He added that his company had, contrary to the accusations, gone out of its way to help the poor African AIDS patients. Talk of skeletons in the closet!

His pleas for forgiveness notwithstanding, he left my office un-forgiven and empty-handed. As I showed him out, he cast a wary eye on Samuel, who was waiting to see me next.

Samuel remembered Don very well, as did some other employees of the hotel whom I talked to later. He said that Ben was unforgettable — mainly for the wrong reasons. He was a memorable guest who stayed for a couple of months before vanishing. It was just after the overthrow of the second regime of President Milton Obote who had succeeded the short-lived post-Idi Amin governments. A horde of businessmen, mainly Kenyans and Ugandans of Asian origin (including many of those who were expelled by Idi Amin in the 1970s), sniffed new business opportunities and rushed to Kampala. They came ready to supply literally anything, as virtually all items were on demand. However, as Ugandans were generally impoverished, it was more lucrative to target government and rich NGOs for business.

One odd man towered above them all. He was an aggressive American businessman specialising in electric typewriters, going by the name of Ben Blockbuster. He had taken up residence in Hotel Diplomate's only VIP suite, which also doubled up as his office. Ben was well liked by both hotel management and waiters because he entertained visitors frequently and tipped waiters generously. His clients were mainly government officials and some Asian middlemen. Other than business, the other habit he had in common with his Asian rivals was his love for green chillies. However, there was no love lost between him and some of his Asian counterparts when he vanished, allegedly without supplying them with the typewriters that they had ordered and paid for.

Samuel could not believe that Ben would ever forget him as he had been in charge of his day-to-day welfare for quite a long time. As to his identity, Samuel was absolutely sure that Don was Ben – one and the same man. He brushed aside Ben's sham amnesia. There was another reason why Samuel would never forget Ben. He used a credit card to settle his huge hotel bill and cleared out of the hotel fast. When the account was presented for payment, the credit card company refused payment. Ben had left an "unreachable" forwarding address, and Samuel had to suffer a lengthy and cumbersome process of claiming the money from insurance. Suddenly bursting into laughter, Samuel said, "Ben, a research scientist! There is just no way I could ever forget him. He was such a unique character. I could even smell chillies in his bag. We used to make special arrangements to get them for him from Nakasero market." But this part of Don's work record, and monkey business, if indeed Don was Ben, did not feature in his CV. But then, again, his CV's major weakness was the unexplained gaps and paucity of details.

At the end of it all, I survived and still held on to my job by the skin of my teeth. Then Don Ben started a long but ultimately fruitless attempt to find an alternative institution to undertake the clinical trial of his drug. Unfortunately for him, wherever he went he was turned down. "Unless you work with Mugyenyi, this kind of research is otherwise not possible in Uganda," he was told repeatedly. A few institutions that accepted Don's incentives to host the trial had grossly constrained facilities. Later, when he finally found one of reasonable competence, he discovered that the more complicated tests had to be referred to the JCRC. "Oh! My Gad!" Don was said to have lamented, "Bloody Mugyenyi is everywhere."

Having made no headway, it was time for Don to pack up and move on. I had a feeling that he was well used to this. I feared that some other poor African country was about to have a chilli-eating visitor and that the melodrama would play out all over again. As Don prepared to leave Uganda, some curious events occurred in and around Kampala. Giant counterfeit Sony television sets turned up in city rubbish dumps fought over by hooligans. The "TVs" were nothing but cheap cardboard boxes apparently used to transport things that needed to be concealed. I had a flashback of "a man who had fought like a lioness to protect his goods" that were declared as foodstuffs. He couldn't possibly have had something to do with this, could he?

Two years later, as the fiasco of Don was beginning to fade from memory, I received a jolt in the form of a rather curious telephone call. It was an apprehensive voice on the line from a medical institution in Kenya. "Do you by any chance know a man by the name of Ben Blockbuster?" Evidently Samuel was absolutely right. Ben and Don were as identical as Dr Jekyll and Mr Hyde. "There we go again!" I instinctively exclaimed on phone, as I listened to a replay.

Mysterious People

He was the kind of man that this often troubled world needed.

I will call him Lionel O'Connell. He was the right person to meet at this time of utter frustration brought about by conmen and disappointing drugs trials. In him I could see a promising breakthrough to resolving the anguish of our nation. Lionel, an Irish PhD holder in chemistry obtained in Australia, was first introduced to me in 1996 by Dr Jerry Noble, an Irish doctor working with a Catholic missionary hospital in Kampala. He described Lionel as a "God-fearing scientist, without commercial interests, whose only wish is to use his expertise in chemistry to develop a drug that would save the poor AIDS patients in Africa."

Lionel had synthesised some anti-AIDS molecules in his laboratory at Cork University, and he was trying to develop this further into candidate AIDS drugs. He was constrained by lack of funds so he solicited help from his better-connected colleagues at the University and wrote to some pharmaceutical research organisations to help him advance his discovery, but all to no avail. He appealed to church and charity organisations but he always ran into a wall of refusal. He even offered to go to AIDS-devastated countries in Africa as a volunteer if this would help raise funds to accelerate the development of what he considered a potential breakthrough in AIDS treatment. But no suitable role would be found for a chemist in any humanitarian organisations working in Africa. Lionel, a devout Catholic, resorted to prayer and meditation. But if this was of any help it was only in mysterious ways. He remained stuck with his molecules. All doors remained shut. He lost hope because whatever he tried seemed to come to a dead end. Disappointed, frustrated and exhausted, he returned to the routine of his poorly-paid job at the college where he worked as a tutor, and continued to get solace from his bible study group and small family in Dublin.

The enemy responsible for most of Lionel's failures was no other than Lionel himself. On first encounter, the very first impression most people got of him was almost always unfavourable. Until someone got to know him better, Lionel tended to come across as a rather naïve and eccentric character. Down-to-earth, simply dressed, and polite to a fault, Lionel at first sight looked more like a peasant than a scientist. He was not a good speaker. He stuttered frequently and, as a result, found it difficult to get his point across. These unfortunate trends masked his brilliance and instead projected him as a rather dithering person. I later found out that these adverse characteristics had worked against him throughout his career. Although he was arguably one of the most brilliant chemists in Ireland, he was always overlooked when it came to promotions. But nobody who took trouble to check on his knowledge of chemistry and his laboratory work would be left with any doubt about his intelligence. For this reason he was retained as a faculty member but relegated to the background. Lionel, who had never known better treatment, had no complaint about his work conditions.

When Lionel first told his colleagues about his discovery, it was not that they did not believe him, but they found his explanations rather difficult to understand. It required patience to understand him and everyone was busy and wanted to get on with their own work. Unfortunately, some staff members who had not bothered to examine the details of his work falsely accused him of concocting results and making false claims in order to make a quick buck. Lionel, a highly ethical man, was deeply upset by these false accusations. He became so depressed that he had to be put on antidepressant medication. However, Dr Noble, who had grown up knowing Lionel, understood his handicap and came to his rescue. Patiently, he convinced some other scientists that his work deserved another look, and persuaded them to investigate his products. That was the turning point for Lionel.

The first drug that he discovered was tested on animals and tissue cultures for safety and was found to be non-toxic. Further tests determine how it would react and be handled in the body (pharmacokinetic studies) were undertaken in Cambridge, U.K., and the findings were encouraging. It seemed as if Lionel's molecules could be developed into an effective AIDS drug for humans. The next step was to carry out clinical trials on AIDS patients and determine whether the product was effective. This is the stage at which Lionel's and my path crossed.

I recall the first time I met Dr Noble, who had come from Rubaga Catholic Hospital to explore the possibility of testing Lionel's drug at the JCRC. It was back in 1996, when claims and counter claims of breakthroughs in AIDS treatment were the order of the day. It was not uncommon to hear two or three drugs discovery claims in a single day. Therefore there was nothing special about this encounter. My interest was aroused when Noble explained that Lionel did not seek to make money out of his discovery but instead wanted his drugs, if found effective, to be made freely accessible to the poor. However, it was not possible to test a new drug and develop it into an approved medicine without substantial funding, pharmaceutical expertise and a well equipped drugs factory. However with people dying around me because life-saving antiretroviral drugs remained prohibitively expensive, I just had to try out any promising lead. When Lionel got the news, he was excited by the prospect of getting his drugs tested. Unfortunately the involved procedures were to open up new demands and challenges that exerted different kinds of pressures on him, which he was ill-suited to handle.

My very first meeting with Lionel was during the winter of 1998. I had travelled with my late wife Christine and children to Dublin for my investiture as a Fellow of the Royal College of Physicians of Ireland. Lionel invited us for dinner at his house. We very much looked forward to some good Irish cuisine. However, on our way to his home, Lionel stopped at a roadside mall and picked up a few pizza takeaways for our dinner. Lionel lived humbly with his wife and teenage daughter in a small but neatly kept apartment. His wife worked as a cleaner in a hotel in Dublin. Three days a week, he commuted to the southern city of Cork and spent the rest of the days doing menial jobs or attending Bible studies and helping his teenage daughter with homework in the evenings.

What Lionel may have not fulfilled in dinner expectations, he more than made up for in humanity. He was unpretentious and kind and with his down-to-earth manners he came across to me as a really pleasant man. He referred to all the peoples of the world as "God's children". Despite his modest means he sought to reach out to those less privileged than himself, especially those who he called "the suffering people of the world". He was particularly appalled by the devastation of AIDS in Africa and repeatedly asked me if there was anything he could personally do to help. Looking around his sparsely furnished house he said, "If there is anything in this house that can be of help to anyone out there please take it to them." There was no doubt that Lionel meant every word he said. "And if my drug can be of any help, please take it free, patent it and use it to save lives," he said, looking up and raising his hands in a prayerful gesture.

"Initially no one showed any interest in my discovery, but since news got out that it may be effective, a number of mysterious people have approached me, wanting me to reveal the formula and sign a contract with them," Lionel said as he shook his head disapprovingly. "This drug is not for sale. It is for humanitarian use and I would prefer that your poor, suffering country takes the formula, manufactures the drug locally and distributes it free to the poor. I am ready to resign my job as long as my daughter's education could be taken care of, and I will go to your country and work as a volunteer to help in this endeavour."

I was later informed that the "mysterious people" resorted to some unscrupulous ways of working around him. All of a sudden they treated the lacklustre Lionel like a luminary. He started getting special invitations to specially arranged scientific conferences to give presentations about his work. Believing that he was talking to bona fide scientific colleagues, he talked of his molecules and the potential for it being developed into AIDS drugs. After he had poured his heart out, his time in the limelight came to a sudden end. Later, when he tried to make applications for patent protection of his "very secret" formulations, he found to his consternation that the formulations were already in the public domain. However, this information was not of immediate use to anyone because the synthetic pathway was not described. This had not been part of Lionel's talk at the conferences. When new invitations to obscure scientific meetings to talk about "current topical issues," started arriving once more and rather unexpectedly, Lionel was aware that he had to be guarded about what he revealed. When it became clear that his presentations would not touch on the "relevant" issues, the invitations once more fizzled out.

I worked closely with Noble trying to arrange Lionel to come and work on the development of his products with us in Uganda. Noble approached the Irish Embassy in Kampala to request help and sponsorship for Lionel to come over on this mission. In the meantime, I made arrangement with the newly built National Enterprise Corporation (NEC) Pharmaceutical plant to take him on as a pharmaceutical consultant for the new product. The Embassy accepted our request but insisted that Lionel, like all other government supported Irish expatriates, had to undergo an aptitude test in Dublin before he could be cleared by the foreign ministry to undertake this job. If successful, it would count as part of Irish development aid to Uganda. When Noble was told of this requirement, he immediately saw red. Having undergone the modus operandi himself, he knew exactly what would be involved. "I am afraid that Lionel will never pass this test," he said, "because he is not right — politically, so to speak. Anyway, let's keep our fingers crossed. I will try to coach him and see whether it helps."

Lionel, as Noble had feared, failed the aptitude test and botched the interview. His application was declined. But the Irish Department of Foreign Affairs appointed a well qualified pharmaceutical chemist as a substitute. This was, however, the one job where a substitute, whether politically right or not just would not do. It was only Lionel who knew the formulation of his still experimental drug and how to synthesise it. The industrial manufacturing process had not yet been developed and furthermore, the drug itself had not undergone all the necessary clinical trials and safety clearances to warrant a go-ahead for industrial production. Only Lionel was suited for this job, which required patience and painstaking hard work in the laboratory. Also the NEC factory was not operational, and needed a project of national urgency, like AIDS treatment to jump-start it.

My original plan had been to recommend Lionel for a job at Makerere University as a chemistry lecturer, for which he was very well qualified. That would have kept him busy during the period needed to get the factory up and running. The teaching position would also provide him with facilities and the opportunity to continue working on the development of the drug while advising on the establishment of the manufacturing process at the NEC plant. I asked Noble to request the Irish embassy to reconsider but they made it very clear that there was just no way that Foreign Affairs would approve Lionel's appointment. He was just not the right person to be sent out as an Irish expatriate. I imagine, they were looking for a person of sophistication and poise who would reflect what would be considered "respectful and elegant Irish character!" Lionel was just not this type. He was just himself, a good chemist, a person who cared about huge numbers of people dying of AIDS and wanted to do something about it. Unfortunately, he was severely handicapped by his plain character. In addition, his inability to express himself in a positive and inspiring way was sure to unnerve people out to project Ireland's good image abroad. Understandably it would be desirable to send out only those Irish expatriates who would not lend any credence to the whimsical English comedians' caricature and stereotype of Irishmen.

The Irish Government went ahead and sent a pharmaceutical chemist to work with NEC. She was introduced to me by the manager of the pharmaceutical plant, Col. Fred Mwesigye. The pleasant young woman was almost everything that Lionel was not. She was smartly dressed, articulate and sophisticated. She appeared to me to be a good team worker most suitable for a routine and established work environment. She found the factory in impeccable condition. For a start, all equipment and buildings were brand new. There was a spacious quality control laboratory where she would presumably work. Despite all this, the factory was not in production. The hitch was that it lacked everything else essential for pharmaceutical production, ranging from human resources to raw materials. The management was searching for an investor to partner with and get the factory going. This is the situation that welcomed the keen and energetic pharmaceutical chemist on her mission to address what she had been told was an urgent need of her expertise. Unfortunately for her, there was no specialised department of pharmaceutical chemistry at Makerere University where she could have been seconded to work while the factory was being readied. She must have been amazed at the folly of the people who had sent her on such a hopeless mission. Frustrated, she resigned and returned to Ireland, thoroughly cheesed off. Yet with Lionel the situation would have been different.

The only alternative left to Lionel was to continue searching for help to support the development of his drugs in Ireland. Judging by his past and recent events it looked like luck and Lionel lived worlds apart. But this time round, it seemed like fortune was smiling on him. A consortium of businessmen in Dublin offered to fund the clinical trials. They also promised that if the trials were successful, they would go on to invest in the manufacture of his drugs. An expert pharmacologist working in Cambridge, UK, was brought on board as a key scientific partner. He started working on the product with Lionel immediately.

In November 2000, while visiting my daughter Michelle who was studying law at the University of Ulster, Lionel's prospective drug trial sponsors took the opportunity to arrange a face-to-face meeting with me in Belfast. During the meeting which included Lionel, sponsors requested reassurance from me that the JCRC would be able to carry out a quality study on the product. After addressing all their concerns, they declared themselves ready to go ahead with the project and Lionel promised to speed up the preparation of the drugs for the trial. As speed is critical in the highly competitive pharmaceutical world, the study sponsors kept pressure on both Lionel and the other scientists to expedite the work. Talking to Lionel on the phone one day, he told me of his frequent long walks to the offices of the sponsors in Dublin to keep them happy and informed about the progress of his work on the drugs.

Approximately two weeks later, I received a call from our switchboard to inform me that there was an impatient man on the line from Dublin insisting that he talk to me right away. By intuition I sensed that something terrible must have happened. Hesitatingly, I reached for the phone. "I am afraid it is very bad news." It was one of the eager sponsors whom I had met in Belfast. "Lionel suffered a massive heart attack while walking along a street in Dublin today," he said. "An ambulance rushed him to hospital, but he was pronounced dead on arrival. I am sorry," he added struggling to contain his emotions. Then there was a moment of silence and I thought he had hung up.

"Is there something I can do to help with the funeral?" I asked, just like any African who remains culturally loyal to his friends even in death. I was mulling over the idea of travelling to Ireland to attend his funeral, but wondering whether I would get a visa in time. "No, thank you – nothing," he said, "except — his wife asked for flowers to be left at the church, and any donation to go to charity. I have already sent the flowers on your behalf," he added.

I found my mind flashing back to my visit to Lionel in Dublin. Oh, how I missed Lionel! "Why Lionel?" This question kept reverberating in my mind. If regular exercise and good physique prevented heart attacks, then Lionel would have been safe. He exercised daily. He once told me that he virtually walked everywhere in Dublin on foot – covering many miles daily. As a result, he had a trim, muscular and athletic figure. His modest lifestyle did not readily place him among the stereotypes of heart attack candidates. Yet the strain associated with his new and unfamiliar work with businessmen wishing to make a profit from his discovery, and who intruded on his quiet lifestyle, and the pressure on him to speed up the procedure could have placed too much of a strain on him. He always strongly objected to commercial exploitation, especially when it involved what he referred to as "a humanitarian product" like the one he was trying to develop. In fact, he had insisted that his drugs would first and foremost be used to help the poor, and made this a condition of his agreement to work with the consortium.

Perhaps the only bright moment during that difficult time was the call I received a month later. It was the pharmacologist from Cambridge University, who informed me that Lionel's wife had given her blessing for Lionel's work to go ahead, and that the sponsors had pledged their continued support for the project.

However, picking up from where Lionel had left off proved to be no easy feat. Apparently, he was working on more than one candidate molecule, but it was not immediately clear which one was the fully developed drug ready for testing. I had some samples which he had sent me just before his death, and I returned it for analysis, but this was not of immediate help. Nobody knew the full synthetic pathway and no notes about it were found anywhere among Lionel's documents, except perhaps the chemical formulations that he had sent me earlier. This did not surprise me because he didn't want to risk his discovery falling into the wrong hands, or be hijacked, patented and denied to the poor. Specialist pharmaceutical chemists had to work backwards, trying to analyse the samples. This task initially proved too unwieldy, I was told. However, I repeatedly heard rumours that some other scientists were following up on Lionel's discoveries. I wondered whether, somehow, the "mysterious people" had picked up Lionel's leads, carried on the work, and left the rest of us in the cold.

Years later, I chanced to meet Dr Noble on 17 March, 2006, at the Kampala Irish Embassy's St Patrick's Day party to which we had been invited. He confirmed some of my suspicions and threw some light on the circumstances surrounding Lionel's death which had always puzzled me. He told me that at the time of his death Lionel was on high-dose antidepressants, which were thought to have induced the heart attack that killed him. With regard to the drugs, Noble informed me that the manufacturing process of Lionel's drug was successfully rediscovered and that work was still going on to develop it into an effective new class of AIDS medicine. It was also being tested for possible use as a vaginal microbicide for the prevention of HIV transmission.

In early January 2008 I was pleasantly surprised by a telephone call from Ireland informing me that Lionel's products were still on course for development into a new generation of AIDS drugs. Apparently, his products had continued to show promise and had reached a stage for first and second levels of testing. If they were eventually successfully developed into an effective and affordable AIDS drug to add to those currently available, it would be a fitting tribute to the life of a wonderful human being.

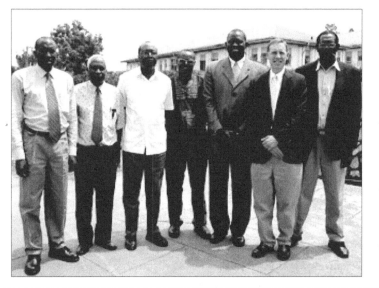

Left: *Grace Zamukama, Fred Mahlu, Peter Mugyenyi, Elly Katabira, Papa Salif Sow, Brooks Jackson, Job Bwayo (Late), after ACRiA meeting in Kampala. 18th January 2003*

Right: *Timothy Brown the only man thought to have cured of HIV.*
Picture for consciouslifenews.com June 2012

Below: *With US Ambassador Jimmy Kolker being welcomed by Karamoja rural community served by JCRC clinic in their area. 8th December 2004*

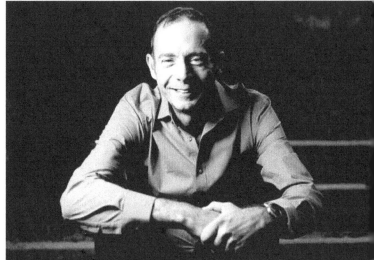

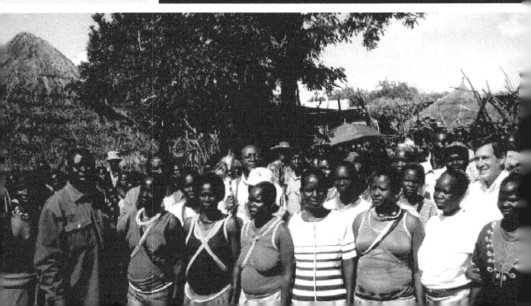

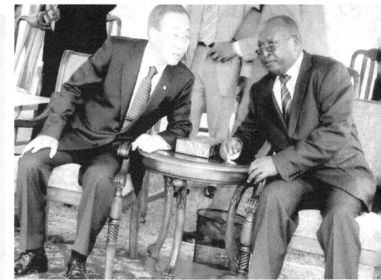

Right: With UN Secretary-General Ban Ki-moon, visiting the JCRC on 31st May 2010

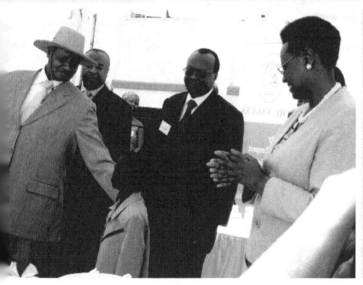

Left: With President and Mrs Museveni meeting a child living with HIV under the care of JCRC. 28th November 2006

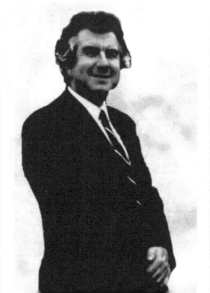

Left: Maurice Rouchy one of the pioneering researchers on AIDS drugs.

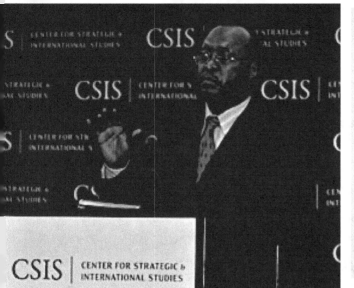

Left: Speaking at Centre for Strategic and International Studies Washington DC. 18th March 2009

Below: With Mark Dybul at Georgetown University in Washingtom USA. 18th March 2009

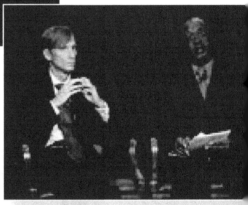

Below Right: With Matt Kavanagh, Jirair Ratevosian meeting with US Rep. McDermott. 19th March 2009

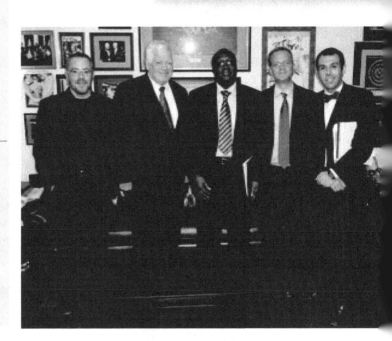

Right: Meeting with
Gayle Smith and Jeff
Crowley. White House.
Washington
on March 20, 2009.

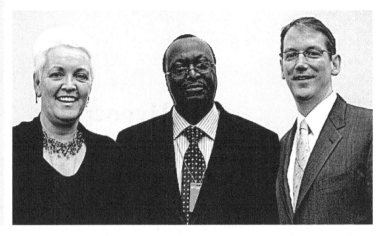

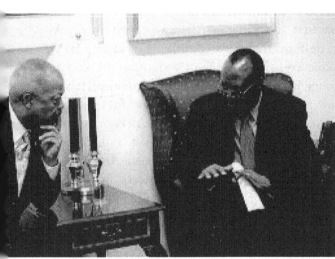

Left: Meeting with
US congressman the
late Donald Pyne in
Washington.
12th February 2010

Below right: With actress
Debra Messing in US
Congress after testimony
about AIDS in Africa.
12th February 2010

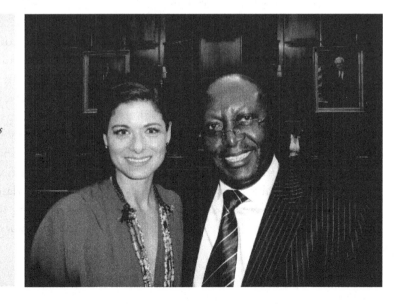

8

Hypocrisy

I am Dead!

By the mid-1990s, Uganda had emerged as a country that had achieved what was then considered to be impossible.

It became the very first sub-Saharan African country to break ranks with the almost uniform trend of a relentlessly escalating HIV epidemic. This was achieved by the launch of a vigorous preventive campaign that was strongly supported by the country's president. It was based on a programme of sexual abstinence, being faithful - dubbed "zero grazing" in Uganda - and the use of condoms. All components were advocated as a package. Indeed, no measure that could in any way help to alleviate the catastrophe would be shunned. And it paid off. Not only did Uganda register an impressive success, but it also defined an effective strategy and methodology for AIDS prevention. As a result, national HIV rates tumbled from a very high prevalence rate that at its peak ranged from 12% to 30%, down to an average rate of 6.4%. Remarkably, this was achieved without access to modern life-saving ARV treatment.

This achievement was the only good news we had received since the outbreak of the epidemic in Uganda. It was a glimmer of hope that the epidemic could be slowed down in other affected countries in Africa too. However, there was a tendency to exaggerate the achievement. For instance, some people suggested that the AIDS epidemic in Africa could be successfully controlled without treatment. While it was being defined as "Uganda's success against AIDS" by UNAIDS and other organisations, the carnage in the country continued unabated, because over one million people were already infected with HIV and unacceptably high numbers were still being infected daily. These grim statistics were set aside as songs of praise were being sung. This was understandable because the world was thirsty for good news in the midst of a bleak situation that had brought only bad news for over a decade.

The success triggered an incredible debate that still rages today. It was about the way the success had been achieved, and which component of prevention was responsible for it. Thus Uganda became the focus of what was to become a highly controversial debate, as some vested interests claimed that Uganda's success was all due to abstinence. It is interesting to note that before PEPFAR funding for Africa there had been no such debate. Uganda's highways were filled with billboards that informed citizens about condoms, faithfulness and abstinence, without triggering the flurry of controversy that arose during PEPFAR implementation.

In retrospect, part of the reason for the epidemic raging out of control throughout the 1990s was that despite the agony and the carnage that constituted a state of dire emergency, crying out for urgent humanitarian relief, all rich countries and donors steadfastly refused to provide any significant funding for AIDS treatment in Africa. The situation was so bad that films about the AIDS epidemic in Uganda, which were often screened on European television, were often preceded by warnings that the footage "contained disturbing scenes".

The first intervention to be funded in Uganda at the AIDS Information Centre was limited to counselling and testing. This was later expanded as the epidemic worsened, to involve a more comprehensive preventive programme that was provided throughout the 1990s and which had condoms as a major component. However, it was clear that, without treatment, the death toll would continue to mount as would people's alarm and anxiety. In response, some donors and charity organisations established terminal care support services or hospice care to ease the pain of dying AIDS patients.

Seriously ill AIDS patients were generally treated the same way as terminal cancer patients. Distraught counsellors were on hand to calm them down. As the condition deteriorated morphine would be administered, to attenuate the distressing end. While nothing could be done for terminal cancer patients except to alleviate the pain and make them as comfortable as possible as the inevitable approached, AIDS, on the other hand, was different. Since 1996 treatment that could save the vast majority of AIDS patients, including those who presented in advanced stages of the disease, had become available.

Their deaths were not necessarily inevitable. Morphine would not have been necessary for the vast majority of them. The right treatment was ARVs but it was denied to them because they could not pay the price.

I felt sorry for the staff who had to help patients die "peacefully" instead of saving their lives – if only they had ARV drugs to give them. But those they gave morphine were the lucky ones. The vast majority who could not access hospice services whimpered and groaned, and some screamed all the way to the end of their consciousness. Meanwhile, elsewhere in the privileged world, close-to-death AIDS patients were daily being revived back to health. Lazarus syndrome, the name coined to describe close to death patients whom ARVs brought back to life, was already well known in medical circles.

The welcome relief, albeit long delayed, finally came in 2003 and 2004, when PEPFAR and Global Fund (GF) programmes started respectively. But the lifesaving programmes came at least ten years late and was not accessible to all in need. Ten years delay that cost millions of lives across Africa. I suppose that we can say, "It's better late than never." But even this was a great favour, considering that there were those who advocated "Never" for Africa on the pretext that Africa would neither properly use nor afford ARVs. Sadly, some people have continued to oppose universal access to ARV on similar pretext.

For the very first time, PEPFAR and GF programmes brought into sub-Saharan Africa substantial money for AIDS treatment. Then, all of a sudden, the previously shunned AIDS work became attractive and even trendy. People of all walks of life and religious persuasions jostled in the queue to follow the money. NGOs and other establishments were formed in developed countries to follow the money all the way to AIDS-battered Africa. Likewise, in Africa, NGOs sprang up, involving individuals and organisations that before 2003 never had anything to do with HIV/AIDS. Even the stigma could not hold them back. Prominent among them were some religious extremists who in the past had never wanted anything to do with AIDS. Some of them held extreme views about the disease and strongly condemned sufferers as "sinners who deserved what they got". Many such characters who jumped on the bandwagon did so not because of a change of heart but for the change in the bank. They needed the money to further their agendas. Accordingly, some used PEPFAR funds to crusade against condoms, describing them as immoral. They were among those who brushed off the Ugandan success story that had condoms as an important component. They lied, saying that condoms played no role whatsoever. Instead, they tried to instil fear in people by claiming that condoms were tainted with HIV, or that they had holes in them that allowed the virus to move freely in and out and therefore were totally useless as a barrier. Worse still, some of them claimed that use of condoms was a sinister scheme to spread the disease.

Some of the religious extremists planned to use AIDS relief money to punish those they perceived as "the sinners". Some lobbied US politicians and decision-makers, insisting that the only preventive intervention PEPFAR should support was abstinence from sex until marriage and thereafter absolute faithfulness. A number of organisations in Uganda which were funded to promote abstinence launched controversial public and media campaigns claiming that abstinence was the only effective way to prevent HIV. The net result was that the preventive agenda suffered a setback.

This regrettable situation triggered a storm of protest. Then, when its folly was exposed by data that showed that all components of prevention were synergistic and played important roles in reducing the rate of HIV in Uganda, some of the people who previously denied that condoms had played no role in HIV prevention changed tactics and in a double denial insisted that – if anything at all - condoms only contributed a very small part.

As described in *Genocide by Denial*, the scenario back in the 1980s and 1990s, when AIDS was at its height, presents an interesting contrast. At the time, almost all the religious leaders in Uganda were stunned by the AIDS carnage. Helplessly, they lived and shared the tragedy with their flocks. A significant number of them were also victims of the scourge. In many of their sermons, they preached abstinence and faithfulness in marriage, but their sermons made no dent in the runaway epidemic because, sex being what it has always been – a strong natural drive – went on for various reasons. These included pleasure, keeping relationships going, holding marriages together, obtaining favours, as a means of income, housing dependants, putting food on the table, begetting children, paying school fees – and, not infrequently, just for the heck of it. No amount of fear or threats, whether deadly or not, has ever been known to completely stop all sex, because sex is a critical natural survival strategy. In one extreme example from

204 A Cure Too Far

the insect kingdom, the male Praying Mantis pays the ultimate price for sex to ensure survival of the next generation. The female partner actually eats the male after mating. Incredibly, more males continue to come forward and actually fight to make the ultimate sacrifice for the sake of sex.

Some among the religious right insisted that God made humans with a higher sense of reason and self control which should prevent the so-called animal-like behaviour that exposes them to HIV. While it is true that equating human sexuality with animals' sexual instincts is misplaced, the kind of sexually motivated crimes committed by humans makes one wonder! Sex in humans is mainly recreational. The only animals that seem to engage in sex for the sheer pleasure are dolphins. There is a declining number of children in Europe, Japan and the USA, yet we are told by authoritative sources that sexual encounters in these countries have not declined.

Unlike the ineffective HIV preventive strategy advocated by religious zealots, the government's AIDS Control Programme fared better because its comprehensive programme of Information, Communication and Education (IEC), empowered people with knowledge for effective self-protection. This consisted of a combination of measures aimed at reduction of the risky behaviours that fuelled the epidemic. Sexual abstinence was advised for those who could manage it but the majority who could not abstain were educated on safer sexuality. Either they had to be faithful to their sexual partners or, if they were not, they had to use condoms. Much later a catchy slogan: ABC (Abstinence, Be faithful, Condoms) was coined to define the scope of the prevention strategy in a captivating fashion.

Religious bigotry with regard to sex is not new. It was even a problem in the biblical times. One vivid example is Jesus's exposure of the hypocrite charade, as narrated in St. John's gospel, Chapter 8:

> The teachers of the law and Pharisees brought in a woman caught in adultery. They made her stand before the group and said to Jesus, 'Teacher this woman was caught in the act of adultery. In the Law Moses commanded us to stone such women. Now what do you say?'

What, indeed, could Jesus say to such hypocrites? These were words from the equivalent of today's "holier than thou" extremists, pretending to occupy the high moral ground, ignoring reality and their own shortcomings and vulnerability. To begin with, the woman was not alone in this act but the "pious" accusers had nothing to say about the "partner in sin". In reply, Jesus simply called their bluff.

> If anyone of you is without sin (in other words, has not committed adultery — in the AIDS era this is equivalent to engaging in risky behaviour), let him be the first to throw a stone at her.

Not only did no-one stone, the woman which is already remarkable, but the accusers melted away in shame! This was a reflection of their disgusting hypocrisy.

On another front, some religious activists took strong exception to sex education in primary schools. They argued that it was a form of moral corruption of children. Yet, many children in Africa do not get the chance to go beyond primary school education and even fewer go beyond secondary school. Nevertheless, the reality is whether children have sex education or not, almost all of them inevitably become sexually active sooner or later.

To have vulnerable children going out to face the world ignorant of the looming dangers and how to protect themselves is similar to playing a sexual version of Russian roulette. The knowledge acquired in primary school may be all that stands between them and HIV. Of course no sensible person advocates the "playboy" version of sex education for primary schools. The misguided opponents of sex education imagine the worst-case scenario. They cannot trust or appreciate that the education system, as with other subjects, would tailor sex education to different age groups' needs. Appropriate sex education is welcomed by many parents who find it difficult to discuss sex with their children. Most parents never got any sex education in their youth and, as a result, some of them make sexual blunders in their adulthood – even in married life! Not surprisingly, some of the parents who try to educate their children fail to do a good job.

If there is any doubt about the necessity of sex education, take a good look at the school dropout figures due to teenage pregnancies in Africa. Fred Ouma, a Ugandan journalist, writing in the *New Vision* daily newspaper of 12 January 2011, in a special section to mark World Population Day, described the dire situation.

Uganda has the highest teenage pregnancy rate in Sub-Saharan Africa, with half of its girls giving birth before the age of 18. Some give birth to healthy children, but for many, pregnancy was unplanned, birth comes too early and the experience is one of fear and pain.

In the same article, he quoted a WHO statement that; "Many times girls marry and start their families before ending their own childhood." This should jolt anyone into recognising the seriousness of a problem that is not unique to Africa.

The survival kit for teenagers who engage in sex in the era of the HIV epidemic should include condoms. This common-sense recommendation is often confused with "encouraging" them to use the condom. It is like saying that arming a night watchman with a gun means he should shoot any passer-by. A condom merely arms someone with protection if he or she runs into temptation, which is never too far away. To quote the late Ugandan Bishop Misaili Kawuma:

> If some people are foolish enough to go ahead and have sex, then to save their own lives they may use a condom.

The bishop knew that as far as sex is concerned, there are very many "foolish" people. They may be the majority. They include the legendary "foolish virgins", though this was in a different context admittedly. To be a virgin and foolish at the same time may lead to virginity being replaced by life-long HIV unless she learns about effective protection methods.

I recall an anti-condom crusader preaching to a youth congregation in December 2004: "A condom cannot save you. If you put it on, every step you take, you should say to yourself: I am dead! I am dead."

Unfortunately humans are such that many are prepared to pay the ultimate price for sex — though not quite deliberately in the normal sense of the word. By the early 2000s, a staggering three million people in Africa were dying of this sex-linked disease every year. Considering the millions of condoms then used in Uganda every year, thousands were right then singing, "I am dead! I am dead!" If this chant was a pop song by the condom users' pop stars band, it would have been a number one hit. In reality, many of those "rebels" who use condoms will not die, as long as they use them properly and consistently. The strategy for effective HIV prevention was of course to inform, educate and persuade as many as possible of those who engage in casual sex or had sex with partners of unknown HIV sero-status, to use condoms. It would be more accurate if they so liked or found it motivating to sing "I am saved! I am saved," instead.

Just as it seemed as if the condom issue was getting settled, His Holiness Pope Benedict XVI was drawn in the debate when, on a visit to Cameroon, he declared on 17 March 2009 that condom use will not help Africa to fight HIV/AIDS and could instead make the problem worse. This, declared on a continent where an estimated 25 million Africans were infected with HIV and upwards of 6,000 people were dying daily, outraged health agencies trying to halt the spread of HIV and cope with the devastating effects of AIDS in sub-Saharan Africa. As the controversy reverberated around the world the unimaginable seemed to happen! Pope Benedict XVI's subsequent comment, that condoms were the lesser of two evils when used to curb the spread of HIV, even if their use also prevents pregnancy, were on 23 November 2009, described by Victor L Simpson and Nicole Winfield in the Associated Press release as "a seismic shift on one of the most profound — and profoundly contentious — Roman Catholic teachings". According to a number of surprised commentators, the acknowledgement by the Pope that condoms help prevent the spread of HIV had ushered in a new era for the Catholic Church and was a major landmark in the fight against AIDS.

However, I realise that this is not the end of the story. I know there are many denialists and religious zealots who will continue to insist that the only acceptable method of HIV prevention is sexual abstinence, despite glaring facts to the contrary.

Virginity Prize

As the sexual abstinence debate spread, some incredible schemes to promote it were announced by some of its zealous advocates.

One of the most interesting was conceived by one Honourable Sulaiman Madada, a Uganda member of parliament (MP). His matchless plan to promote sexual abstinence received wide coverage in a Ugandan independent newspaper, *The Sunday Monitor* on 24 July 2005. It was indeed timely since all other methods to stop young people from engaging in sex seemed to have failed. He proposed a form of monetary inducement of up to one million shillings in scholarships to every adult female who could prove that she was a virgin.

Of course, numerous poor parents struggling to pay their daughters' school fees wished that their daughters could emerge as winners but it appeared that not many were holding their breaths. Simple arithmetic would have shown that if this generous offer was taken up by millions of girls then the Honourable MP would have been presented with a huge cheque to settle. Therefore to come up with such a clever scheme, the MP must have considered it a very low-risk gamble. However, the newspaper article weighed the merits of this outlandish offer. Not surprisingly, the newspaper did not encourage anyone to keep watching the space for photographs of smiling virgins at a specially called press conference, receiving Madada's coveted virginity prize. Amazingly, this rather far-fetched plan was, against all conventional wisdom, not entirely ignored. The same article reported that some serious contenders for the virginity prize had come forward. They were confident that they could prove their virginity and claim the coveted prize. So which group of women could possibly be so confident about proving their virginity? Wait for it ... They were prostitutes!

So how would the prostitutes, or sex workers, as they are called these days, go about proving the impossible to the Honourable MP, and wrestle out of his grip a small fortune that he seemingly never intended to part with? The key was the burden of proof. Proof, the sex workers figured, would most likely be provided by doctors, in which case, they said, they were in the best position to come to some understanding. One sex worker was quoted as saying that they would be open to *kitu kidogo*, a Swahili language term for inducement — a variant on Honourable Madada's own strategy.

Interestingly, top among their reasons for the desire to win the virginity prize, the sex workers explained, that they wanted to go back to school and pursue studies that would give them better and more honourable prospects in life. This throws some light on yet another aspect of the abstinence debate. Some young girls who would rather abstain from sex find themselves forced by adverse social economic conditions to engage in it for money. Others are forced into risky marriages for cultural, religious or economic reasons. Some girls fall under the powerful grip of men who dominate society. Thus a considerable number of women, especially married women, find themselves in situations where they are powerless to refuse sex. Sometimes even state laws do not protect them. On the contrary, some laws actually ensure the sexual subservience of women. For instance, in 2009 the Afghan government caused worldwide controversy when it sought to legislate that married women could not legally deny their husbands sex! In many other situations, even when not written in law, many women take it as their obligation to consent to their husbands' sexual demands. Yet some men, including those infected with AIDS, refuse to use condoms. In such instances, the best that can be done to empower women in their sexuality is to teach them sex-negotiating skills, and to strengthen their legal protection. In addition, the introduction of affirmative action to increase educational opportunities as a prelude to increased female employment would help reduce dependence on men.

In the same paper that carried Madada's controversial proposal, there was a letter written by one Edwin, a self-declared born-again Christian, under the heading "Sex must be sacred". In this letter, Edwin commits himself to abstinence until marriage but at the same time laments about his friends who fail or refuse to abstain. In AIDS prevention, the likes of Edwin should be encouraged to uphold their abstinence choice. However, experience shows that they still need to be educated about alternative preventive strategies, as many abstinence candidates fall by the wayside. For instance, it was found in studies carried out in Texas, USA, that few of the youths who commit themselves to abstinence succeed. Edwin's friends, engaged in potentially risky sex, urgently need to know about the proper use of a condom. It is not that Madada and Edwin are wrong about the power of abstinence to stop the spread of HIV. However, being right and being applicable are two different propositions. The point is that abstinence alone does not work for the majority of people. For many of those that cannot abstain, the very thin layer of rubber might be all that stands between them and death.

The life survival kit and the most useful preventive strategy against AIDS is the package of ABCD and not merely ABC. ABC was coined by Americans in the PEPFAR era to make the prevention message sound sexy. Otherwise it would have been AFC Abstinence, Faithfulness, and Condoms. B(e) substituted F to make it rhyme and catchy. D standing for Drugs—more specifically ARVs, is an important component of AIDS prevention.

Some people have another meaning for D that was coined before the introduction of ARVs. D then stood for Death. If this has to be included in the abbreviation it should only come after D for drugs as a small "d". We now know that drugs have powerful AIDS-preventive properties. ARVs have almost eliminated mother-to-child transmission in the USA and Europe. Breastfeeding women on ARVs rarely transmit HIV to their babies. People using ARVs properly do not transmit HIV to their sexual partners as readily as those who are not on therapy. The realisation that ARVs restore the health of ailing AIDS patients has resulted in unprecedented numbers of people undertaking HIV testing. People who know their sero-status are more motivated to change their behaviour than those who don't.

The Mildmay Centre, an AIDS treatment centre in Uganda, carried out a study in early 2000s to find out what it would cost to treat AIDS with ARVs instead of just treating opportunistic infections and symptoms. Surprisingly, it was found out that it was cheaper to treat AIDS patients with the combination ARV drugs than to treat them for opportunistic infections only. The reason for this was quite obvious to those of us who had been treating AIDS patients for a long time. When you treat an opportunistic infection (OI), it is just a matter of time before a new infection attacks the patient. Treatment is endless, as more and more serious infections emerge. Some of the OIs, like an infection that could lead to irreversible blindness, called cytomegalovirus infection, require very expensive drugs to treat them. On the other hand, the use of ARVs stops the emergence of almost all OIs. The patient goes back to becoming a productive member of society and, unlike those severely affected by some OIs, will not strain usually scarce family resources. That is why universal access to ART, when it finally arrives, will be one of the most effective preventive tools against AIDS. People will wonder why it was not used right from the start.

Why has there been silence on the D, especially with regard to recommendations for resource-constrained countries? The most important reason for the silence was obviously the exorbitant cost of the drugs. Cost meant that they were inaccessible to the majority of those who needed them in poor countries. If Western donors and governments were too vocal about the preventive potential of ARVs, they would have been morally obliged to provide them as part of the public health strategy for the control of AIDS which was recognised as a catastrophic state of emergency. Also, there were concerns that it might encourage people on AIDS drugs to abandon preventive measures like the use of condoms, or lead them to become more promiscuous, trusting in ARVs for protection. However, this was pure speculation because at the time there was no concrete evidence to support this school of thought. Certainly, experience among patients does not support this view.

Another concern was that the use of ARVs for HIV prevention would increase the likelihood of HIV virus developing resistance to drugs. It was further feared that if people with resistant virus engaged in promiscuous sex they could spread resistant strains to their sex partners thus increasing the prevalence of resistant virus in their community. Therefore some people believed that the easy way out was to drop D from the catchphrase. However, this was ill-advised. People always need to be told the truth. It is, indeed, reasonable that lay people expect ARVs to offer some protection from HIV. They already know that it protects most babies whose mothers are HIV positive from being born with the virus. They also know that ARVs are used for prophylaxis after accidental exposure to HIV. Certainly, many healthcare providers have used ARVs after accidentally being stuck with needles contaminated with HIV-infected blood. Women who are victims of rape are encouraged to report very early for treatment with ARVs. Instead of dropping the D altogether, it is better to explain that while there is some degree of protection, HIV can still be transmitted because ARVs are not a cure, and that the prevention offered by ARVs is not 100% effective in every case. This is not just a matter of the truth setting people free from ignorance, but it would also save numerous lives. It is a more prudent approach - and, moreover, is the truth - and better than leaving people to take uninformed decisions based on intuition. The ABCD package is a scientifically proven strategy for the prevention of AIDS, and not just a single component of it. Another C standing for male Circumcision' has since been added to make it ABCCD. Meanwhile, we wait for V for Vaccine to be added – when, not if, an HIV vaccine is finally discovered.

Despite recent scientific advances, AIDS remains a formidable and vicious enemy. I have witnessed it torture victims to unbearable stages. I have seen children suffer untold hardships because it killed their parents. I have witnessed the devastation it caused to my country and continent. It still threatens countries like Swaziland with mass extermination of its citizens. Therefore there is no room for a softly-softly approach to this hideous killer! It is abundantly clear that advocating abstinence only as the sole strategy for prevention of HIV was just obstinate.

Total defeat of HIV/AIDS requires that while we await a vaccine and a possible cure, all currently proven preventive armaments must be harnessed and unleashed against this century's most devastating enemy of mankind, even if all the weapons do not necessarily conform to all people's revered dogmas.

9

The Ultimate Solution?

Speckled Monster

Way back in 1978 I was once caught up in a dramatic incident in my clinic at Queen Elizabeth II Hospital, Maseru, Lesotho, where I was employed as a medical officer. About 11.00 pm on that fateful day a teenager, his head covered with a traditional Basotho blanket, arrived at the outpatient reception area. His condition was so serious that he was allowed to jump the long queue of patients, and he was led shuffling slowly into my busy outpatient clinic room. He was accompanied by his evidently worried parents.

When his mother pulled off the blanket, his face was a sight to behold! Just one look and the diagnosis immediately flashed into my mind. Remarkably, I had never seen a real case, but old medical textbook pictures I had seen resembled the patient right in front of me. The extensive pus-filled eruptions all over his face were so severe that he could hardly open his eyes. A milder form of the rash covered the rest of his body. He was also running a high fever and looked ill. To reassure the patient and his parents, I tried my best to remain calm as I mulled over various courses of action, but unfortunately the clinic nurse was not doing a good job of concealing her distress, and to add to that she was itching to say something.

"Are you thinking the same thing Doctor?" she asked nervously as she slowly retreated to the door.

"Yes," I had to admit, "but we need a second opinion to be sure," I added as calmly as I could.

But it was apparently ineffectual, because she immediately bolted out of the room. I am not sure whom she consulted, but whoever it was, he organised for her to be bundled back into the consultation room immediately. I could read terror on her face as she entered. She had a message for me which she conveyed nervously.

"I was instructed to inform you that the patient, his parents, you and I, are not allowed to leave the room under any circumstances until the World Health Organisation country representative has cleared us," she said nervously. "They said if anyone needs to pee, just do it in the room," she added, as she moved to take her position as far from the patient as she could. We were virtually under quarantine — prisoners of fear.

Over two long hours of sweat, as the windows had been partially closed from the outside, concern about the increasingly fretful patient, and anxiety made worse by pangs of hunger, had passed agonisingly slowly. Then, finally, some sort of a spaceman clad in a theatre gown, surgical gloves, head cap, face mask and goggles finally entered the room. He slowly examined the patient but periodically stopped to compare his findings with a manual of signs, check lists and illustrations that he had brought with him. Then after what looked like eternity, he finally removed his face mask and gloves and smiled. It was a beautiful smile – or so it seemed.

"At first, I also thought it was smallpox," the infectious disease consultant who had been rushed in from a nearby South African town said reassuringly, "but on closer examination I find that this is a severe form of chickenpox. The severest I have ever seen," he added. I vaguely recall that he tried to lecture to the nurse and I on what we ought to have done if it had been a real case of smallpox. By that time, over three hours after our ordeal had started, he could as well have been talking Latin to the walls.

Fear of smallpox goes back many centuries. Mere mention of it used to send people fleeing in utter terror. Nothing could be done to either stop or slow it down as it relentlessly spread across the world, maiming and killing millions in the process. Hitherto, no cure has ever been found. But it is no more. It was wiped off the surface of the earth by a low-cost, simple to make and easy to administer jab — a vaccine. Nowadays it is unknown to almost an entire generation of people. What a simple vaccine was able to accomplish for humanity in eliminating this killer disease is nothing short of a miracle. The story itself is mesmerising. The question is, could the same eventually turn out to be the case for HIV?

For thousands of years smallpox, dubbed the "speckled monster" in Europe, was one of the world's most frightening diseases, which over millennia and across continents, had killed countless millions of people, in some cases wiping out entire races and civilizations. The end of this disease came when the WHO started a worldwide vaccination initiative against it in 1967. The mission extended from the richest to the world's poorest countries and from the most urban to the remotest places on earth. Planes delivered the delicate vaccines to airports all over the world, as did ships to ports and on to all accessible vaccination stations by trucks. Where road accessibility was a problem, like the rugged mountain areas of northern Pakistan and India, donkeys came in handy, as did mountain horses to carry the vaccinators and vaccines to the remote mountainous areas of Lesotho. Healthcare providers on bicycles, on foot and various other means of transport crossed jungles, lakes, high seas, deserts and mountain ranges, and reached almost all major populations on earth, thus completing a medical miracle of the modern era. Within a mere ten years, smallpox– the speckled monster that had killed and maimed and scared millions for thousands of years – had been eliminated!

Two years after that haunting incident in a Lesotho hospital clinic, on 8 May 1980 to be precise, the WHO assembly declared the world free of smallpox. Despite a number of scares, the last known case of naturally transmitted smallpox had occurred in Somalia in 1977. A hefty reward was offered to anyone who reported a new case and hitherto the prize remains unclaimed. These days the smallpox virus is only found in heavily fortified research laboratories in Atlanta, Georgia, USA, and Siberia in the Russian Federation – where it is kept deeply frozen in liquid nitrogen for possible future scientific purposes, including making new vaccines, if the need would ever arise.

To a slightly less dramatic extent but no less frightening were diseases such as measles, whooping cough and poliomyelitis, which used to wreak havoc on children—a nightmare to parents all over the world. Once devastating epidemics of these diseases swept across villages throughout sub-Saharan Africa. The fear inducing polio was on the verge of being eliminated from the world when fear instigated by a few religious bigots in the northern Nigerian state of Kano claimed that the vaccine was laced with HIV. In organised campaigns that quickly spread to neighbouring states these scare mongers warned that vaccines would cause infertility and were a sinister Western plot to harm Muslims. The consequence of this unfortunate propaganda was a resurgence of debilitating polio outbreaks that resulted in a number of children suffering permanent limb paralysis, not only in Nigeria and neighbouring countries but as far away as the Middle East and Indonesia. When scientific tests (genetic fingerprinting) were carried out to determine the origin of the resurged polio outbreaks in different places, it was found that the spreading polio virus strain was of the same type as that in Kano. But, if you think that this only happens in Africa or with some peculiar religious zealots, think again.

The British early childhood vaccination programme also suffered a severe setback following the publication of a paper in February 1998 (which has since come under severe criticism and has been partially retracted) that suggested a link between measles, mumps and rubella (MMR) vaccine with autism—a feared pervasive developmental disorder. The media took up this disconcerting story and blew it out of proportion, causing a nationwide scare that quickly gained momentum. This gave birth to a formidable anti-vaccination vigilante group that carried out a widely publicised campaign against MMR vaccination programme. Many distressed and fearful parents, in response to unfounded rumours of a clandestine plot, refused to have their children vaccinated. Their fears seemed to be vindicated when the prime minister at the time, Tony Blair, was asked whether Leo, his newborn baby had been given MMR vaccine. Citing the right of his child to privacy, he ignored the escalating public health crisis, and steadfastly refused to answer. The result was a fall in the numbers of children being vaccinated in the UK, from a high of 92% in 1996 to 73% in 2008. It was reported that between 2004 and 2005, only 38% of children in the city of Westminster received all the recommended shots of the vaccine. Inevitably resurgence of cases of measles and mumps and the complications that go with them followed.

Despite these setbacks, vaccines have reduced the incidence of these serious diseases drastically even in the poorest of countries, to a stage that any new case is reported as headline breaking news. Likewise, a safe and effective HIV vaccine, once found, would be the ideal solution for poor, AIDS-battered countries. Millions of lives would be saved and the prospect of stopping this century's most catastrophic epidemic in its tracks would be a distinct possibility. However, this is still only a dream.

The excitement about ARV drugs (though fully justified in terms of lives saved), has tended to push the thrust for vaccine development out of the limelight. Yet a permanent solution to HIV/AIDS requires both effective treatment and a robust preventive intervention. Use of an effective vaccine, once it was discovered, would be the ultimate preventive strategy.

Of all the currently available vaccines for various diseases, none has presented with such scientific and technological challenge as has the still ongoing quest for the development of a vaccine against HIV. These complex challenges are as old as the discovery of the HIV virus itself. However, it is not only scientific issues that have dogged the development of a HIV vaccine. Some social and cultural issues have been just as daunting. In fact, a variety of concerns, some of them bizarre and others just amazing, were being expressed long before the earliest work started on a HIV vaccine.

Such controversies were not at all new to vaccine discovery, even though vaccines have been used successfully for centuries. Some of the controversies associated with them have been as fear-provoking as the diseases they were supposed to prevent. I was to learn that inherent fear of vaccines is as bad today as it was centuries ago. For instance, the development of the polio vaccine in 1950s whipped up enormous fear and controversy among scientists and ordinary people especially parents of at-risk children. The astonishing story of the obstacles that shadowed the polio vaccine discovery in the USA has been well described by Jeffrey Kruger in his remarkable book entitled *Splendid Solution* which is about Dr Salk, the discover of the polio vaccine.

The fear of the HIV vaccine, especially among the elite, was even more intense. The main concern with regard to polio before the discovery of a vaccine was the paralysis that occurred in about one percent of infected children, and the smaller number of fatalities. HIV, on the other hand, killed everyone who got infected. It was therefore deemed imperative that any HIV vaccines would need to ensure a much higher standard of safety than that of polio and any other existing vaccines.

Phantom Scare

In the late 1980s, when AIDS deaths were mounting rapidly, many, especially members of the educated class, were afraid of HIV vaccines – the intervention that had the best chance of protecting them. Incredibly, the vaccine they were so terrified of did not even exist anywhere in the world. If a phantom HIV vaccine could whip up so much fear, what would a real one do?

The fear of HIV vaccines could be traced back to the time when some quacks, (including an Egyptian working with a Congolese mentioned in *Genocide by Denial*), tried to sell dangerous concoctions claiming that they were HIV vaccines, and suspicions that early researchers were harbouring ulterior motives. Some rumour mongers whispered that some rich countries in collaboration with the big pharma had conspired to use Africans as guinea pigs for the development of HIV vaccines for the West. This and other concerns were discussed at a special emergency meeting of Ugandan scientists and various interest groups convened in 1989 to brainstorm the future of HIV vaccine development. At the time, the complexity associated with HIV vaccine development was not fully appreciated. Many people naively expected that it would be developed within a couple of years.

The meeting came out with some far-fetched guidelines and recommendations that were mainly fear-inspired. When I looked at the guidelines I worried that they would, if left unchanged, kill any chance of Uganda ever testing an HIV vaccine if it became available. The guidelines included a requirement that for any HIV vaccine to be used or tested in Uganda, it must have first been tested in the country of its origin. Though I could understand the underlying anxiety, I was dismayed by this unfortunate decision, as it had retrogressive and unfavourable implications for our country. I considered it intellectually defeatist. Good science on which safety was to be based did not need to be location-specific. All that was required was to insist on conformity with exacting universal standards. Any safety concerns could have been better addressed by ensuring a thorough scientific assessment of any candidate vaccine - each one on its own merit. An additional safeguard could have been a requirement that any clinical trial involving vaccines be strictly supervised to make sure that safety standards were not compromised. I therefore set out to discuss the shortcomings of the 1989 recommendations and how they could be revised.

To illustrate the futility of the proposed guidelines, I frequently invoked the example of malaria, a mostly tropical disease. If, for instance, scientists in Alaska or Norway were to discover a malaria vaccine, would it be reasonable to insist that they must first test it on their populations? Though HIV was different in that it affected all regions of the world, it was Sub-Saharan Africa that was on fire with a huge number of our people dying every day. Therefore it was in our people's vital interest to expeditiously test any promising new HIV vaccine. All we needed to do was to ensure that the latest scientific procedures were followed in the development of any vaccine to be tested, that it had exhibited a reasonable preliminary safety profile and had a good chance of success. It would be irresponsible of African scientists to stand by while millions of Africans continued to die every year, with a hope that some other countries' citizens would be kind enough to be the first to undertake the risky research on our behalf.

By the early 1990s, technology for the development of a safe HIV vaccine was still in its infancy. The sophistication of the HIV virus and exceptional safety concerns necessitated new scientific and technological approaches in order to produce a safe and effective vaccine. At the time only a few candidate vaccines were undergoing animal and safety tests in preliminary stages (phase one and two). However, there was growing, though cautious, optimism that one of the candidate vaccines would eventually succeed. Understandably, any suggestion of progress raised unrealistic expectations. It was similar to a weary, thirsty traveller seeing mirages of water in the desert.

I remained absolutely convinced that it was imperative for Africa, and Uganda in particular, to start preparations for the HIV vaccine so that no time would be wasted before its launch once it had been discovered. We needed to be part of a scientific solution instead of passive spectators and expectant recipients. To begin with, it was imperative to study and internalise public perceptions and attitudes towards HIV vaccines well in advance.

Vaccine safety and acceptability concerns, however, were not the only issues of public concern. There were questions regarding the impact an HIV vaccine would have on behaviour. Some people worried that HIV vaccine trials would mislead people into a false sense of security, thus reversing any gains in preventive strategies that had been achieved. "As soon as a new vaccine is announced people will go on rampage, reverting back to risky sexual behaviour, and make the situation worse than before," one delegate said at one of the vaccine preparatory seminars.

With so many misconceptions and controversies it was imperative that these issues be resolved ahead of any vaccine development in Uganda. But nobody knew whether it would be possible to do so.

Be Prepared

I was determined to play my part in ensuring that no chance of testing an HIV vaccine would bypass Uganda on account of us being unprepared to receive it. But we almost missed a rare opportunity to test a promising candidate HIV vaccine because of some dumbfounding controversies.

As I discussed the issue with professional and lay friends, it emerged that persuading people that HIV vaccines were desirable would be an uphill task. Some of my friends echoed the old fears that participants risked being vaccinated with a tainted HIV vaccine which would transmit the deadly HIV virus to them. I had taken HIV vaccine acceptability for granted, but it became clear that we needed to involve the community representatives including opinion makers, scientists and religious leaders, in a dialogue regarding the future of HIV vaccine trials.

We started working on this early in 1993, by looking for financial support to carry out a study to determine what people thought of an HIV vaccine and whether our society would welcome it if it became available. I solicited the help of Jerry Elner, an American professor of medicine who was then on a visit in Uganda. On 13 May 1993, I held a meeting with him to discuss the possibility of working together on a research project involving young soldiers. We wanted to determine their attitude to HIV vaccines, study their sexual behaviour, and find out whether such vaccines would be acceptable to them. The suitability of the military as a study cohort was based on results of an earlier pilot study involving almost 500 soldiers, which found that the military was a high-risk group for HIV. In addition, the Uganda military was supportive of HIV prevention programmes.

At a follow up meeting on 19 May 1993 that involved Prof Roy Mugerwa from Makerere University, we agreed to apply to the WHO for possible funding. Elner contacted Dr Jose Esperza who was then chief vaccine development research and intervention development officer for Global programme on AIDS at the WHO in Geneva, and asked him to support our budding plans. Esperza encouraged us to submit a proposal to study the acceptability of HIV vaccines and any other associated factors in Uganda for consideration by a WHO technical committee of experts. I spent long hours, sometimes until very late hours in the night, in my office working, with Mugerwa and Dr Edward Mbidde, a senior physician, developing the proposal. Elner, who had since returned to the States, communicated with us by telephone and fax. I recall that by the time we agreed on a final version for submission, the dustbin in my office was overflowing with discarded draft fax papers. And I suspect the same was the case in Elner's office.

In planning for the study, we faced a number of obstacles. The very first one concerned our selection of the military as a source of research subjects. We were obliged to ensure that individual soldiers, who, by and large, work on orders, would be free to choose whether or not to participate in the trial without coercion. We also had to guarantee that the soldiers' careers would not be jeopardised by their participation. Another concern was that soldiers participating would be stigmatised by their comrades in the mistaken belief that they had HIV. We worried that those found to be HIV positive at the screening stage would suffer psychologically, since we had no ARV treatment to offer them.

The other tricky issue concerned the accuracy of the methods to measure the real level of vaccination acceptability. We realised that it would be easy for any study participants to report that they would accept HIV vaccination as long as they were sure that it would not happen in reality. To get around this, we planned to offer a surrogate vaccine that was already approved for some other disease to all those who reported acceptability, to see whether they would go all the way. For ethical reasons, the selected surrogate vaccine had to be safe and be of known benefit to the recipients. It would have been unethical to offer them a placebo when we had no trial vaccine to test.

Not surprisingly, when our application was reviewed by WHO in Geneva, the same concerns were raised. On 15 March 1994, William Heyward, the WHO vaccine development programme officer, wrote to me seeking clarification about the way we planned to address these important issues. To ensure that there would be no coercion, we explained, only civilian JCRC counsellors and personnel would be involved in counselling and recruitment of study subjects from the army. We undertook to ensure confidentiality of the soldiers by identifying them only with a code number, no senior military officers would be involved in this allocation, and individuals would not be able to be linked to data. Although we needed to enrol only HIV negative people, we planned that both HIV-positive and negative soldiers would undergo exactly the same general screening procedures in order to minimise stigma. We also received assurances from the military authorities that participants would not be discriminated against or suffer any disadvantage as a result of participating in the study.

With regard to the choice of a surrogate vaccine, we chose the meningococcal vaccine, because meningococcal meningitis is a dreaded killer disease. It was well known that soldiers were at risk. Therefore use of such a vaccine known to offer protection, would be fully justified and ethical. Our explanations were duly accepted by the steering committee of the WHO Vaccine Development Global AIDS Programme. This cleared the way for our pioneer study in Preparation for HIV Vaccine Evaluation (PAVE), the first one in Africa. It started in May 1994.

The aim of the study was to establish a group of over 1,000 uninfected people aged between 23 – 26 years, suitable for future vaccine trials, and follow them up for a period of three years. The study involved imparting intensive HIV information, educating and communicating to them other risk-reduction messages (IEC). Free condoms were provided to those who asked for them. The effect of IEC on HIV risk behaviour was then measured. The parameters that were measured included whether numbers of sexual partners and the incidence of HIV changed over the three-year period of follow-up. Both questionnaires and actual numbers who would accept meningococcal vaccination would give a reasonable overall indication of the level of vaccine acceptability.

As part of initial assessment, we studied the sexual activity of participants in an effort to identify any risk factors that would need to be addressed in future preventive strategies. Working with WHO experts, we also set out to find the kind of HIV subtypes infecting our participants during the trial. The information would indicate the kind of HIV virus circulating among the population and help in targeting future HIV vaccines if HIV subtype-specific vaccine formulations were found to be necessary.

The approved budget for the study was small and therefore we had to devise some cost-saving measures. As the Uganda lead investigator, I offered my services free, as did all our American partners, including Jerry Elner, Chris Whalen, John Johnson, all of them physicians, David Hom, an expert on data, and Estelle Piwower, a laboratory specialist. This meant that the money saved could be ploughed back into the study.

As preparations started on 20 June 1994, I wondered whether my then inexperienced Centre would be able to recruit all the subjects successfully, carry out a quality study, and achieve our objectives. My research team then consisted of one junior doctor, a few counsellors and laboratory technologists. They fanned out into the military barracks explaining the purpose of the study and assuring the soldiers of their full confidentiality as well as full freedom to choose whether to join. The concept of volunteerism in research was explained to them, emphasising that it had to be on their free will, and was not associated with any inducements or special benefits. They were also assured that they retained the freedom to withdraw from the study at any time.

By 13 July 1994 enrolment in the study had started and by 23 December, over 650 volunteer participants were already on board, well ahead of schedule. This was a remarkable achievement considering the time it takes to fully recruit one participant.

At each visit, participants were screened for HIV and other sexually transmitted diseases and asked about risk behaviours. The prevalence and incidence of HIV were measured among the whole group. Behavioural changes were assessed using such indicators as condom use and other parameters indicative of high-risk behaviour including the incidence of new sexually transmitted infections (STI). Being infected with a new STI suggested that the concerned individual had engaged in high-risk sex even if he reported otherwise. Logistical issues important for future vaccine trials and successful follow-up of study participants were also evaluated.

As we made our first-year report to WHO, I was amazed at the wealth of new information emerging from the study. We were astonished to find that about 26% of the young soldiers had become infected with HIV in the first year, despite intensive HIV preventive messages about ABC and regular counselling. This rate was much higher than previously thought. We also found that more young soldiers were still getting infected at the high rate of 2.62% per year. However, these rates were not dissimilar to those of the other youths of the same age. Uganda at that time had the highest HIV incidence and prevalence in the world. In fact, in some Ministry of Health antenatal sentinel sites, the rates were even higher. The military was clearly a very high-risk group to target for a future HIV vaccine. In an unprecedented move, the Ugandan military allowed us to publish the high incidence rate that we found. Some other armies would have considered such data a military secret. This level of openness was part of the reason why Uganda did relatively well in the control of HIV.

We were able to make other discoveries that had implications for better planning of future HIV-preventive strategies. For instance, we found that on average in this male cohort, the age of sexual debut was 18 years. By the age of 23 to 26, past sexual partners would have risen to the middling of eight, though the numbers ranged from 1 to 400. As would be expected, those with a higher number of sexual partners, whom some referred to as "conquests", were more likely to be HIV-infected and therefore fail to qualify for the study.

Assessment of participants' attitudes to vaccines revealed interesting findings. Contrary to the gossip, the vast majority—up to 70% did not believe that vaccines would harm them. An even higher number – over 80% did not believe that vaccines cause HIV or any other disease. As only 4% of the participants had attained higher education and about half had only primary-level education, it may be that perceived fear and scepticism about HIV vaccine safety was fuelled by the elite.

When participants were asked what would motivate them to accept HIV vaccines, the overwhelming majority of up to 90% said they would have the vaccine if a loved one had AIDS. At the time the majority of Ugandans knew at least one person who had AIDS and many were close relatives or friends. More surprisingly, 97.2% of the participants said they wished to be the first to have an HIV vaccine if it was discovered. We wondered whether it was due to the fact that participants were soldiers, who by profession expect to take risks, that acceptance was so high, but we found no evidence to support this. It appeared to be a true reflection of society's fear about the devastation of AIDS. We also found a high level of AIDS awareness in the cohort.

Of the participants 84% reported that they trusted condoms for protection against AIDS.

One of the beneficial effects of IEC was clearly demonstrated by condom use, which was initially very low but increased the longer they spent in the study. However, despite intensive counselling there were still a relatively high number of participants taking risks with new sexual partners. In fact, no preventive strategy has ever entirely succeeded in eliminating risky behaviour. Worse still, we later found out that the preventive messages were, in the long term, not being taken as seriously as at the beginning. I called this phenomenon, "message fatigue". Clearly, HIV-preventive messages, like all adverts, needed continuous review and revision if they were to remain effective.

Among other findings were five study participants who admitted being practising homosexuals. This was remarkable because some people previously asserted that the practice was nonexistent in indigenous Ugandan society. Besides, homosexuality in Uganda is taboo and illegal. Anyway, the study demonstrated that it existed though in very small numbers and it was certainly not contributing significantly to HIV spread in Uganda.

Meanwhile, national and international interest in the data emerging from the study was high. I was invited to present our data to a number of international scientific conferences. I made presentations at a number of vaccine meetings organised by the WHO in Geneva, and others in USA and at the AIDS in Africa conference in Kampala, among others. I also had the honour to present the data to Her Majesty the Queen of Sweden at a conference she attended in Stockholm. My colleagues also were equally busy, presenting our findings in other countries, including Japan and Thailand, and at other scientific meetings.

Recognising the importance of our pioneer study (PAVE), we agreed with our American partners to expand the study in order to get more comprehensive data. This resulted in a linked study known as HIVNET PAVE. The National Institute of Health (NIH) of the United States agreed to fund it and hence it was also known as NIH PAVE. This was a very exciting development for me. There were many side advantages that the planned study would bring to the JCRC in particular and Uganda in general. The resources for the study were substantial, allowing an addition of another 1,200 participants. Both studies extended the age range from 19 to 26. In addition, the study aimed at strengthening the technical capacity of the JCRC, to undertake future research projects.

The JCRC expert workforce was reinforced by the addition of two pleasant American experts, Anita Loughlin and Cathy George. Another advantage of the new study was that it brought on board a wider range of other experts that also included Dr Janet McGrath, an anthropologist. Janet studied the reasons behind such high acceptability of vaccines. She found that willingness to participate in vaccine studies was to a considerable extent based on the expectation that future HIV vaccines would be protective. This indicated the need for future vaccine study participants to be better educated to appreciate that trials do not necessarily guarantee or aim at providing protection. Secondly, Janet noted that the perception of participants of "treatment" versus "prevention" did not "always match those of Western researchers". However, this information was not new to practitioners of medicine in Uganda, where the difference between a vaccine and treatment is not always clear to people with low or no formal education. This underscored the need to always include local experts in HIV vaccine study designs and implementation.

Other interesting findings were the widespread misunderstanding by participants about the basic principles of clinical trial design, including study objectives and the kind of results expected at the end. For instance, they didn't understand why one volunteer would qualify to participate in the trial while another would fail. Use of a dummy drug or placebo as a control needed to be explained, otherwise some participants would assume that all of them were taking the same vaccine or drug. Later we had to coin words for participants to understand the scientific research methodologies better. For instance, "air supply" was used to explain placebo, "wrapping" was used to explain blinding that ensures that the doctors and participants do not know what an individual patient is taking until the trial is over, and "lottery" explained the method of randomisation, whereby participants are randomly allocated into various groups to be compared. We soon found out that the choice of "air supply" to mean placebo was spot on. It readily captured lay peoples' imagination because it was widely used at the time by radio, television and newspaper journalists to refer to exorbitant promises made by politicians during their campaigns, that they never deliver on when elected.

The overall conclusion from both HIV vaccine preparatory studies was that HIV vaccine acceptability was very high. Important issues to be taken into account as far as vaccine acceptability was concerned had been identified and to a considerable extent addressed. My institution, the JCRC, had passed the test. The next step was to go ahead and test a real HIV vaccine. We were prepared, confident and motivated. However, there was one simple snag in our way.

No HIV vaccine ready for testing existed anywhere in the world.

Shooting a Moving Target

"I commend JCRC for the work that you have been able to do so far," a visibly surprised visiting American scientist said to me. "But I must be frank with you. What you are envisioning is just not possible at this time in Uganda."

He was responding to my invitation to partner with us in a joint venture to develop an HIV vaccine.

"My own institution in USA has not yet started on the kind of HIV vaccine testing that you are talking about," he elaborated. "With the current technological challenges the continent currently faces, it will be many years before Africa sees her first HIV vaccine trial," he said. "With respect, in your case it's just like a dream."

An opportunity to move my dream forward occurred almost by chance. It arose when Jose Esperza, the WHO chief of HIV vaccine development, visited the JCRC in 1995 as part of a delegation to assess research capabilities in Uganda. During the break I took him aside to pick his brains on the state of HIV vaccine development and to inquire about our possible future role since we had proved the feasibility of such studies in our Centre.

"We need a vaccine to test; otherwise we will lose all the groundwork that we have achieved in PAVE," I said. "As Uganda is the most AIDS-affected country, it is crucial that we take the initiative to test an HIV vaccine." "That's exactly what I was thinking too," he said in his usual engaging rapid-fire way of talking. "I think I know of a candidate vaccine that might be just right for you. The French scientists at Pasteur Institute in Paris have discovered a promising vaccine known as ALVAC," he said. He explained that the scientists had ensured that the vaccine could not possibly transmit HIV by excluding live or whole dead HIV from it.

As Jose explained, it became clear that a novel way to stimulate the body to produce antibodies against HIV without risking use of the HIV had indeed been found. In cases of some other vaccines, for instance the polio vaccine, one component of it consists of a live virus but it is artificially weakened so that it is not able to cause the full-blown disease when used for vaccination. The body's immune system produces antibodies against it, which protects it against the infective form of polio. In the case of HIV, this type of vaccine could not be used for fear that it could transmit HIV disease.

In simple terms the ALVAC vaccine was made using a limited number of HIV fragments technically known as gene sequences. As these disjointed fragments or pieces of HIV could not exist as a viable virus and yet needed to be conveyed to the body by a live virus, they were inserted into the genome of a bird virus known as canarypox. The role of the bird virus was to carry and present the non-infectious HIV pieces to the human body's immune system.

The canarypox virus was chosen because it is harmless to humans. When injected into the body, it initially takes hold and actually starts to multiply like it does in birds, but the vigilant human immune system quickly recognises it as an "invader" and successfully eliminates it before completing its cycle of reproduction. However, the fact that it survives for a while made it a good candidate for delivery of the "payload" (in this case HIV fragments) to the body and to give the body's defence system enough time to react by generating antibodies before dying off. Scientists hoped that the antibodies generated against incorporated HIV disjointed genes would be robust enough to protect against HIV, without the need to use potentially risky live or killed intact virus. The hypothesis was a good one but no one knew whether it would succeed in stimulating sufficient specific and strong antibodies to actually protect against real HIV. The only way to find out was to test it on people.

"The new vaccine has already undergone a couple of tests in both France and the USA, mainly to determine safety and early indication of immunogenicity. But these tests were not conclusive," Jose said. "I will introduce you to Dr Michel Klein, the scientist concerned at Pasteur, and then you can take it on from there." As if to warn me not to be carried away, he added: "It's not going to be easy to pull this one off. But it is worth a try." Jose must have meant it as a reality check and, indeed, I found out later that his warning statement was a gross understatement.

The sobering reality was that preparing for a hypothetical HIV vaccine trial, as we did for PAVE, was a far cry from carrying out a real one, especially if it was still in very early stages of development. One of the problems was that in our HIV vaccines preparatory studies we had more or less studied the acceptability of a fully developed HIV vaccine. The reality was that no fully developed HIV vaccine suitable for efficacy testing was in existence at the time. The ALVAC construct that Jose referred to was still at an early stage of development. HIV vaccine testing at such an early stage was thought to be unfeasible in Africa. The then Ugandan scientists' recommendation was that no HIV vaccine should be accepted for testing in Uganda unless it had passed through all the early stages of its development.

The early stages of vaccine trial normally involve only a small number of volunteers. It entails intensive and extensive laboratory tests and animal studies. The main aims are to find out whether the candidate vaccine is safe for human use, and whether it generates within the body the required specific immune properties (immunogenicity) in a sufficient amount to potentially protect against HIV infection. To measure immunogenicity required expensive equipment including blood scanners to identify the HIV targeting killer cells known as Cytotoxic T lymphocytes (CTL). The necessary technology for CTL assays was new to east and central Africa, and yet without it the landmark study could not proceed.

Besides equipment, highly trained scientists and technologists were required to carry out the work and they were not available in Uganda. To make matters worse there was no apparent donor to provide us with the necessary funds. Some of the possible donors we approached were put off by the seemingly hopeless circumstances. All in all, it looked like the scientist who had warned that the proposed study was only a dream had been right. The problems associated with such a study seemed to be insurmountable.

However, at the time, the complexity of the project was not my immediate concern. This was a project that just needed to be undertaken in an attempt to find a way to alleviate the AIDS crisis. To sit back in limbo moaning that the work was too difficult was not an option. I had no doubt in my mind that the right thing to do, regardless, was to persist. It was preferable to fail in the attempt than to throw in the towel, as one of my patients had taught me when she faced a similar dilemma. I was encouraged by Jose's unwavering support despite the glaring odds. He knew very well that to hire and train the necessary staff as well as acquiring the necessary equipment required funds over and above the WHO budget allocation that he had under his vote. Unlike the low-budget PAVE study, anything that WHO could possibly provide would not be anywhere near enough. However, Jose, a highly respected scientist with wide connections, was all I had to build my dreams on.

True to Jose's word I was invited to France to hold discussions with the staff of the Pasteur Institute about the proposal. I was later told that the first reaction of the Pasteur Institute staff when they heard of my request to study their state-of-the-art vaccine was total surprise that anyone in Africa thought that such advanced research on the frontiers of science, and still not totally free of controversy, could be possible there. ALVAC had only recently been developed with the very latest of technology and only been tested on a small number of participants in France and the USA. The technology necessary for testing the vaccine was so new that some research centres in developed countries had not yet acquired it. No scientific work of this kind on HIV vaccine had ever been undertaken in Africa. Yet here was some Ugandan, requesting to be allowed to test the latest high-tech vaccine! However, when you are recommended by the likes of Jose Esperza, chief vaccine programme officer of the WHO, you cannot just be dismissed outright. I think they were obliged to be polite to him and, accordingly, sent me an invitation. However, they did not offer any funding to enable me to travel to France or offer any other logistical assistance like accommodation. Nevertheless, I was most grateful for the invitation. They had done their part. Mine was to find my way to Paris and, harder still, convince them that I knew what I was talking about.

I first thought of the French Embassy in Kampala as a possible sponsor for no other reason than that the candidate vaccine was French. Accordingly, I contacted the French envoy to Uganda (1994-1998), Ambassador Francois Descoueyte, who invited me to meet him. There was an immediate rapport between us. This started a friendly relationship that resulted in a number of invitations to French Embassy functions and parties, which involved dinners of exquisite meals accompanied by the fine wines for which France is renowned. I found the remarkable ambassador very well versed in virtually anything that ticked in Uganda, in such amazing details that I was often left in awe. Whenever he recounted stories including serious political issues about Uganda and other countries where he had served, he did it with such a remarkable sense of humour that I would often be left totally captivated. It was obvious that he was very well suited for his role as an envoy of his country. He seemed to genuinely care for the peoples of the countries where he served. He had all essential facts about the AIDS epidemic in Uganda at his fingertips. Therefore, I did not have to explain the seriousness of our HIV vaccine need. However, I am not sure if he fully appreciated the complexity and scientific challenges surrounding HIV vaccine development that I faced at the time. To my delight and profound appreciation, the compassionate man offered not only to help with the ticket but also to cover other expenses. In fact, he arranged for the French Ministry of Foreign Affairs to host me in Paris.

Though I was overjoyed that this hurdle was overcome, at the back of my mind I realised that the main battle was yet to be won. My challenge was to convince the Pasteur Institute scientists that I was a worthy scientific partner to advance their state-of-the-art vaccine development. I realised that the minimum requirement for them to take my request seriously was for me to demonstrate that I had a well organised and disciplined laboratory. Jose had warned me that it would be an absolute necessity. He had toured our laboratories, seen our work practice and felt that with a little help we could do it. He was also kind enough to give me a favourable recommendation to Michel Klein. Without it, I don't think I would have been allowed through the front gate of the world renowned Pasteur Institute.

The meetings were scheduled for May 1995. In Paris I was met by a pleasant woman from the French Ministry of Foreign Affairs. She took me to my hotel in the centre of Paris and briefed me on the details and logistics of my official meetings. The next morning I was picked up by an official who gave me   directions to the Pasteur Institute. As we were waiting for the taxi, I was surprised when he asked me why my country was obstructive to French policies in Africa. I am not sure whether the official was asking out of personal curiosity or whether it was an official inquiry. Anyway, I replied something to the effect that as a scientist I was not competent to respond to political questions. I also expressed surprise that Uganda's relation with France were anything but friendly.

At the Pasteur Institute the questions were more relevant to my mission. Still, I was initially asked about the political situation in Uganda, and whether the conditions were conducive to collaborative scientific work. I assured them that Uganda was stable and that the government was highly supportive of AIDS research. Thanks to the respect the French seemed to have for President Museveni and his role in the fight against AIDS, my assurances were readily accepted. The rest of the discussion was almost like an interview. All in all I think I convinced a good number of them that, at the very least, Uganda and my centre in particular was worth investigating as a possible research partner. However, I had no assurances that any funding would be forthcoming for the study. In fact, Pasteur did not promise any. No other specific commitments were made except promises that scientists from the Institute would visit the JCRC and assess the facilities in the near future. To me, this was as successful an outcome as could be expected in the circumstances. I had dreaded outright rejection, which earlier that very morning had looked like a distinct possibility. I left the meeting cautiously optimistic.

After that I touched base with my old friend Pierre Lys (my link with Mr Rouchy), who had been collecting unwanted but still usable medicines returned to pharmacists in Paris for poor patients in Uganda. The drugs were to help treat opportunistic infections. As I gleefully departed for home, I was already planning for the crucial visit of the Pasteur scientists to the JCRC.

Back home, in a more sombre mood, I kept my fingers crossed until after the inspection carried out by Dr Jean L Excler, who gave my centre a tentative thumbs up. The next item on the programme was to find the funds and to address other challenges before this pioneer study could start. A lot of money was needed to purchase the equipment, renovate and remodel the laboratory to accommodate the delicate machines, and to recruit and train the technologists and scientists. We also needed to set up the necessary logistics to deliver the highly temperature-sensitive vaccine and reagents in an unbroken cold chain voyage from France to Uganda.

We also needed to establish partnerships with reputable scientific institutions to work with us on the project. This was the most challenging undertaking I had faced since I became the head of the JCRC, but it was so important because it would, if successful, signal the beginning of effective prevention and ultimately control of AIDS. Admittedly, my zest for finding a solution to HIV was running far ahead of the reality on the ground.

With regard to the need for collaboration with technologically advanced experts, I turned to Jerry Elner, and he immediately agreed to help. Locally, I mobilised senior Ugandan professionals, including Edward Mbidde and Roy Mugerwa. Elner contacted NIH for possible funding and arranged a series of trips to Washington to present our proposal. With Esperza's support, we began to make inroads. The study started looking more and more as if it would become a reality.

Next, we needed to set up a steering committee, establish a full project leadership and a research team to start serious preparations. However, despite all that I had done to initiate and get the project started, Prof. Elner who had been instrumental in getting the necessary funds, putting together a team of American scientific partners, training Ugandans and helping with the necessary logistics, did not appoint me to lead the steering committee as virtually everybody had assumed he would. I very much wanted the project to succeed and did not want any egos to get in the way. Therefore I promptly agreed to the arrangement, ignoring colleagues who raised objections insisting that I should continue to lead the entire initiative since I had started it. In the end Elner's foresight was vindicated, as it later turned out to be the best possible arrangement, because it freed me to take on a number of critical challenges that arose. Some of these challenges became so highly volatile and controversial that they threatened to undermine the study long before it got under way.

Tight Spot

The most serious challenge that we faced before the groundbreaking trial could begin was not technological in nature, but the same old nagging problem that many scientists of the past faced while trying to develop vaccines. For instance, way back in 1797, when Edward Jenner first presented his landmark finding that cowpox vaccination provided protection against smallpox, to the Royal Society of London, it was contemptuously rejected. As is still the case today, the extremist religious factions, who have never accepted that science is beyond their religious control, took strong exception. An imaginative cartoon of 1802 still brings to life the prevalent mood of the time. It depicts Edward Jenner vaccinating people who would then immediately transform into humanoids complete with horns and hooves! The original cynical caption read, "The treatment had wonderful effects."

We also had our share of modern-day controversies. It was actually like a replay, as some of the controversies were the same as those Jenner faced. Some scientists strongly objected to the use of bird virus as a carrier of HIV genes in humans. Others questioned the scientific merits of the vaccine, wondering whether it was suitable for testing. It became clear that first and foremost, these concerns needed to be addressed before embarking on the trial. It was important to reassure all stakeholders that ALVAC vaccine was selected for testing because it was developed on sound scientific principles, and was manufactured under good manufacturing practice by a highly reputable organisation. Uganda was undertaking the pioneer HIV vaccine study based on its scientific credentials and purely in her own interest, and was not merely being used as a guinea pig. But this was not easy to explain to the habitual sceptics.

A series of meetings and workshops were arranged to precede the trial. Some were requested by our external partners and some potential sponsors who insisted that specific issues needed to be resolved first. In particular, they wanted to be reassured that the proposed study had local support. In addition, some sought to protect themselves against possible future litigation and to be in tune with their home countries' regulations. As a result, the project was almost flawed by over vigilance and misconceptions. At one point I worried that this vital project would be ruined altogether as some of our foreign partners brought to the forefront farfetched issues that I considered irrelevant to our local situation. For instance, the fear was raised that some of the participants could temporarily test falsely HIV-positive not as a result of HIV infection, but because they had developed antibodies to the vaccine.

"You know, people can lose their insurance cover," one foreign colleague said to me. "Nobody insures an HIV positive person," he added.

The common HIV test just determines whether one is HIV positive by detection of antibodies against HIV in the blood. The fear was that the common HIV tests would fail to differentiate whether antibodies were due to infection or merely induced by a vaccine. The scaremongers talked about health insurance companies refusing to ensure study participants on account of a false HIV positive test results, employers refusing them jobs, and women refusing to marry men mistakenly thinking that they were HIV infected. It was not that these issues were not worth discussing. The point was that the emphasis was exaggerated. For instance, with regard to the issue of health insurance very few participants had ever heard of health insurance, let alone had insurance. The participants did not have jobs that discriminated against HIV positive people. In reality, it was already well known that any positive reaction brought about by the vaccine would be very temporary, as earlier studies in France and the USA had shown.

If it became absolutely necessary to determine whether someone tested positive because of HIV infection or merely a false HIV positive due to vaccine induced antibodies, it was possible to do so. We also had in place another safeguard. We planned to offer all volunteers who tested positive for antibodies to HIV because of the vaccine special cards explaining that they were participants in the study, just in case this was needed for work, immigration or insurance purposes. For that reason, a false test was the least of our participants' fears. The threat they faced and worried about more was "real" HIV infection that was rampant at the time. Therefore it was much ado about little. Yet it bogged us down for a while, until the concerned vigilantes had been thoroughly overindulged. However this caused unnecessary delay that many people faced with the threat of HIV could have done without.

Besides people living with HIV, mainstream religious leaders, politicians, scientists, doctors, civil society and others with various agendas were also invited to attend the consensus-building workshops. Weekly meetings of focus discussion groups were arranged for the benefit of potential volunteers so that they could ask questions and internalise the issues to better understand what the vaccine trial was all about. What a fiasco that it almost turned out to be!

It was the very first time that some of the scientists and doctors had heard of the new science and technology in vaccine development. Unfortunately, many had not received the relevant literature in advance to enable them to internalise these rather complex advances. Therefore, inadvertently, some of them ended up causing considerable confusion to themselves and, in turn, to lay participants who looked to them for guidance. Some of them painted frightening scenarios that made the proposed new vaccine study look like a very dangerous undertaking that would harm Ugandans. As for the lay people, we were amazed by the wide range of misconceptions and incredible fears which they expressed. Some thought that the candidate HIV vaccine would protect against unsafe sex while others feared that volunteers would be injected with HIV.

Most of the unfounded fears were fuelled by widespread rumours and the equally confused media, which reported some scary stories about the vaccine, questioning its safety. The Ministry of Health children's polio vaccination programme suffered a serious setback, fuelled by allegations that the polio vaccine was tainted with HIV, partly because some people confused the two vaccines despite the fact that they were totally unrelated. This misconception almost caused havoc. One of the people who made the volatile situation worse was a man described as a communication mogul, but better known in southwestern Uganda as Kaihura Nkuba, which means "one who handcuffs lightning and puts thunder in jail". Kaihura Nkuba, a highly sensational radio broadcaster and founder of Greater African Radio, aired scary stories about polio vaccine in Uganda and linked it with HIV. As a result the successful national vaccination programme suffered a devastating setback as scared parents feared that their children would be harmed by the vaccine. The Ministry of Health scrambled together a damage control team of medical experts who rushed to the area to reassure the community.

In an article in the *New Vision* of 22 September 1996, the HIV "candidate vaccine" was mistakably referred to as a "candidate drug" leading some people to believe that the vaccine was some sort of ARV drug. Some misled HIV-infected people desperate for treatment launched a campaign demanding to join the vaccine trial, because ARVs were at the time not accessible to the vast majority of Ugandans. Yet the trial vaccine was to be tested only among the uninfected.

Perhaps not surprisingly some opportunistic politicians tried to gain political advantage from the controversy. They amplified the fears that Ugandans were being used as "guinea pigs" in a study that they falsely alleged had been rejected in United States and Europe. One controversial member of parliament went as far as organising a noisy rally which received wide publicity through a local radio station that broadcast it live. "This vaccine should be tried on animals in the national parks. President Museveni has sanctioned its use on Ugandans in exchange for money to finance his war in the Congo," the politician declared, amid wild applause of his hoodwinked supporters.

As time passed it became increasingly clear to me that not all stakeholders raised issues in good faith. However, everyone was entitled to their opinion, free speech and enjoyment of the full benefit of the doubt. At the end of it all, I hoped that some good would come out of the consultation process, though I could not foresee the price that we had to pay.

The Great Debate

It was the hottest debate that I had ever been involved in. The architects of the main contentious issues at the HIV vaccine workshop were three participants, but two of them, whom I will call Jasper Bampa and Gregory Nuhasi, were so vehement that their third counterpart's disruptive role was eclipsed.

The meeting was certainly a great opportunity for the elderly Bampa to make a post-retirement comeback to the centre stage. There was no doubt that he had had a distinguished career. For the benefit of those who were unaware of it, he used the occasion to remind them of his heydays when he was a firebrand who solved complicated scientific problems. However, he could not discern that times had changed dramatically. There had never been anything in his entire career as complex as the new science of HIV vaccines. Some of the methods applied to the manufacture of the older vaccines for less sophisticated infections like polio or measles were not only obsolete but also outright unacceptable at that time for HIV because of the fear of infection.

Based on outdated knowledge, Bampa incited fear among the participants. "This HIV vaccine is highly dangerous," he cautioned. "It will infect the study volunteers, who would in turn infect their spouses and then go on to start a new type of catastrophic HIV epidemic. The new epidemic will make the current HIV/AIDS scourge look like child's play by comparison." And what was his evidence that this apocalypse that he predicted with such confidence would come to pass? His vast experience.

"What's wrong with the man? For heavens sake, this is a new generation of vaccines, resulting from new science that we are all struggling to understand," I recall one scientist whispering to me. Bampa's colleague Nuhasi, on the other hand, was more up to speed with scientific advances in biotechnology, and the challenges of HIV vaccine development. He readily understood the advanced innovations that were used in the development of ALVAC in order to circumvent having to use live or killed HIV, so as to produce a safer and more acceptable vaccine. He basically acknowledged that the canarypox virus that had been genetically modified to carry some HIV genes could not be infective because it did not carry complete sets of HIV virus genes. However, in a strange twist of his imagination, he warned that the HIV genes introduced into another virus (canarypox virus) could cause it to reconstitute into a new monster infection. He ignored the fact that canarypox virus does not fully thrive in humans, but went on to cause unfounded fear.

Nuhasi went further and caused chills down the spines of some of the delegates by warning that the purity of the vaccine was suspect. "It is likely that, during the manufacturing process involving removal of genes from the real HIV virus and instilling them within the canarypox virus, that some HIV virus may have inadvertently persisted as a contaminant and would readily infect the volunteers." Obviously, he was unaware of the painstaking technical details involved in the new vaccine manufacture, or if he was, he chose to ignore them. He also referred to the whispers, albeit unproven, that HIV itself was in the first place introduced to Africa by laced polio vaccine. Nuhasi was beginning to gain ground in the debate by flaring up fears and doubts about the vaccine's safety in an increasing number of delegates. In the end, he seemed to offer a way out.

"We must first check out the vaccine for purity ourselves before we allow it to be researched on in Uganda," Nuhasi said. Never mind that, at the time, there were no facilities for testing the vaccine in the country. I strongly disagreed, pointing out that the prudent way forward was to make sure that the choice of vaccine for testing was based on good science with reasonable safety profile, and that it was manufactured under good manufacturing practices (GMP) in compliance with international standards. The rate at which our people were dying constituted a state of emergency. This did not afford us the luxury of waiting for our own advanced vaccine manufacturing facilities to be set up to double-check the quality of a vaccine. In this case, it had already been tested by highly reputable world-class laboratories. Moreover the vaccine had undergone further preliminary tests in the US and France. Their findings indicated that the vaccine was safe.

However, what was becoming clearer by the minute was that Nuhasi and Bampa would never be influenced by such arguments. Yet they had absolutely no expertise or special skills in that particular area of research to offer. However, they succeeded in propelling to the top of the agenda the issue of safety of volunteers. I agreed with them that this was important but I was of the opinion that they had deliberately and grossly exaggerated the perceived risks for reasons best known to themselves. This led some participants, especially lay people, to get very concerned. It raised the issues of compensation of the participants in case of death or harm including HIV infection. Then a barrage of questions arose. Who would compensate the victims? What form would the compensation take? If anyone got infected how would we tell whether the vaccine had done it or the participants had become infected the usual way? If the participants were infected by a new recombinant HIV infection, how would it be stopped from spreading into the community before starting a new parallel epidemic?

Confused participants talked of preventing vaccinated participants from having sex with their spouses or sexual partners until safety was established. With a disease of such a long incubation period how long were they to abstain from sex until they were cleared to have a normal sex life? Who would police whether they had or did not have sex? The second possible scenario had to do with HIV infection from possible vaccine contamination. Who would pay for a lifetime of the then extremely expensive ARVs? At the time, both the state and study sponsors considered ARV treatment in Africa unaffordable and too cumbersome. The problems that needed to be addressed seemed to be overwhelming and insurmountable. And yet the rate at which Nuhasi and Bampa were identifying new scares about the vaccine was showing no sign of abating.

In the heat of the discussions, one of our American partners took me aside and whispered: "By the look of things this study is not going to be possible in Uganda. These guys are hell bent on ruining it for you."

I assured him that since I could not see any convincing reason to stop the study we just had to keep on repeating the facts until they were clearly understood by everyone. We owed it to Uganda and Africa to keep trying. "It is our cardinal duty as African scientists to actively participate in finding a scientific solution to a scourge that is annihilating our own people," I said to him, "and no scaremonger should divert us from this noble goal."

"But the tide of opinion seems to be turning against the study," he replied.

"We shall overcome," I replied. "Too many people have died. Many more are in the pipeline of death. Any possible risk as we try to find an AIDS vaccine needs to be measured against the current carnage," I argued.

"Then we must bring the two ringleaders to join us, as they seem to be determined to spoil it for everyone unless they are brought on board," he whispered.

"That would be like bribing them," I said heatedly. "No," I insisted. "It would set a bad precedent. We must not be blackmailed. We win or lose on facts. This study is so crucial that only scientists who have the necessary knowledge and who are ready to make scientifically applicable contributions must be involved."

"I am glad you think like that," he said, "but keeping those guys out there in the cold and not liking it may mess it up for you."

"I don't think so," I reassured him, "Lets allow free debate. The truth will emerge in the end, and see us through."

The truth was that the Europeans and Americans were not being annihilated by AIDS the same way as the Africans were. They already had access to ARV drugs that stopped their infected people from dying. On the contrary, Africa could not afford ARVs for the millions of their dying patients. Worse still, millions of Africa's young people were still being infected and joining the conveyer belt of death. In such dire circumstances, prevention was a crucial health measure that would help reduce the rates of new infections. If a vaccine was discovered, even if it was not one hundred percent effective, it would be a much more effective tool in the control of AIDS than other current preventive measures. Therefore it was wrong to leave this crucial work to other nations and people who were not facing such a disastrous problem. We could not expect them to be the ones to take all the risks. Being resource constrained and technically challenged did not mean that we could not find some important scientific answers that would constitute an important part of a solution to AIDS. At least we had it in our power to help by speedily testing promising vaccines. The sooner a vaccine was found, the earlier would the carnage of our people end.

If, on the other hand the candidate vaccine failed, it would not all be in vain. The lessons learnt would inform scientists that no more valuable time should be wasted on that kind of vaccine or line of research. It would be a signal for a quick return to the drawing board to look for an alternative, thus saving time and resources.

But as Nuhasi and Bampa raised more and more questions, the impression that some delegates got was that we had been duped by unscrupulous foreign scientists with ulterior motives or possibly even been compromised to jeopardise the lives of our fellow citizens. While this false accusation was bad enough, the situation in the meeting was rapidly getting worse as new and even more contentious issues were raised. The new bone of contention was that the ALVAC vaccine was based on Clade B HIV subtype which was the predominant subtype found in Europe and the USA. This was fuel for the already volatile situation. It became a rallying issue for all kinds of sceptics, including those who, for various other reasons did not support an HIV vaccine trial in the first place.

"If ALVAC, which is based on HIV Subtype B, which is found predominantly in Europe and USA, is tested here, then surely Ugandans are just guinea pigs," one delegate remarked, as a number of others nodded in agreement. Bampa and Nuhasi now had their smoking gun, which all delegates including non-scientists thought they could understand. "This is irrefutable proof," another participant echoed the concern.

Admittedly, it was true that the HIV in Uganda was almost exclusively of the subtypes A and D, while the ALVAC vaccine was based on subtype B. Therefore the opponents of the proposed study had a valid point. Not surprisingly, the general mood was now swinging decisively in their favour. I became anxious. It was much easier for people to understand that there was a difference between the HIV subtypes in Uganda and USA than the complexities of recombinant and molecular technology used for making the vaccine. Therefore this relatively easy-to-grasp concern captured most lay people's imaginations and, for a while, took centre stage. Understandably, a few of my colleagues who had hitherto supported me started having second thoughts too. Some were jolted into changing their minds because of the perceived irrelevance of the type of candidate vaccine for our country.

The earlier concerns were by and large relegated to the background. Some moderate delegates tried to help find a way forward. They suggested that if the vaccine trial went ahead, the study sponsors had to provide assurances that any participant who got harmed would be adequately compensated. Among these critics were those who erroneously believed that there were many Western study sponsors out there with plenty of money and vested interests in the vaccine ready to pay any price to ensure that the study went ahead. I knew that such participants were unaware of the tortuous journey to get the vaccine to Uganda. Looking back at everything I had been through, and what still lay ahead made me more determined to fight on. The reality was that we were having a very tough time finding sponsors for the study. In fact, at that point, none had made a firm commitment to provide funding for the study. And the controversy was certainly not helping.

Adding an extra requirement that the sponsors also become the study participants' safety guarantors was sure to bring the initiative to a screeching halt. I argued that we owned the study because it aimed at finding a solution to a scourge that was devastating our own people. Therefore, we too had a responsibility to share in the risk, if any. And if no one would take up the job of insuring participants, then our government needed to do it. What right did we have to expect others to undertake all the risks on our behalf and unashamedly turn up at the end of it all to reap the benefits of their sacrifice? In any case, it is the cardinal duty of any government worth its salt to provide medical care and protection to its citizens. The alternative would be to sit back and await future discovery of the subtype A and D-based candidate vaccines. But this, to me, would have been irresponsible, and a missed opportunity because there were some important scientific questions to be answered using a subtype B vaccine, even though it was based on a subtype that was not found in Uganda.

With regard to use of HIV subtype B-based vaccine, the example of the cowpox vaccine which provides protection against human smallpox came in handy. This was a clear case of one type of a virus disease being used to protect against a different but related virus infection. This scientific fact of cross reactivity to different subclasses of viruses was discovered centuries ago and it is for that reason that we still remember Edward Jenner. Therefore there was at least some basic scientific merit in trying to find out whether the subtype B-based vaccine would be protective against other HIV subtypes. After all, the relationship between the HIV subtypes that affect humans is much closer than that between cowpox and smallpox that affect different species. HIV subtypes are the same group of viruses that only differ slightly in limited numbers of genetic constitutions. Almost all subtypes are diagnosed using the same antibody tests and they are all treated by the same drugs with the exception of HIV2 found only in the minority of cases in West Africa. It would therefore be important to find out whether a subtype B vaccine provided protection against other HIV subtypes. The only way to find out whether this was the case was to test it. If no cross-protective properties were found, it would still provide vital data that would inform future scientific strategy in HIV vaccine development. We still did not know whether each subtype of HIV would need its own special vaccine. Perhaps, as is the case of polio vaccine, a cocktail based on a number of sub-types would be the answer.

There was another reason why we had opted to test this particular vaccine. At the time, there were just no subtype A or D vaccine constructs. The only available candidate HIV vaccines were all subtype B-based. The candidate vaccine we sought to test was called ALVAC (HIV vCP205) that had at that time only undergone testing in France and the USA – the subtype B areas. The findings from Europe and America could not be assumed to apply to Africa in general and Uganda in particular. Other additional advantages of going ahead with the research involved the fact that we would in the process be building our own capacity for future vaccine trials.

Fortunately, we did not have to belabour the issue of compensation as the Ugandan government was very supportive of AIDS alleviation initiatives and agreed to take responsibility for the participants in case the study caused them harm. With the issue of compensation and testing of HIV Clade B-based vaccine out of the way, any feeling of accomplishment was short-lived, as a new issue arose.

"As the aim of the study is to find out whether the vaccine can protect against AIDS, how would you know that it would give such protection unless you either injected the uninfected people with HIV or encouraged them to undertake risky behaviour?" one lay person asked. "This study is unethical. You plan to infect people with HIV," he cried out and others joined him in expressing their alarm. Not surprisingly, someone wrote a letter to the editor in the *New Vision* demanding that the scientists, including Mugerwa, Mbidde and myself, be the first to be vaccinated if we were so confident that it was safe.

It was difficult to make all lay people understand, especially those determined to find objections, that no participant would be exposed to HIV in this study. The only role of the participants involved injecting about half of the volunteers with the ALVAC vaccine construct, and the other half with a placebo or an approved safe vaccine. Thereafter, the study involved almost exclusively laboratory tests. It was a question of taking blood samples at regular intervals and measuring in the laboratory the amount of vaccine-induced antibodies, in the vaccinated volunteers as compared to those who had received the placebo. Secondly, only the cells of the participants would be exposed to the HIV virus in the laboratory, to check whether cells of those vaccinated with the trial vaccine were protected against HIV. In any case only HIV-low-risk participants were to be selected for the study and they would all be regularly counselled to reduce the chances of engaging in HIV-risky behaviour.

The ALVAC vaccine trial was to be the very first HIV vaccine ever to be tested in Africa, and we hoped it would break the ice and open a way for other trials on the continent. Africa would no longer be seen as a technologically challenged continent. Indeed, if a complicated high-tech AIDS vaccine trial could be carried out in Uganda, it could, by implication, be done in other resource-constrained countries. Above all, it would be a small step in the direction of ending the carnage. If it failed, it would be a long wait before Africa got another chance to test an HIV vaccine.

In hindsight, I must confess that I felt very disappointed that some of our own people did not appreciate the desperate situation and the urgent need to try and find a vaccine. Of course I appreciated the importance of consensus building and the need for dialogue. I have never had any problem with genuine discussion and alternative views, even if they conflicted with my own as long as this is done in good faith. And it was understandable that people may harbour misconceptions as the science of HIV vaccines was new to all of us.

At the end of the day there was a broad consensus that cleared the way for the pioneer vaccine study to go ahead. Further good news followed. The NIH of USA agreed to provide funds for the study through Family Health International, and a partnership with other scientists was also established. History was in the making.

However, I had no illusions regarding the challenge that still lay ahead.

Mount the Insurmountable

As the dust raised by the consensus building meetings and workshops started settling, I was relieved that, at long last, we could start on the nitty gritty of the trial itself. I soon realised that the optimism was, at best, premature. There, staring at me, was yet another mountain to surmount.

First a meticulously scientific research protocol needed to be written. This was in anticipation of a thorough review by both the Institutional Review Board (IRB), which consists of a group of independent scientists, non-scientists and community representatives, and the Uganda National Council for Science and Technology (UNCST). This was a prerequisite for the study to be carried out in the country. The UNCST is the overall authority in charge of scientific research in Uganda. The ALVAC vaccine research proposal was the most controversial and challenging UNCST had ever been presented with in its entire existence. As would be expected, the protocol was to be thoroughly scrutinised to ensure that there were no risks or mistakes. Therefore tough questions had to be anticipated, and answers prepared well in advance, otherwise queries would delay the already long held-up project further. With our national and international partnership of scientists on board, preparing a meticulous protocol that would pass assessment of a scientific review board was, perhaps, the easy part. The problem was that JCRC had no IRB. It was not only the JCRC that had no IRB at that crucial time; no other institution in Uganda had one either. Instead, there was an AIDS Research Subcommittee (ARS) that had been set up by the UNCST which mandated it to review and provide provisional approval of all AIDS research to be conducted in Uganda. It was established mainly to check some wearisome quacks like Gasket and unethical researchers who had started targeting Uganda because of the high rates of HIV/AIDS.

The volunteer subcommittee, of which I was a member, was headed by Edward Mbidde. It conducted business on a needs basis in the board room of Mulago National Referral and Teaching Hospital. The ARS had done a tremendous job of reviewing a variety of AIDS research proposals that ranged from AIDS herbal medicine protocols and Western drugs trials to epidemiological surveys. But never in its history had it faced such a highly complicated and controversial research proposal as was the case with the ALVAC vaccine trial.

Among the issues and queries that had arisen during the rather querulous vaccine preparatory consensus-building workshops was the urgent need for legal safeguards. In response, UNCST felt it had to establish a special independent committee to review the protocol over and above the review by the AIDS research subcommittee. Accordingly, a specially constituted committee reviewed the protocol, paying special attention to ethical and scientific merits of the proposed study. Among its final recommendations was the establishment of a Data and Safety Monitoring Board (DSMB) to oversee the study, especially the safety aspects.

As there was no specific law governing research on HIV vaccines in Uganda, it was also considered prudent to seek political approval, a usually cumbersome process even at the very best of times. Accordingly, a request seeking the approval of the cabinet and the national parliament was sent. Cabinet and parliament debated the pros and cons of conducting HIV vaccination in Uganda. It is difficult to express fully the impatience and frustration I felt about the long delay it caused. It seemed as if senior government role players did not feel the same urgency we in the scientific community did. The whole approval process took almost two years, which seemed to me like forever.

Some people argued that the delay was worthwhile because it allowed due diligence to be done, thus avoiding any dangerous mistakes, and that it would also help dispel the notion that Ugandans were being used as guinea pigs. Some of our foreign partners supporting the trial felt that the approval from the highest level of government was crucial because it would protect them from possible legal entanglements. In hindsight the silver lining was that one major obstacle to future vaccine trials in Uganda had been removed. The ice had been broken, and future trials would be able to proceed expeditiously.

After all that, it was time to start the intricate task of identifying suitable study participants. The delay had also given us time to make preliminary preparations. The priority was to educate potential participants and the community at large about the study, its benefits, possible risks involved and what it meant to be a volunteer on such studies. Education of and communication with the volunteers and the community about the proposed vaccine started right away. Information was disseminated directly to individuals and indirectly through community representatives and the mass media. In turn, the local media discussed, debated and disseminated the issues extensively. To keep the public updated and to handle any queries, an information desk was established with the help of the WHO in the Ministry of Health and a media liaison person was appointed. Although a few controversies arose, as was perhaps inevitable, the media on the whole did a good job. Media reports involved interviews with scientists and community representatives which helped explain some of the sophisticated science and other salient issues involved in testing HIV vaccines. The public asked questions regarding the risks involved in such trials, the benefits to individual participants and the community at large. Their views were respectfully considered and their questions and concerns addressed. It was realised that issues of public concern would keep popping up throughout the trial period and perhaps beyond.

Also identified during the workshops was the need for a special community advisory board (CAB). The main task of the CAB was to represent community interests and act as a link between the community and scientists. Consequently, the first Uganda CAB, also one of the first in Africa, was set up. Among the members were a community educator, an ALVAC vaccine trial volunteer, a parish priest, a journalist, an administrative officer, a nursing officer with the Uganda Police and a counsellor from the women's prison in Kampala. In preparation for their role as community watchdogs, CAB members discussed vaccine trial issues with scientists and also held their own workshops.

It was acknowledged that for the vaccine trial to succeed, a variety of experts from diverse institutions would be needed. We succeeded in forming unprecedented partnerships that had never before been thought possible. The consortium consisted of the JCRC, Makerere University, the Uganda Virus Research Institute (UVRI), and two American institutions, namely Massachusetts General Hospital and Case Western Reserve University (CWRU). The next task was to identify, recruit and train local technologists and scientists to work on the trial. The JCRC staff underwent an intensive crash course in the science of HIV/AIDS vaccine research. Hands-on training conducted by experts from the USA took place on site. At the same time, a number of our staff were sent abroad for advanced short-term training.

Among the scientists who were identified for the advanced scientific work was a brilliant medical doctor, Catherine Othieno, who was sent for training in the USA. She was among the very first Ugandans to be trained in advanced laboratory techniques crucial for measurement of vaccine response. All the clinicians, scientists and other staff involved in the study received training in good clinical and laboratory practices.

While all the pieces seemed to start falling into place, and as the seemingly insurmountable problems were being overcome, one nagging predicament still haunted me. In between all the discussions, debates and meetings that were held as part of intensive lobbying to get the vaccine trial going at the JCRC, I paced up and down the narrow corridors of our main laboratory. The more I paced in and around the former residence of the Buganda Kingdom's prime minister that we had converted into laboratories and an AIDS clinic, the more I worried. I could clearly see that there was no room in the neat but battered old building to accommodate the vaccine trial laboratory. None at all!

Ready at Last

Having come this far, there was no turning back. Room for the vaccine laboratory just had to be conjured up somewhere, somehow. But the reality was that all the space in the clinic was fully occupied and, in most cases, crammed. Our two doctors had only a small office room each, in which they examined patients, and there was no other space.

I strolled into one of the rooms, looked around and then surprised the doctor when I told him that I was going to convert his office into a new HIV vaccine laboratory. He thought I was joking until a few days later, when he found his desk and examination couch missing from his office. However, one clinic space was not enough. The doctor next door who had began to celebrate the survival of his clinic space, suffered the same fate. His office had to be sacrificed too.

At the risk of destabilising the structure of the battered old building, we demolished the wall in between the two clinics to create space for the laboratory. I then pitched a large tent in the clinic compound, and relocated the doctors' consultation clinics there. I hoped that this would not affect their self-esteem, having to work in such makeshift surroundings.

Having somehow come up with the precious space, though hardly sufficient, I faced another dilemma. I had no inkling of what a vaccine trial laboratory looked like. I had never seen one. I turned to our US partners who identified Bruce Walker, a clinical trials' expert who knew much more than I would ever know about laboratories. He came up with a simple but highly practical design. With the help of our study sponsors we acquired the state-of-the-art equipment and soon we were all set to evaluate the very first HIV vaccine on the African continent. The laboratory was also the first of its kind in the region. We developed it to acceptable international standards, incorporating strict quality assurance and quality control practices.

Having set up the laboratory, the next requirement was to standardise the laboratory procedures, carry out test runs and establish normal baseline parameters among normal HIV-negative Ugandans. Obviously, if we did not know the "normal" we could not accurately measure the changes brought about by the vaccine. Everything had to be arranged meticulously, and tested out so that when the actual trial started it would run smoothly.

Even the logistics for delivery of the vaccine from France to Uganda were tested out. We needed to be absolutely sure that the priceless vaccine would remain safe and effective during shipment. We were told that there was so little of it that every drop mattered. A slight rise in temperature would destroy the precious cargo and set the project back for a long time. A dry run from Paris in a container similar to the one that would be used for the actual vaccine but containing a placebo and a thermometer was done. On arrival at the JCRC laboratory, the container was thoroughly examined and the temperature measured. It was smiles all around. The package had arrived in pristine condition and the temperature inside the container was just right.

Meanwhile, in the laboratory things were going well. It was quite evident that Dr Catherine Othieno, whom we had hired as our laboratory scientist, was equal to the exacting task ahead. All local and international monitors judged us ready to go ahead.

The groundbreaking study involved recruitment of HIV-negative adults. Volunteers were pre-screened for appropriate social and behavioural history to make sure that people found to exhibit risky behaviour which could expose them to HIV were excluded. This study needed participants who had the highest possible chance of remaining HIV negative. Any participant who got infected would compromise the objectives of the trial. It was also vital that the participants fully understood what the study was all about, and that their decision to participate was truly voluntary. Therefore qualifying volunteers were extensively educated about the study purpose, procedures, and HIV risk reduction behaviour by our specially trained counsellors.

It was explained in simple language that the trial vaccine was not known to provide protection against HIV, and that not every participant was being vaccinated with a real test vaccine. Some were only getting air supply, we elaborated. It was further explained that the trial was a very early test to assess the vaccine safety, and to check whether it caused special cells in the body to react by producing protective antibodies against HIV. Besides individual counselling, volunteers participated in group counselling. In these sessions they were encouraged to ask questions and to bring a relative along if they so wished. A copy of the consent form was given to the participant to take home and discuss with his family before finally deciding whether to join or not. At the end of it all, they were tested for their knowledge about the trial by an independent group of social scientists. Only those who passed the test were allowed to proceed.

I kept my fingers crossed – anxious and vigilant that nothing went wrong. I was anxious to avoid giving credence or justification to sceptics who never see anything good done in or coming out of Africa. These included the likes of Bampa and Nuhasi. I realised that there would be no shortage of people who would cry, "I warned you," if anything went wrong.

The Bridge over River Mayanja

Just as I was beginning to think that we were home and dry, something did go wrong — seriously wrong! It was my worst nightmare came true.

On the evening of 29 March 1998 the disaster that threatened to halt the study struck. That fateful day, Dr Catherine Othieno, our key laboratory scientist, her husband Dr Michael Sempa, and a number of their close friends including Dr Francis Xavier Mubiru and Dr James Nalumenya, all dressed to the nines, left Kampala early in the morning in a taxi minibus. Their destination was the town of Hoima, the capital of the ancient Kingdom of Bunyoro situated about 200 km west of Kampala. The purpose of their journey was to attend an engagement ceremony, known in one of the Ugandan language as *kwanjula*, of their colleague. As is usually the case, everyone must have been in a party mood and the atmosphere euphoric. The joy, excitement and anticipation must have been even more for the bridegroom to be who travelled in a different car. He must have looked forward to the traditional ceremonies, I presume, with some curiosity and awe since he was not Ugandan.

The journey to the home of the parents of the to-be-bride passed uneventfully, except for a heavy downpour as the party crossed River Mayanja, almost halfway to the venue. At that time Uganda was experiencing torrential El Niño rains that had flooded many areas, destroyed crops and swept away many homes. The colourful ceremony full of traditional rituals and festivities was a spectacular success. Traditional dancers sang and performed for the guests while they feasted. Entertainment interspersed with engagement ceremonies and speeches went on until evening.

On their way back, obviously still in a festive mood, the driver ignored frenzied hand waves of children and some adults who tried to stop him as he concentrated on manoeuvring the vehicle along the waterlogged, uneven gravel road as he descended towards the narrow bridge over River Mayanja, at a place called Wamika. As he sped on, he ignored more people who frantically brandished tree branches and anything they could lay their hands on in a futile effort to flag him down. No one can really be sure what was on the driver's mind, but by the time he realised what the frantic waves were all about, it was far too late!

Unknown to them, while they were celebrating in Hoima, torrential rain in the area had swollen the River Mayanja, bursting its banks and washing away the bridge. There were no survivors! Early the next morning, news of the tragedy hit us hard at the JCRC. We were devastated. It took an agonising two days to find Catherine's body. Fortunately, Catherine and Michael's newborn baby had been left back home.

The country, especially JCRC and the Ministry of Health, had lost highly trained scientists and healthcare providers that Uganda needed desperately. Catherine, in whom we had invested so much, had already proven her worth by winning the trust of all our partners in this crucial pioneer research initiative. We relied on her to carry out the complicated tests in the newly established vaccine laboratory. Our HIV vaccine trial preparations had been dealt a devastating blow.

At that late stage, it was virtually impossible to identify and train another high-calibre Ugandan to take her laboratory leadership role in time to keep the trial on schedule. I was left with two Ugandan technologists, Steven Mutalya and Martin Okello, who had been trained to assist Catherine in her work. After consultation with our American partners, an interim solution that allowed the study to proceed as scheduled was found. An American expert Norman Jones from Massachusetts General Hospital was identified to fill the gap left by Catherine and to continue the training of the two Ugandan technologists. Jones returned from time to time to support our team and we were able to keep the project on track.

The recruitment of study participants on trial started in February 1999. In total 40 volunteers were recruited, of whom 20 received the real HIV vaccine, and of the rest, ten received a placebo and another ten received rabies vaccine that was made using the same ALVAC technology used for the HIV vaccine. The inclusion of rabies vaccine also triggered a debate of its own. Some scientists expressed concern about its inclusion as a control since it appeared that the information coming out of the rabies vaccine part of the trial would be solely for the benefit of the manufacturer. However, it was justified on the grounds that it involved a beneficial vaccine for a lethal disease that was also endemic in our region. If indeed some information came out, the findings would be in our interests too.

That memorable day of 8 February 1999 will go down in history as the day when the first volunteer received the very first HIV test vaccine on the African continent. The occasion was attended by some of our American partners.

In contrast to the hullabaloo of the preparatory stages of the study, the actual vaccine trial was characterised by quiet hard work. It involved intensive follow-up of participants and careful attention to details. When it finally got going it ran almost like clockwork. Considering all that we had to go through, including the untimely death of our key scientist, it had looked like the study would never start. But six months later on 30 August 1999, it was a great relief and a time for celebrations to witness the last vaccination of the fortieth volunteer. "At long last," I said to myself, "it is finally over. We did it!"

Our success in completing the study on schedule not only silenced the prophets of doom but sent a clear message to announce to the scientific community and the world at large. First of all, no participants defaulted on clinic visits. A staggering 95% of visits and vaccinations were completed on the exact scheduled clinic visit dates. What made this achievement even more remarkable was the fact that the study participants included soldiers, some of whom were highly mobile. Our research team followed them all up, in some cases to as far as the border with the Democratic Republic of Congo. This in itself, the results notwithstanding, was a great achievement.

It was a triumph for Africa as a whole, and Uganda in particular because it demonstrated the feasibility of the state-of-the-art vaccine trials in Africa. It proved that the usual excuses for denial of research opportunities to Africa, including inadequate infrastructure and lack of human resources, are either red herrings or obstacles that can be overcome. It also showed that seemingly complicated ethical and socio-political issues regarding vaccine trials and other scientific challenges in Africa are not, as often believed, insurmountable.

In addition, we learnt that developing and developed countries can work together to overcome mutual constraints and harness joint strengths in order to find solutions to mankind's scientific challenges and world emergencies. The ALVAC trial was a small demonstration of what could be achieved if such partnerships were part of the new world order.

Successful conduct of a pioneer HIV vaccine trial in Sub-Saharan Africa also defined a way forward by opening many other doors for future HIV vaccine trials. Indeed, preparations for more HIV vaccine trials followed immediately, in Kenya, South Africa and other countries. Scientists started to develop new HIV vaccines tailored to HIV clades predominant in Africa. These included clades A, D constructs tailored to East Africa, and Clade C vaccine constructs aimed at southern Africa. In Uganda, it paved the way for another vaccine trial that followed at the Uganda Virus Research Institute and Makerere University College of Health Sciences. Meanwhile, several different international groups and organisations, including IAVI, Walter Reed, and National Institute of Health, considered new vaccine trials in partnerships with African countries.

However, more work still lies ahead before Africa can be accepted fully into the elite scientific circles of the world. However, this successful HIV vaccine trial in Uganda was a step towards that goal.

Results

The long awaited trial results were sweet and bitter.

In summary, the trial findings raised more questions than answers but it was not a failure in any sense of the word. A negative result from a scientific experiment or trial is often taken as synonymous with failure. The finding that an experimental drug or vaccine did not work as expected does not mean that no new scientific lesson was learnt. In the case of the ALVAC vaccine, no serious scientist had expected that it would be robust enough to be immediately usable as a public HIV-preventive vaccine. At this early stage of its development it was only suitable for testing and to answer a few basic questions including whether it was safe and if it was able to elicit sufficient antibodies against HIV. Only if it passed this primary phase would it be appropriate to take it forward for testing on a wider scale to determine its effectiveness. If on the other hand it showed that it was poor at inducing protective antibodies, then scientists would go back to design alternative strategies to overcome that deficiency.

With regard to the specific objectives of the ALVAC trial, we were delighted to find that the safety profile of the vaccine was excellent. Other than mild inflammation on the site of vaccination, no adverse side effects of any concern occurred in any participant. But we were disappointed to find that it did not induce sufficient protective antibodies against HIV. It did indeed provoke some production of HIV-specific antibodies but these were not robust enough to protect against HIV infection. However, there was evidence that a subtype B-based vaccine was able to induce antibodies that could cross-react against the HIV subtype A and D viruses, which are the predominant in Uganda. However, once again, the antibodies were not in adequate amounts to offer any protection.

The information that was provided by the ALVAC study was important and made a significant contribution to our knowledge in the continuing search for an HIV vaccine. It also informed the urgent need to widen the search by investigating other novel approaches, including the then emerging science of DNA-based vaccines.

Soon after the trial I received many enquiries from all over world about how we were able to do what had a few years earlier been considered almost impossible. I was invited by *Elsevier*, a reputable science peer-reviewed periodical, to write an article about our experience. This was an opportunity to answer many questions, and I did so in an article entitled *HIV Vaccines: The Uganda Experience*, in which I reported my personal perspectives of HIV vaccines. However, a more comprehensive account of what transpired was published in the *British Medical Journal* by the entire research team on 26 January 2002.

Whenever I reflect on this groundbreaking vaccine trial, I remember the tragic event of 29 March 1998. Perhaps the only semblance of a consolation out of this debacle was the summons that I was served to the High Court to give evidence in support of the families of the victims of the accident who had sued the government for compensation. I saw this as an opportunity to do something, though small, for Catherine, her husband and especially their young child. As I sat on a bench outside the high court awaiting my turn in the witness box, I asked the child's grandfather how the child was doing. I shouldn't have. A tear materialised from the corner of his eye. I had gathered from other sources that the child was doing well. Many of Catherine's friends in Uganda and US had pulled together to ensure that the child was taken care of, at least in the short term.

It took a whole decade before justice was done. The morning of 2 September 2009, I woke to the headline in the Ugandan daily, *New Vision; Government to Pay Sh500 Million for Doctors' Deaths*. Apparently the High Court had on the previous day finally ruled that the doctors perished due to the negligence of the police who failed to warn motorists or block the road leading to the bridge and divert the traffic. It was revealed at the trial that the police were aware that the bridge had been washed away but failed to act.

In recent years the relief brought about by increased access to ARV drugs is certainly justified because of the millions of lives that are being saved. However, finding a safe and effective HIV vaccine remains one of the most promising strategies for HIV prevention, especially in Africa the, the main victim of this pandemic.

Step Down

In the midst of frustrations resulting from repeated failures of HIV vaccine trials, we were suddenly pleasantly surprised by the announcement of a breakthrough from an unexpected and, some would say, a most unlikely source.

The new beacon of hope that promised to be an amazing scientific breakthrough came not from the most advanced laboratories in the world; incredibly, it came from brothels in the Kenyan capital, Nairobi! Implausibly, it was a special group of commercial sex workers (CSWs) who, against all logic, seemed to hold the key to the mysterious puzzle of an HIV vaccine. Initially, mesmerised scientists could not quite believe their eyes, as they observed that some sex workers were apparently immune despite repeated exposure to their HIV-infected clients. In effect, this special group of prostitutes had demonstrated the existence of highly effective protective immunity against HIV. At that time, all that was known about prostitution with any certainty was the very opposite — that it was one of the biggest risk factor for HIV, and that CSWs had the highest rates of HIV infection in the community.

Scientists set out to determine why this group of CSWs had a unique protective advantage against HIV that other fellow CSWs or, indeed, other HIV-exposed people lacked. Their blood was examined intensively to try and identify whatever it was that gave them this extraordinary defence against the dreaded disease which was daily infecting their fellow CSWs and thousands of other people including those with much less risky exposure. Finally, scientists found that these particular CSWs had an increased number of special defensive cells (T lymphocytes) that had been activated by repeated exposure to target HIV. This finding suggested that if a vaccine which could similarly boost the specific T lymphocyte responses was found, it could likewise protect against HIV infection.

The pharmaceutical company Merck followed up this lead, among others, in an effort to develop a vaccine that could imitate the kind of protection the sex workers seemed to have. Merck scientists took in account all lessons learned from long observation of AIDS infectivity in nature and all previous vaccine trials, and came up with novel ways to stimulate the body to produce more anti-HIV antibodies than ever before. Indeed, in its early stages of development, their candidate vaccine was remarkably promising. By 2003, after years of research and a number of small pilot studies, Merck reckoned that their vaccine was ready for final testing.

When news about the Merck breakthrough reached us, the spontaneous excitement we felt was only dampened by scientific prudence that necessitated caution until D-day, when its efficacy would be announced officially. The technology used by Merck to develop the new vaccine and ensure its safety was based on the same principle as the ALVAC vaccine that we had tested earlier at JCRC, whereby a bird virus was used as a conveyor of the HIV genes. Merck used a deactivated type of common cold virus called adenovirus instead of canarypox to carry and transport into the body the synthetically produced genes or the tiny fragment of HIV that were inserted into it. Merck selected the adenovirus hoping that it would do a better job of stimulating the body to generate a potent immune response to HIV than the canarypox did. It was expected that this would lead to the production of an "army" of killer T cells that would recognise, target and kill HIV-infected cells, thus preventing the establishment of HIV as an infection. Indeed, the preliminary data had been so impressive that many people had taken its subsequent success in a wider trial for granted. If it was successful, the countdown to the utopia of an AIDS-free world would begin to be seen as a possibility.

Meanwhile, Merck searched for sites that could participate in the landmark trial. I held discussions with some Merck representatives trying to secure a slot for the JCRC among the network of trial sites.

However, despite my intensive efforts, we were, to my profound disappointment, unsuccessful. This was explained to me as having been due to HIV epidemiological considerations. I agreed with their choice of South Africa as one of the main trial sites because, at the time the epicentre of HIV was in southern Africa and it was their predominant HIV subtype C that was spreading fastest on the continent.

The start of Merck's vaccine study was announced on 19 September 2003. In a widely quoted media release Merck stated that the trial was to begin in 18 cities in the United States, Puerto Rico, Brazil, Haiti, Malawi, Peru, South Africa and Thailand. The trial was innovative in several aspects. It was the very first trial of an HIV candidate vaccine to take place in so many global locations simultaneously. The statement further exalted the benefits of the unique partnership:

> This effort is an example of the type of public/private partnership that brings collective strengths to bear on one of the world's most serious health problem. With approximately 14,000 new HIV infections each day, 95 percent of which occur in developing countries, testing vaccine candidates in all affected regions, and in locations in which there are different viral strains, is of crucial importance.

The trial came to be known as the STEP trial. It began enrolling participants at 28 sites all over the world in December 2004 and ultimately signed up 3,000 people. Merck hoped that besides protecting uninfected people from getting HIV, the vaccine would also be beneficial to people already infected with HIV. The expectation was that the HIV-specific T-cell response would offer enough protection to slow down the infection by suppressing the viral load, with no or little need for antiretroviral therapy.

Meanwhile, to us healthcare providers in Sub-Saharan Africa where HIV was continuing to spread like wildfire, this announcement was good news. We hoped for the success of the vaccine and, indeed, waited for a favourable outcome with bated breath as the study continued. For over three years, all we heard was that the trial was proceeding well. Then suddenly the failure of what had promised to be the most important breakthrough since the outbreak of the AIDS pandemic was announced on 21 September 2007. In part the announcement stated:

The Data Safety and Monitoring Board concluded that the vaccine cannot be shown in this trial to prevent HIV infection or affect the course of the disease in those who become infected with HIV. Therefore, Merck instructed all study sites to cease administering the investigational vaccine. The same candidate HIV vaccine is also being tested in South Africa, in a clinical trial known as the Phambili study. The Phambili study has now been paused.

The news dealt a devastating blow to HIV vaccine development initiatives, and was a great setback to HIV prevention. The news was announced under such headings as: Merck abandons HIV vaccine trials. A step backwards. Vaccine study brought to a screeching halt, and so on.

Some people in the scientific community pessimistically voiced their frustration going as far as stating that an effective HIV vaccine would "never be discovered", while others said that an entirely new scientific approach would be needed and would require the involvement of young and more open-minded scientists. Once again, it was back to the drawing board. If this was a sad day for industry, to the anxiously waiting public health professionals and millions of people in Sub-Saharan Africa, especially the young generation whose lives remained at stake, this was shattering news.

Some of the findings were particularly unsettling. In the uncircumcised group of participants, the vaccine inexplicably seemed to increase infectivity. But in contrast, among the circumcised, it seemed to offer some degree of protection. What did this mean? Scientists started looking more closely at men's prepuces, trying to find out what it was that seemed to increase HIV infectivity.

When the dust settled and a more reasoned look was taken at the data it started to emerge that the gloom expressed about the STEP study failure was perhaps not the whole story. Statements to the effect that HIV vaccine would never be discovered reminded me of the pre-ARV days, when it was also said that effective AIDS treatment would never be found but only three years later Highly Active Antiretroviral Therapy (HAART), which was to revolutionise the treatment of AIDS, was discovered.

I shared the sentiments of Richard Jefferys, an HIV vaccine activist affiliated with the New York Treatment Action Group, who said at the time, "I think that disappointment is certainly justified, while despair would be premature." Reassuringly, some others also viewed the findings with measured optimism. "A trial is only a failure if we don't learn anything from it," said Seth Berkley, then the President of the International AIDS Vaccine Initiative (IAVI). It was indeed true that there was a lot to learn from the STEP study that would advance vaccine development efforts. Lessons learnt extended beyond mere HIV vaccine development and included learning something about how HIV causes disease (pathogenesis), especially during the very early stages of HIV infection; the mechanisms of protection; how the body's immune system responds to it; and why it fails to control it.

It emerged that HIV causes most substantial damage within the first weeks of infection and yet this crucial early stage is not widely studied in humans because infection is usually detected only when it has been established awhile, by which time it has caused substantial damage to the immune system. Secondly, the gut, especially the mucosal areas, seem to be where most HIV immune activation takes place. This implies that the gut plays a bigger role in HIV infection than previously realised. Further research involving long-term non-progressors (HIV-infected people whose infection progresses slower than expected), and discordant couples (where only one partner is infected), may help to unlock the mysteries of the role of the mucosal and systemic immune responses. The science involved is beyond the scope of this book.

In retrospect, the reaction to the announcement of vaccine failure should not have been so despondent. For almost three decades, the science of HIV had been a long frustrating story of endless challenges, despite the input of some of the best of scientific brains and the very latest technological advances. We should remember that many great scientific discoveries come about against the background of infamous failures.

Thai Success

Never giving up finally paid off — sort of.

The announcement made on 24 September 2009 at a special media conference, called jointly by the US army, the main sponsor of the HIV vaccine trial, and the Thai Ministry of Public Health, caused great excitement the world over. At long last, after twenty years of frustrating failures, an HIV vaccine that worked had been found. It was carried as a major story in virtually every print and electronic news media. *The Daily Monitor*, a Ugandan independent daily, surprised me with a call before I got the full details of the still developing story, and wanted me to comment on the newsflash. I just could not conceal my enthusiasm, but regretted that I could not make any comment before I had reviewed the whole study report.

Earlier on, I had learned that the landmark study that involved over 16,000 participants in eight sites in Thailand, took six years to complete and had cost a whopping US$105 million. Unlike the Merck study, not many scientists had paid attention to this vaccine trial because it was expected to flop, just like all the others before it. The failure of the STEP study was still ringing loudly in many peoples' ears. Added to this, the two main components that constituted the Thai vaccine were not new. One of them was a canarypox carrier in which HIV genes were inserted to make the candidate vaccine. This concept was similar to the first vaccine we tested at the JCRC, when, as described above, the results fell short of expectation. Therefore, as far as some scientists were concerned, failure was almost guaranteed. In fact, the US National Institute of Allergy and Infectious Diseases had turned down support for another similar study in 2002. As the study was starting in 2004, 22 leading AIDS researchers gave it the thumbs down. They published their views in an editorial in *Science Magazine*, pouring cold water on any hope of a breakthrough.

Interestingly, I found out later that controversial issues not dissimilar to the ones that arose when we prepared for our first HIV vaccine had surfaced in Thailand. Whispers that the vaccine would infect participants with HIV and that they would go on to infect others were rife. The media quoted a 36 year-old volunteer by the name of Saichon Booncharoen, explaining the dilemma: "At first, I was scared I would become a guinea pig and that they would inject us with AIDS." Some others feared losing their jobs or girlfriends if word spread that they were involved in an AIDS vaccine study.

As I learned of the issues that arose in Thailand, I kept nodding at each one as I recognised the similarity to those that bogged down our first trial. I could even imagine the Thai versions of Bampa and Nuhasi predicting all kinds of disasters if the study went ahead. But I also realised that the issues raised in Thailand were not entirely of Thai origin. The uncanny similarities with some of those raised in our trial were too much of a coincidence. During our trial I had been

262   *A Cure Too Far*

concerned about donors bringing to the forefront some issues which were not always applicable in our circumstances.

The devastation of AIDS was very well known to those who volunteered for the study. Thailand was the first country in Asia to be hit hard by AIDS, just as Uganda was the first in Africa. One of the participants by the name of Tanad Yomaha, who had lost a sister and a brother-in-law to AIDS, summed up the dire situation.

"In the 1980s, the coffin business was booming around here," she said. "The temple here had at least one cremation ceremony every night and people were in perpetual mourning."

Therefore volunteers, 16,402 from diverse backgrounds, many with personal sad stories of their own, ignored the false rumours and enrolled on the study. By so doing, they sought to be part of the solution to their national disaster, as Saichom elaborated further on his reasons for participation in the trial. "I spoke to my parents and local doctors and thought about it for months. Eventually I decided I wanted to do this to be part of something bigger, something beyond myself."

Successful participation in vaccine trials is no mean feat. It involves significant intrusion on volunteers' time and privacy. It involves exposure of very personal information, including sexual and behavioural details, to the scientists. It commits the participant to undertake frequent visits to the clinics where numerous blood samples are taken. Volunteers are subjected to regular HIV and sexually transmitted disease tests. In the case of the Thai study, this went on for six years. Despite all this, an incredible 90% of the participants persisted to the very end of the study.

Considering the disappointment associated with all previous HIV vaccine trials, the media extravaganza surrounding the announcement of the Thai success on that memorable Thursday, 24 September 2009, is understandable. When the excitement calmed down, attention shifted to the details. It was soon realised that the success was not entirely what it appeared to be. What followed were different descriptions and interpretations of the results.

Basically, the researchers had set the goal of success at 50% protection. But the trial vaccine did not meet this goal or even come close to it! So what was the hullabaloo all about? The justification for the enthusiastic reception of the results is perhaps better understood if it is considered from a broader perspective. The trial vaccine cut the risk of HIV infection by 31.2%, which was statistically significant, but only just. At the time an estimated 7,500 people were being infected by HIV daily. UNAIDS had estimated that two million people had died of AIDS in 2007. When considered from this viewpoint, the 31%, though small, still meant significant numbers in terms of lives that would be saved.

Perhaps the best person to put all this in context was one of the world's recognised experts, Tony Fauci, the director of the National Institute of Allergy and Infectious Diseases, which was one of the trial's backers. Fauci had this to say:

> I don't want to use a word like 'breakthrough' but I don't think there's any doubt that this is a very important result. For more than twenty years now, vaccine trials have essentially been failures. Now it's like we were groping down an unlit path and a door has been opened. We can start asking some very important questions.

It is however true that the publicity was disproportionate. When the results were subjected to sombre scrutiny, the true picture emerged. Seventy-four of the participants in the placebo arm of the study got infected, compared to 51 in the vaccine arm. That small difference is basically what the excitement was all about. Incongruously, it was found out that the infected people in both arms of the study had the same numbers of viruses in their blood, suggesting that the vaccine had no effect on the course of HIV disease. If it was not for the previous 20 years of grim news, it is doubtful that such marginal results would have been newsworthy. But dismissing the study outright would have been wrong too. Vaccines remain one of the most effective ways of disease control known to science. And vaccines are one of the most effective ways to end a vicious viral epidemic. Therefore all participants who took part in all previous vaccine trials and all of those who will do so in future are genuine heroes for volunteering for such a noble cause. It is therefore crucial to ponder the important questions, that Fauci referred to in order to map out the way forward. Among them is need to study the immunological pathway for the protection that was observed, albeit modest. However, what has since become abundantly clear is that this vaccine is not the one that will end the epidemic. The greatest value of the findings is perhaps the renewed faith in the feasibility of HIV vaccines that it inspired.

If science could build on this, a process that would take years, and combine it with lessons learnt from other vaccine trials and emerging knowledge, and add on other preventive measures, including universal treatment, then the end of the vicious epidemic that has killed over thirty million people and has left another thirty million living with the virus, could be contemplated.

Despite all the setbacks and this one glimmer of hope that was not as strong as desired, it is undeniable that progress has been made. It is now no longer a question of "if", but of "when" an effective HIV vaccine will finally be discovered.

10

Interim Cure

Mission of Mercy

Although Highly Active Antiretroviral Therapy (HAART) was not a cure, it was powerful enough to save millions of lives, prevent millions of new infections, including some dreadful cancers — and do all this without coming anywhere near to curing the dreaded disease. Considering the then dire circumstances — when virtually all AIDS patients died - it was a great interim cure!

HAART first became available in 1995. As described in *Genocide by Denial*, the breakthrough came at a time when hope for an effective treatment was fading. It was being said quite openly and even by some high ranking scientists that effective AIDS treatment would never be found. By then, a handful of ARV drugs had been discovered but each had individually failed to effectively control the HIV virus. It was then found that in triple combination they were so effective that the treatment was dubbed Highly Active Antiretroviral Therapy (HAART). It looked like nothing would ever surpass the power of this new therapy. In fact some authorities initially thought that it would end up as an AIDS cure if used correctly and for long enough but within a short time this hope was dimmed. The search for safer, more user-friendly and effective drugs against emerging resistant viruses has been going on.

While the rest of the world quickly adopted HAART as the standard of care for their AIDS patients, it was too expensive for the people in Sub-Saharan Africa who were in desperate need. This was the main reason why we kept on trying to reinvent the wheel while the carriages were out there running. Sometimes I felt as if we lived on a different planet with a different terrain, necessitating a special wheel!

By the year 2002, seven years after the discovery of HAART, which President George W. Bush later described as "miraculous medicines", millions of Africans were still dying from what in developed countries had become an easily treatable chronic disease. Worse still, there were no prospects on the horizon for AIDS-afflicted Africa to access HAART. The absurd excuses given to explain this appalling situation would be laughable if they had not contributed to the prolongation of the AIDS bloodbath in Africa.

Fortunately, the bleak AIDS situation in Africa was changed, by the pronouncement at the annual US State of the Union address on 28 January 2003. Within a few years, virtually all Sub-Saharan African countries were successfully using combination ARV drugs that were previously alleged to be unfeasible to use in Africa's public health sector. As numbers of patients on ARV Therapy soared, the death rates declined, and it became evident within a relatively short period that the carnage in Uganda and other parts of Africa was being alleviated.

Although I briefly covered the case of South Africa in *Genocide by Denial*, it is necessary to revisit the topic because the country has the biggest number of PLWHIV in the world today. South Africa, the richest country in Africa, delayed introducing ARVs because of leadership flaws and denial. Even when the efficacy of HAART was abundantly clear, the late Mantombazana 'Manto' Edmie Tshabalala-Msimang, South Africa's minister of health from 1999 to 2008, continued to amaze the world by her refusal to embrace ARVs. Her boss, President Mbeki was alleged to have been misled by so-called AIDS dissidents, who included David Rasnick and Peter Duesberg, whom Mbeki sought out to provide him with their views on AIDS. Even as late as 2002, when the cause of HIV was no longer in any doubt, the devastation it had caused in Africa was being decried the world over, and the effective role of ARVs proven beyond any reasonable doubt, David Rasnick was still unrepentant.

"I don't think there is any such thing as AIDS going on in South Africa. Its just the same old things that Africans have been suffering and dying from for generations due to poverty, malnutrition, poor sanitation, bad water, that sort of thing. We are calling it AIDS now instead of by the old-fashioned names that were more honest," Rasnick said.

He did not bother to explain why the death rate had, since mid 1980's, suddenly accelerated to such a devastating scale. "It is not a disease, and HIV is an Orwellian deception. It is not an immune deficiency virus. It is just one of thousands of retroviruses. First of all you can't even find it in a human being," Rasnick, who went as far as suggesting that "all HIV testing should be banned on principle and that South Africa should stop screening supplies of blood," added. When challenged to explain the AIDS epidemic in America and Europe Rasnick had this to say: "Peter Duesberg and I are convinced that AIDS in USA and Europe is the clinical manifestation of the drug epidemic in both places," he explained. With advisors like this, it is no wonder that President Mbeki went on record as expressing doubt as to whether HIV caused AIDS.

Tshabalala-Msimang, echoing the frequent assertions of AIDS dissidents and especially vitamin and so called immune booster peddlers, frequently referred to ARVs as very toxic and ineffective. Her tenure as minister became highly controversial because of her much publicised initial reluctance to accept public sector use of antiretroviral drugs. Instead, she preached treatment of AIDS with vegetables and was nicknamed Dr Beetroot for promoting beetroot, garlic, lemon peel and so-called African potatoes, as effective and non-toxic treatment for AIDS. Yet among the studies carried out at the University of Stelenbosch in South Africa on her chosen African potato, it was found that its extract was toxic to bone marrow, and lowered immunity as evidenced by a drop in CD4 cell count. This caused the study to be abandoned hastily to protect participants. But "Dr Beetroot" ignored this evidence and in addition, promoted vitamins and other kinds of food supplements. She was also accused of acting as an advocate of Mathias Rath, a German doctor who was in turn accused of discouraging the use of ARVs in order to promote his huge vitamin business.

Rath launched a protracted campaign against the South African Treatment Action Campaign group (TAC), which was trying to stop the carnage in South Africa by increasing access to life saving ARVs. To their dismay, advertisements alleged to be linked to Rath suddenly appeared and were widely distributed in South Africa stating: "TAC medicines are killing you. Stop AIDS genocide by the drug cartel." But this did not end there. The head of TAC Zackie Achmat was dragged to the International Criminal Court in The Hague accused of genocide for successfully campaigning to increase access to ARVs for the people of South Africa and demanding that he be "severely punished with the highest sentence provided for under the Rome Statute".

The outrage that Tshabalala-Msimang's policies and her tolerance of dissident views against the background of an estimated hundreds of thousands of deaths during her tenure as minister of health was so intense that by the time she died on 16 December 2009, many activists were calling for her to face genocide charges. Certainly the majority of deaths could have been avoided by timely and proper use of ARVs, which her misguided policies denied the people of South Africa for so long.

To the relief of millions of South African AIDS sufferers, the situation changed for the better after the Mbeki regime. Hundreds of thousands of lives have been saved, as the country has since become the biggest user of ARVs in the world. By 2010, well over a million South Africans were receiving ARVs. However, much more is still needed to be done because over five million people in South Africa are living with HIV and the infection continues to spread.

By 2008, with US$18.8 billion spent and millions of lives saved, PEPFAR, that President Bush called "a humanitarian mission of mercy", was already in the record books as the largest donor programme for mass treatment of a chronic disease. President Bush who deserves credit for this life-saving initiative was kind to acknowledge in his book, *Decision Points*, the part I played in the formative stages of PEPFAR.

When I got another chance to meet President Bush on World AIDS Day, 1 December 2007, in the Oval Office, I had the opportunity to personally thank this man I consider to be a hero of Africa for the millions of lives that his PEPFAR initiative has saved. His reply was that he wished to do more to help. I could see that this was coming from his heart. Later, after President Bush's tenure, Ambassador Mark Dybul, who did a great job as PEPFAR global coordinator, told me that he too believed that President Bush personally felt for the AIDS sufferers and passionately wanted to do all he could to put a stop to the carnage.

Thorny Issues

Other unsung heroes also played vital roles in the formative days of PEPFAR and in its implementation. I mentioned some of those that I came to know about in *Genocide by Denial*, but others, including all PEPFAR staff, led by Ambassadors Randy Tobias, Mark Dybul and Eric Goosby, are heroes. Credit must be given to the caring staff of

USAID and CDC, who did a great job at the forefront of PEPFAR implementation.

However PEPFAR almost got derailed, just as it was becoming clear that it was destined to exceed its original goals and emerge as one of the most successful humanitarian rescue missions in history. Sadly, it became embroiled in a highly controversial debate over obscure ideological views. The controversy seems to have stemmed partly from opposition by some conservatives and religious fundamentalists to the supply of condoms (see Chapter 8) and opposition to any support for anything to do with family planning. It was alleged that both were repugnant, morally wrong and an endorsement of premarital sex and abortion.

To address these concerns, which were fronted by a powerful lobby in the US, legislation that enforced the need for one-third of the overall prevention budget to be allocated to abstinence education was enacted. It also became a requirement that for organisations to qualify to receive aid from PEPFAR, they must first pledge their unequivocal opposition to prostitution. Being among the highest HIV risk groups, prostitutes would obviously have been among the very first to be targeted for help by any serious programme aimed at eradicating HIV, not only for their own good, but for the sake of the entire community. In the jaundiced eyes of some dyed-in-the-wool conservatives it was as if people who become prostitutes ceased to be human – and to borrow from Shakespeare – if you pricked them they would not bleed. This implied that, by virtue of their line of work, they forfeited their human rights, including access to life-saving drugs. There was an attempt to rationalise this callous rule, saying that prostitutes get AIDS because of their own "disgusting behaviour", or lifestyle.

Some schools of thought have attributed the wide spread of HIV in Sub-Saharan Africa to multiple concurrent sexual relationships calling it "Sexual networking" and attributed the low prevalence of HIV in the West to the practice of "serial sexual relationships". But this was a gross oversimplification of a complex multi-factorial problem.

While new poor critically ill AIDS patients could not access ART in Uganda as a result of decreased donor funding, we saw proportionally more funds being allocated to reducing sexual networking. It was mind-boggling that those who believed that reduction of the spread of HIV through sexual networks was such a critical preventive strategy were at the same time denying funding to support risk reduction among the prostitutes, who were recognised as the most at-risk group, and one of the main sources of new infection spreading through sexual networks.

It was also declared that none of the money could go to groups that support abortion. PEPFAR, which President Bush presented as a mission of mercy, was to some extent being hijacked by ideological considerations. This provoked Thomas Coates, director of the Program in Global Health at the David Geffen School of Medicine, California, to comment: "It was like – there they go again – being generous on the one hand and then earmarking these moral dictates on the other." Some plain-speaking American AIDS activists dubbed these directives "moral hypocrisy".

These were not the only controversies. The programme also came under criticism for not addressing the severe deficiency of human resources within the public health sector, which was one of the main constraints to proper delivery of health services throughout sub-Saharan Africa. On the contrary, the new projects inadvertently made it worse by "poaching" on the very scarce trained public health workers by luring them with higher pay. Many PEPFAR programme implementers were disconcerted by the insistence that no donor funds could be used to pay salary supplements or allowances that could be construed as salary top up to any public sector health workers. The plight of public sector workers especially their dire working conditions were not taken in account, yet the long term sustainability strategy of the programme very much depended on strengthening the very weak Health Sector of which human resource support was a crucial component. The reality was that it was virtually impossible to implement a sustainable treatment programme within the public sector without the participation of public sector health workers.

The participation of the overstretched and poorly paid public sector workers over and above their heavy daily work loads, without any extra compensation was just taken for granted. To make matters worse, junior staff employed by donor-funded projects were paid much more than senior and longer-serving public health workers who were often their supervisors. Donor-funded projects also provided much better facilities and work conditions for their employees, providing them with extra allowances and health insurance while their public sector counterparts toiled in poor and often unsafe facilities. This resulted in an internal brain drain, as many public health sector workers resigned or just absconded to seek better-paying project jobs, making the conditions of the dwindling public sector staff even much more miserable. In fact one PEPFAR project worker I know of, did not even bother to resign from his previous public sector work. It took almost three years for the public sector health facility to discover that one of their workers was missing!

The brain drain was not only restricted to the public sector workers. Various rival donor projects grantees poached workers from each other. This was because project grants were awarded on a competitive basis. As a result newer organisations trying to win advertised grants lured experienced workers from established organisations with promises of higher pay to help run their newly established projects, doing the same job. This resulted in ever escalating salaries offered by many organisations trying to fend off the competition, making public sector salaries look abysmal by comparison. This situation inevitably led to envy and conflict, especially when the two sets of workers interacted in course of their work.

In Uganda, this inequitable situation triggered a series of strikes and heightened agitation by public health workers demanding better pay. It presented the government with a special predicament. If only health sector workers were given special consideration, the entire poorly paid national civil and military service would inevitably rise up in "alms" or in arms. The country was too poor to substantially increase salaries across the board, especially at a time when the government had undertaken the highly expensive free universal primary and secondary education.

The competitive bidding method of awarding grants created another problem. More or less the same bureaucratic ways that public sector purchases are made were employed to determine the organisations to be awarded some of the PEPFAR grants. Basically, it was on the basis of a written proposal that best responded to the terms specified within the Request for Applications (RFAs). The terms set out in RFAs raised a number of issues and concerns. First, there was the requirement that any PEPFAR grantee must cost-share by providing 10% of the project's total amount. Secondly, the proposal had to demonstrate proven past experience in providing HIV/AIDS services in developing countries and present a list of experts, with specified qualifications to carry out the work, among other requirements. In some cases it was prescribed that the required personnel had to be expatriates or people who had worked abroad for a number of years.

Foreign organisations were invited to compete with local organisations for the grants on equal terms. The former with their vast resources obviously had unchallengeable advantages because they would easily demonstrate the source of their 10% cost share and provide the list of experts. I never ceased to be amazed by the African experience claimed by some of the foreign organisations competing with indigenous ones for grants. It was as if they had worked in Africa all their lives! I saw many pamphlets and write-ups describing incredible experience and enormous work that they had successfully accomplished in Africa. I wondered why they had been invisible at the height of the AIDS bloodbath, during those terrible pre-PEPFAR days. Other than MSF, Oxfam, UNCEF, Red Cross and a number of well known organisations that have long partnered with Africa and other poor parts of the world, I never heard the voices of the many new ones that had suddenly jumped on board. I recall how frustrated we had felt in the 1990s, when many of those that were in Africa took special care to avoid any work to do with the treatment of AIDS using ARVs. Some of them are on record as insisting that the only practical intervention appropriate for Africa was prevention. Throughout the 1990s and early 2000s, it was almost taboo to talk about public sector use of ART in Africa. Across the continent there were very few charitable organisations that offered any kind of help, let alone 10% of their own resources at a time of Africa's critical need. I cannot even begin to enumerate the numbers of children who would not have become orphans; the number of teachers, health care providers, artisans, and others of all walks of life whose lives would have been saved if such organisations had donated 10% or even less of what was now readily available.

But this did not mean that the competitive process itself was ill intentioned. I think that people who contrived it were trying to ensure, transparency, and the selection of the best possible service providers for a cost-effective outcome. I also know that many foreign organisations and individuals had absolutely no other intention other than to help alleviate the catastrophe of AIDS. I know of those that came to provide critically needed capacity building and technology transfer. I know a number of people who gave their services entirely free to Africa and some others who used their personal resources to help us. To these humanitarian partners we are eternally grateful, and we need their continued participation as the work ahead is still enormous.

Sadly, a few individuals, who came ostensibly to rescue Africa from AIDS, exposed their true intentions when they quoted their so-called "African experience" to campaign against any increase in funding for AIDS treatment. I listened with disbelief as one former expatriate, who had worked for a brief period in Uganda without treating any single case of AIDS, (and was still considered to be an expert on AIDS in Africa), strongly advising against increasing funding for AIDS treatment. He advised that it would be futile to try and treat the big numbers of infected people, perhaps implying that it would be cost-effective to let them die.

The PEPFAR programme, by its definition, was responding to a state of emergency and from the start it was understood that it would be a long-term initiative that included capacity building of recipient countries' public sector and local organisations so that they would play an increasingly crucial role and eventually take it over. Therefore local organisations should have been given the benefit of affirmative action, and should have been supported to prepare for eventual sustainability of the programme. International experts should have been funded to come in as capacity building experts to train and strengthen public and private sector health care organisations to prepare them for the task of managing their countries' health programmes in the long term.

The competitive RFAs were, of course, designed by hired professionals, most of them expatriates. I was concerned because some parts of the competitive process appeared to me to be lopsided. In terms of writing a highly professional bid and ability to provide the necessary experts, the outcome was almost always predictable. Well endowed foreign organisations would present their team of experts and, if they did not have them, they were in the best position to hire them from anywhere in the world. If there was any need for local people to be involved, for instance, to demonstrate local participation, they would offer available staff in the public or private sector terms and conditions that they were not in position to refuse. Then they would hire professional writers — targeting former employees of the awarding agencies - to write a state-of-the-art proposal. Language was very important and was not infrequently the pitfall of some local organisations. Often the local organisations had good ideas but used the wrong words to express them. This enabled those with second best-ideas expressed in better language to win — fairly. These were some of the circumstances under which local and foreign organisations would compete on "equal" terms. It was explained that foreign organisations had a right to sue if they could demonstrate that special consideration was "unfairly" given to any local organisation.

Concerns were expressed by activists and even some PEPFAR officials, questioning whether this was an effective way of strengthening the in-country systems for long-term sustainability. Then some local agencies came out with two kinds of RFAs – (a) free for all to apply, and (b) local organisations only to apply.

Many foreign organisations that put up the 10% cost share had negotiated overheads based on foreign rates, which would ensure that substantial amounts from the award were returned to their organisations abroad. Some overheads could be as high as 50% and occasionally beyond. Such an organisation would in reality contribute nothing from their own resources towards the required 10% cost contribution. It would all be covered for them by the grant. Meanwhile, the local organisations were not always allowed to charge overheads. They were mainly allowed direct cost reimbursements. Those who sought overheads found tight regulations which very few were able to meet. It was the weak local organisations that were left to pay the real 10% cost share from their minuscule resources. No wonder some of those who would probably have done a good job did not even contemplate applying on their own. Later when it became clear that local organisations could not raise the money, this requirement was relaxed, making it possible for local organisations to make in-kind contributions. For instance, your staff could contribute free labour to the programme or value their assets that the project would use and count it as cost-share contribution.

A few foreign organisations secured donor grants using an indirect approach. They would form a collaborative arrangement with local organisations—which was later re-named partnership because it sounded less patronising. Years of deprivation would have taught locals how to manage with little and many of them were able to accomplish much more than they would otherwise be compensated for under the partnership.

Another drawback was that, no funds were provided for building of new infrastructure. Only renovations, remodelling and minor extensions to existing facilities were allowed. With the big numbers of patients, all facilities in Uganda were overwhelmed with the influx of new AIDS patients. I improvised by pitching tents – turning our small JCRC campus in Kampala into a tent village. Meanwhile, in Kakira, a small town in eastern Uganda, where JCRC had established a satellite centre, we initially counselled AIDS patients under trees. Several times I had to vacate my own office so that it could be used for a clinic or a laboratory as we expanded.

As we rolled out the treatment programme, it became clear to me that it was absolutely essential to establish quality laboratories closer to the people. Way back in 2003 there were no laboratories outside Kampala that could carry out CD4 and viral load tests then considered in the West as absolutely essential for proper treatment and monitoring of AIDS. According to the WHO guidelines, CD4 tests are needed to determine when to start therapy and when to change. Yet because of misinformation, it was widely believed at the time that establishment of laboratories capable of carrying out such tests were impossible in African rural areas. Besides, the kind of tents I had set up for clinics could not accommodate advanced laboratories which needed air-conditioned and dust-free spaces. Additional requirements included highly trained technologists, uninterrupted power supply, expensive laboratory equipment and reagents that needed to be kept at constant low temperature.

One day, during a combined meeting of PEPFAR, Global Fund, Clinton Foundation and other HIV/AIDS programme implementers (described officially as "Development Partners"), I let it drop that we planned to establish at least one referral laboratory in each of the five regions of Uganda. I explained that this would make it possible to carry out all the essential tests in the regions where the vast majority of patients lived, instead of referring patients or sending samples all the way to the capital city Kampala where the few laboratories were already overwhelmed. Besides being highly expensive and time-consuming, results for some of the crucial tests that needed to be carried out on fresh samples would be unreliable—a wastage. Establishing quality laboratories in the provinces was surely a sound development and sustainability strategy based on capacity building of vital infrastructure for the country. To my dismay, this proposal was met with naked hostility. It was described as a dream which would be impossible to implement outside Kampala. Various foreign "experts" explained that this has never been done anywhere in eastern Africa and, therefore, it would inevitably flop. "Good money would be just flushed down the drain," they said, but I begged to disagree. Surprisingly, without any functioning quality laboratory in any of the provincial hospitals, a few misguided Ministry of Health officials concurred. One expatriate, who had a long experience in Africa, took such a strong exception to my suggestion that he did not consider it worthy of comment. After the meeting he took me aside to give me a word of advice. "Though in theory the laboratories are needed in the districts, in practice it is virtually impossible to run state-of-the-art tests in areas where they don't even have clean water and reliable power supply." I could clearly see that the level of opposition to my proposal was so intense that winning them over needed action rather than words. I was not only convinced that we could do it, but I considered not doing it a betrayal of the hundreds of thousands of Ugandans who needed this service for their very survival. I therefore started working on it in the background with my colleagues at JCRC.

Almost 18 months later, need for laboratories had become critical, because the numbers of people testing for HIV had increased dramatically, thanks to PEPFAR and Global Fund that made it possible for those in need of treatment to access it. As a result demand for CD4 and others tests, by thousands who tested HIV positive, including pregnant HIV positive women in need of treatment for Prevention of Mother to Child Transmission (PMTCT) of HIV, had shot up. There was also, urgent need for DNA PCR, a special diagnostic test for newborns of HIV infected mothers (HIV tests used in adults are unreliable in infancy), which would make it possible for infected babies to be started early on treatment.

An urgent meeting called to find a solution to the crisis, resolved that one central laboratory should be established in Kampala to handle all the national samples, but due to the state of emergency, it was feared that it would take too long to establish while the need was immediate. I was happy to allay their fears by reporting that the JCRC had established a regional centre of excellence (RCE) in each of the main regions of the country with the capacity to do all essential tests.

Some of those who had thought that such laboratories would be too cumbersome to establish in the districts had to go and see them in full operation. Pleasantly, the major opponent of my initial proposal to set up the laboratories, changed his mind, and started referring samples for analysis to them. However, I later found out that the main reason why he initially sent us samples for analysis was to check whether we were doing it right.

However, lack of infrastructure remained a major constraint in virtually all health facilities across the country. Concerned about the dilemma, I approached PEPFAR officials to find out whether there was any alternative way of addressing this constraint. It was explained that if there was, for instance, an existing building that needed to be renovated or expanded, a partly finished building needed for the AIDS care and treatment, then there would be no objection to use the funds to do the work.

Besides the seven regional centres of excellence that housed the advanced laboratories (situated in Gulu in the north, Kabale and Mbarara in the south, Kampala and Mubende in the central region, Fort Portal in the west and Kakira and Mbale in the east), we also renovated fifty main satellite clinics, mainly within public hospitals, to accommodate the surging numbers of AIDS patients. In addition, we established an additional twenty outreach clinics to serve remote areas where the need for AIDS services was most acute. We built new clinic extensions with laboratory spaces in Kalangala (the biggest island in Lake Victoria, to serve the big fishing community, known to have very high HIV prevalence), Masindi, in western Uganda, and Kapchorwa in the far eastern part of the country, where doctors had no space to accommodate AIDS patients. In the war-torn northern region, where HIV was on a steep rise, we built a clinic in remote Patongo in Gulu district. My aim was to ensure that services were extended to the public sector and that they were continually strengthened to eventually establish and manage their own laboratories and treatment centres. We also extended our services to private, NGO and faith-based organisation hospitals, including Rushere Community Hospital in southern Uganda, where we also built a clinic and laboratory extension.

Besides PEPFAR, we raised funds from our programme income, and support from other partners, including, International AIDS Vaccine Initiative (IAVI), which helped us build Kakira RCE, REALTA Global AIDS Foundation under Professor Ceppie Mary which supported us to build Gulu RCE. These initiatives helped us to exceed our original targets. Within the first five years of PEPFAR, JCRC had started over 70,000 AIDS patients on ART, and was caring for over three times that number in all the regions of the country. Many of those we started on therapy were, later referred for continuing care to centres jointly established by government and other partner organisations closer to their homes or workplaces. Our plan envisaged improving all the clinics that we established, ensuring best practices and then gradually transitioning them back to Ministry of Health for continuity.

The Great Rescue

In the midst of the AIDS disaster in sub Saharan Africa, PEPFAR was the rescue programme. Within a short time after its establishment, with millions of African lives saved, the success of PEPFAR was evident.

The image of America transformed from that of a world policeman to that of Africa's friend. In Sub-Saharan Africa people had more positive things to say about America than ever before. As HIV/AIDS touched on the lives of millions on daily basis, it was inevitably one of the commonest topics for discussion — and America as the main benefactor became the centre point of praise. Where AIDS was discussed as a mass killer, US was talked about as the saviour. Whenever the issue of millions of AIDS orphans and vulnerable children arose, America stood out as the caretaker of helpless little ones. Where AIDS was perceived as a security risk, USA on the other hand was seen as the peacemaker. USA was seen as a compassionate and generous donor – a friend of the world. This was the kind of image that the rest of the world needed to know about.

When the first five years of PEPFAR officially ended in September 2008, it was announced that well over 2.1 million people were receiving AIDS drugs. The vast majority of these people would have died if it was not for PEPFAR. The remarkable success is particularly impressive when it is taken into account that the programme started at the time when only a very small number of AIDS patients in Africa were able to access ART. Further, despite strong opposition by religious extremists, PEPFAR successfully supplied 2.2 billion condoms, with all the immeasurable rounds of pleasure and safety that go with it, to millions of users.

The programme also reached 16 million pregnant women. Among them were 1.2 million who were found to be HIV positive. These were helped to access PMTCT services, thus saving about a quarter million infants who, without PMTCT, would have been born infected with HIV. PEPFAR also reported that 57 million people were counselled and tested for HIV, and about 10.1 million people found to be infected by HIV, but not yet in need of AIDS drugs received care and regular monitoring. These included over 4 million children. It was also reported that nearly 400,000 dually infected clients, with HIV and tuberculosis (TB), received TB therapy, while 58.3 million people received HIV-preventive messages mainly through PEPFAR-supported community programmes. In addition PEPFAR supported 3.7 million training encounters with healthcare workers. In the process, collaborative relationships were established with 2,667 organisations.

Impressive as these achievements may be, they were still not enough, but it was a good beginning. The epidemic had been ignored for far too long for PEPFAR to repair all the damage and reverse the trend within a mere five years. Much more funds were still needed and for a much longer time to bring the epidemic under effective control. It was estimated that PEPFAR and a sister programme, Global AIDS Fund, were able to provide treatment for only about a quarter of the people in immediate need.

With some reforms and cost-saving initiatives introduced in both PEPFAR and Global AIDS Fund, the two programmes had the potential to deliver universal access to care and treatment services in Africa. At this stage, PEPFAR had taken Africa to the mountain and pointed to a land free of AIDS. However, to get there PEPFAR and Global AIDS Fund needed to expand and keep growing to reach out to millions who were still in dire need. Having come this far, turning back was unthinkable.

As the end of the first round of PEPFAR approached, so did the second term of Africa's benefactor President George W. Bush's presidency. In the twilight of his second and final term in the White House, newspaper columnists, book publishers, historians and various commentators geared to review Bush's eight years in power. As usual, the opinions varied depending on people's ideological leanings, other biases and perceptions. On the one side, there were a number of people, including some senators, who could not fault Bush on virtually anything. For instance, Fred Barnes, writing in *The Weekly Standard*, had this to say: "Time and time again, Bush did what other presidents, even Ronald Reagan, would not have done … That — defiantly doing the right thing — is what distinguished his presidency."

As far as the scourge of AIDS was concerned, there is absolutely no doubt that he took a bold step in the right direction. It is difficult to envision any other president being so courageous. The carnage of AIDS was at its peak during President Clinton's presidency and during the campaign for his second term he promised much regarding AIDS relief but when it came to implementation he was no better than his predecessor. However, after leaving office, President Clinton redeemed himself to a considerable extent by establishing a foundation that has done a lot to help HIV-infected children.

President Bush's audacious action went against a tide of disapproval by many infectious disease experts who insisted that AIDS treatment in Africa was virtually impossible. Pharmaceutical companies were also fighting to maintain their ARV monopoly to protect their profits. Yet, without the more affordable generic ARV drugs it was difficult to envision how millions of people in immediate need of ARVs could be successfully treated. Bush's initiative pulled down the barriers against generic AIDS drugs. For the first time there was fast tracking of approvals for some of them to be allowed for use in PEPFAR programmes. It also changed the perception people had of the quality of generic medicines.

The same article also listed the ten greatest achievements of the Bush presidency. When I scrolled down the list, I was surprised to find that PEPFAR was not among them. Many humanitarian activists and most Africans, especially those affected or infected by the killer HIV/AIDS, were justifiably indebted to the saviour of millions of their parents, brothers, sisters and children. Without PEPFAR the majority of the beneficiaries who include parents, teachers, politicians, and peasant farmers, would have died by the time he left office. The dead would have left behind millions of orphans who, in addition to their misery, would have no alternative guidance because of the death of their teachers. There would have been increased hunger and a severe fall in household income because of the demise of breadwinners. Society would have been destabilised as a result of the loss of their leaders. And this list mentions just a few of the devastating effects such a loss would have added to a continent already badly battered by AIDS. Bush averted many of these calamities. Where is the expression of gratitude from Africa's leaders to a man who did so much for the continent?

One remarkable philanthropist who did what African leaders should have done is Bob Geldof, an Irish musician-cum-social activist, who once organised the Band Aid concert to raise funds for starving Ethiopians. He paid tribute to Bush and appreciated what he did for Africa. "Mr Bush has done more for Africa than any other president so far," he said.

Among others that paid tribute to President Bush for the PEPFAR programme were former US President Bill Clinton, United Nations Secretary-General Ban Ki-Moon, and Barack Obama then President-Elect. Writing in Nature, Erika Check Hayden, had this to say about their tribute to Bush: "This was not dutiful lip-service. They were heaping praise on Bush's signature programme to fight AIDS, and what many view as his most significant positive achievement of the past eight years". I have often wondered whether the millions of African lives that President Bush's PEPFAR programme had saved, would not have been enough to qualify him for the Nobel Prize. As mentioned above, I had an occasion to personally thank President Bush for saving millions of my fellow Africans. Remembering the bleak pre-PEPFAR days when I used to watch helplessly as numerous numbers perished, I meant it from the bottom of my heart.

On his part, before his final adieu, President Bush planned a great farewell gift for Africa in particular and humanity as a whole. He planned to more than double the amount of money for PEPFAR. He must have been pleasantly surprised when the US Congress passed his request and approved US$48 billion for five years. Obviously, this would not even have been considered if PEPFAR had been a flop. With this in the bag, it started looking like universal ART access would one day become a reality.

Encouragingly, the approved amount was to build on lessons learned from the first round of PEPFAR, make appropriate amendments and extend beyond AIDS to include other killer diseases, as well as assisting in building health systems in Africa. US$12.6 billion was to go towards malaria and TB programmes, $2 billion was earmarked for the Global Fund to Fight AIDS, TB and Malaria in 2009, all of which marked a substantial increase in US support. The new bill required that gender-based violence and legal protection for women and girls should be addressed among preventive activities. This was spot on, because over the years, a worrying trend towards feminisation of HIV had emerged in Africa.

On a rather negative note, the Bill was silent on the issue of integrating family planning into HIV prevention measures. However, it removed the controversial requirement that at least one-third of prevention expenditure had to go to programmes that promoted abstinence and faithfulness. As the Bill passed through the senate an amendment was inserted that ended the ban on HIV-infected people entering the US as visitors, refugees or asylum seekers which made it possible for USA to host the 2012 international AIDS conference in Washington DC. Previously, all HIV-infected people had to seek a special waiver to be allowed to enter the US. All in all, the entire Bill was applauded throughout Sub-Saharan Africa.

The importance that President Bush attached to the PEPFAR reauthorisation was underscored by the grand ceremony that he presented on 30 July 2008 in the East Room of the White House to mark the occasion. I was among the select group that included US dignitaries, African and Caribbean ambassadors in Washington, and others from all over the world who were invited to witness the ceremony. I had the rare honour of witnessing the president signing this important Bill into law. It was a very satisfying moment. Mohamed Kalyesubula, a Ugandan living with AIDS, was among specially invited guests, representing the key beneficiaries of the donation, and a Ugandan AIDS orphan's choir was in attendance to entertain the guests.

As I left the White House on my way to Mexico City, where I was to make a series of presentations at the AIDS International Conference, I had a spring in my step, reassured that more lives of people in Africa would be saved for at least the next five years. So I thought, but it was not long before things fell apart.

11

Back and Forth

The Crunch

At the time of the PEPFAR reauthorisation in Washington, history was in the making. The talk in the US capital and all over the world was "Obama!"

The charismatic black Democratic Party frontrunner was attracting mammoth crowds at his presidential campaign rallies. Gallup polls had him way ahead of his Republican rival, Senator McCain. Many people I met were trying to clear the centuries' old prejudice from their eyes, and visualise a black man in the White House. It was clear that Obama had long risen above race and prejudice and emerged as a leader that people of all races could identify with. He had also run a brilliant campaign. He talked of change but not merely any change or just the usual rhetoric, but the type that "we could believe in"— a statement that many people felt they owned. He recognised the odds against him and coined a counter slogan "Yes, we can," that also captured many people's imaginations, as individuals of all races set to do it.

Soon the miracle was complete. The night the results were announced, I was in London. Despite an early-morning meeting scheduled for the next day, I stayed awake all night waiting to witness the magic moment that will remain engraved on my mind. The rest, as the saying goes, is history.

However, President Bush's last two months in office were marred by ever escalating global financial problems. Banks were threatened with closure, and some actually closed. Big business enterprises were brought to their knees and many people lost their jobs and mortgages, leaving many homeless. As the crisis spread like wildfire, virtually all the major economies of the world were gripped by the same crisis, reminding me of the saying that when America sneezes the rest of the world catches a cold. It was a vicious crisis with no easy solution

When President Obama took over the presidency, PEPFAR was still operating under the so-called "Continuing Resolution", while formal authorisation to release funds was awaited. Under the new president PEPFAR looked safe, as he had demonstrated the same commitment as his predecessor did to fighting AIDS. As President Obama took office in January 2009, with a mammoth crowd braving the cold winter evening to witness the historic event, it was clear that the first test of his presidency would be how effectively he handled the financial emergency that he inherited. As the new president's men and other US policymakers grappled with it as a matter of urgency, matters to do with the crisis of AIDS in Africa and international aid were eclipsed by the unfolding financial crisis that was deteriorating by the day in the USA. Meanwhile, in Africa, the threat of the resurgence of the AIDS carnage, which only a few months earlier had been unthinkable, hovered

In March 2009, I was back in Washington DC on a joint mission with the Physicians for Human Rights. Our undertaking was to plead for the full release of the funds that Congress had approved for AIDS in the last days of George Bush's presidency, and which was needed to keep the world's most successful humanitarian life saving programme on course. But as I lobbied congress and senate, I was repeatedly reminded, and not always politely, that the USA had a crisis of their own to address.

"This is not the right time to increase foreign aid, even for humanitarian causes while our own house is on fire. AIDS in the eyes of the majority of American people is a remote problem of other nations. This can wait. Our priority is to attend to the very urgent domestic crisis and other more deserving international strategic issues, like the Afghanistan war, where American lives are at stake," one aide to a prominent senator told me, "and I'm sure you can understand that."

This was a far cry from Bush's 28 January 2003 State of the Union address. The mood and the language were different. President Bush had received a standing ovation from both the Democrats and Republicans. In an eloquent speech President Bush had vividly described the bleak situation in Africa brought about by the AIDS crisis. It was a moving oration. "Because the AIDS diagnosis is considered a death sentence, many do not seek treatment. Almost all who do are turned away," he had said. "Ladies and gentlemen, seldom has history offered a greater opportunity to do so much for so many. This nation can lead the world in sparing innocent people from a plague of nature." Since those historic statements much water had passed under the bridge. PEPFAR and the generosity of the American people was the best part of it.

When President Obama took over, he immediately addressed the global financial crisis. The new President successfully secured Congress's approval of an unprecedented stimulus fund to the value of US$792 billion to resuscitate the US economy. In this atmosphere, foreign aid and programmes like PEPFAR were not an immediate priority. The promised PEPFAR funds that President Bush signed into law in a grand ceremony were not immediately released. We received directives that no new patients should be started on ARVs on PEPFAR programme. A crisis started brewing again, and I feared that the nightmare of mass deaths would return to haunt us once more.

In Uganda, it did not take long for the bad times to return. Crowds of patients desperate for the life-saving drugs, for the first time since PEPFAR started in 2003, besieged my centre pleading for their lives. Many of them told us that they had been visiting clinic after clinic and being told the same sad news: "We are not taking on new patients. Try somewhere else."

I started to see an increase in horrific opportunistic infections because people could not start life-saving treatment in time. Then the telephone calls from patients and their relatives inquiring where they could get help started again. The last time I had been bombarded with such frantic calls was in the 1990s and early 2000s, before PEPFAR. I knew from bitter experience that unless something was done fast the situation would soon be out of control again. The bodies would pile up, and endless funerals would once again bring business to a standstill. This was the background and circumstances that forced me to return to Washington DC to try and explain the dire situation that was once more unfolding in Africa. It was the kind of scenario that I had hoped never to see again.

Before PEPFAR, when the carnage was at its height, most AIDS sufferers accepted their fate with gracious resignation. A lot of money had been spent spreading the word that nothing could be done about AIDS. All that AIDS patients were advised to do was to live positively by accepting to die peacefully. The difference this time round, was that the patients knew that death was not inevitable. Many members of their own families whose lives had been all but given up, had been restored back to good health and were back at their work of taking care of their families, and playing their roles in their community and country.

The life of healthcare providers had also changed over the years. Way back in the 1990s they had to convey the frightening news to dying patients and their relatives. To attenuate the anguish of it, they coined comforting words and phrases to calm scared patients. Healthcare providers had become experts in their role as bearers of bad news. But by 2008, many had forgotten how to do it. Surely, they would look ridiculous if they once more started advising patients with the hackneyed phrases, "Live positively, die with dignity." We had experienced more than six years of hope when, once more, doctors could be doctors who prescribed medicines to patients – medicines that worked. Medicines that were in stock.

Patients' confidence in healthcare providers had been restored. They were once again visiting hospitals and health centres. The quacks, including the likes of Gasket, Blockbuster, Pastor Mululu, and the infamous Haji were out of business. The death rates had declined as many sick people moved from their death beds to their work places. Funerals were no longer the order of the day. The orphan factory was operating at a lower production level as deaths of parents slowed down. The previously booming coffin-making business had burst as carpenters had turned to making furniture which survivors needed to sit on instead of being laid out in.

However, it was not only Uganda that I thought about, because the devastation of AIDS affected most parts of the continent. I realised that some other African countries, especially Zimbabwe and Swaziland in southern Africa, were in a worse situation. Therefore I was back in Washington DC not only for Uganda but for Africa as a whole.

When I arrived in the US capital on Sunday 15 March 2009 I was surprised to find that AIDS was the hot topic! "HIV/AIDS Rate in D.C. Hits 3%" screamed the Washington Post headline. This was as surprising to me as it was to many Americans who had long considered AIDS a problem of Africa and backward countries. The director of HIV/AIDS administration in DC, Dr Shannon Hader, who once worked in Africa, was quoted expressing her concern. "Our rates are higher than West Africa," she said, "they're on a par with Uganda and some parts of Kenya. We have every mode of transmission going up, all on the rise, and we have to deal with them."

The coincidence provided me with arguments to use in explaining that AIDS was not only a vicious epidemic in Africa but remained a global threat, which if ignored even for a short time would resurge with devastating consequences. Indeed part of the reason why HIV/AIDS had risen in Washington was attributed to "a city that for years has stumbled in combating HIV/AIDS". In fact the identified risk factors in DC followed a familiar pattern, including overlapping sexual partners, which has been dubbed "sexual network" in Uganda, and failure to use condoms, as only three out of ten sexually active people in DC said they had used condoms when they last had sex.

Overall, the report found a 22% increase since 2006, and identified black men, with an infection rate of about 7% (which at the time was higher than Uganda), as the most affected racial group.

When some DC journalists got wind of my presence in Washington, they sought to interview me. "The AIDS epidemic in the US capital is being compared with the African one," one journalist said to me. "We would like to hear your point of view as an African from a poor country looking at America, a rich country, and tell us what you think of it," he said. One journalist repeatedly asked me on camera: "Isn't it a shame that USA has the same rate of HIV as Uganda?" I repeatedly refused to answer this question, because it was as inaccurate as it was misleading. The journalist persisted, asking the same question in different words, but I refused to reply.

The reality was that, bad as the HIV/AIDS situation was projected to be in Washington, it was nowhere near the catastrophic levels of Sub-Saharan Africa. The reported increase in DC translated into a rise from 12,428 cases in 2006 to 15,120 in 2008. In Uganda and many parts of Africa, the increase in the same period was by hundreds of thousands – and some estimates put it in millions. Secondly, the USA, the world's richest country, was able to tackle the problem, while Africa, the poorest continent, was overwhelmed by the sheer magnitude of the still-unfolding disaster. Therefore it would have been ill-advised for me to say on American TV that the situation in their capital was as bad as Uganda's while I was at the same time lobbying for continued help for Africa. However, it was appropriate to refer to the data without engaging in misleading comparisons, as I emphasised the need for increased funds to fight AIDS globally. Indeed, the timely Washington Post HIV/AIDS story helped me to present my case to members of congress, senate and their technical assistants at a time when increased foreign assistance was not among their priorities.

My meetings in Washington included lectures at prestigious universities and institutions that had influence on policy. On Monday 16 March 2009 I gave a presentation at the Washington Centre for Strategic and International Studies. The following day I gave a talk at George Washington University on the topic, 'PEPFAR What is Working, and What Isn't.' Then on 18 March I went to the famous Georgetown University where I gave a presentation entitled, 'It's not over: Global Funding in an Era of Uncertainty.'

In all my presentations I expressed Africa's gratitude for PEPFAR to the American people. I explained that, contrary to earlier concerns, ARVs had been successfully used in rural and urban parts of Uganda and other African countries. I happily reported that adherence and treatment outcome were comparable to that in the West. I showed how treatment was going on hand in hand with capacity building and I also enumerated many other critical achievements of PEPFAR, which included a marked decrease in mortality and assistance to over 4 million vulnerable children. After taking stock of all these achievements I explained that despite this, the crisis was still far from over. Africa had over 25 million people living with HIV. Each year hundreds of thousands of Africans got infected. All these people would eventually need treatment and the demand would inevitably keep on increasing for well over a decade. Across Africa only about 3 million people were on treatment, leaving more than twice the number in immediate need of therapy. In subsequent years the demand would surpass 15 million people. Therefore in undertaking global relief work it was always prudent to take a broad perspective with a view to solving the problem permanently. This implied spending more in the short term in order to manage the problem in the long term.

Repeatedly during discussions, legislators would retort that although they understood the seriousness of the situation, this was not the USA's responsibility. "Certainly not," I would unreservedly agree, "alleviating the AIDS crisis, that UN had declared a catastrophic state of emergency, was a responsibility of all nations – and all mankind." The USA as a more prosperous member of the global community should take the leadership in trying to alleviate the humanitarian disaster brought about by AIDS. It was therefore the wrong time to scale down support for PEPFAR, or to use Capitol Hill jargon, to "implement a level budget". On the contrary, it was during the financial crunch that the HIV/AIDS budget needed to increase to avoid making a bad situation worse.

I came across a number of policy makers in Washington who believed that the best option during the financial crisis was to freeze the funding and provide only for patients already on treatment until the crunch ended — if it ended. After the domestic crisis had been addressed, additional funding could be considered. In my submissions and presentations in Washington, I explained that ignoring the HIV/AIDS scourge even for a short time was a recipe for chaos.

PEPFAR was about life and it could not be frozen or scaled down unless it was decided that people's lives would be sacrificed. This however did not mean that by undertaking to help the world's poor, USA had painted itself into a corner. The action was justified because it was an ongoing emergency. Also, it was the kind of emergency that everyone knew would require long-term commitment for the simple reason that it concerned a vicious chronic infection that, if allowed room, would resurge, with devastating consequences. In addition, successful AIDS treatment is determined by strict adherence and it would be virtually impossible to have a successful AIDS treatment programme where some people received the lifesaving therapy while others, also in dire need, did not. The result would not only be treatment failure but a much more serious outcome would include the possible emergence of resistant HIV virus.

If resistance became widespread, low-cost and user-friendly AIDS drugs would fail. Alternative drugs would be more expensive and their efficacy could not be guaranteed, because long-term use of failed first line AIDS drugs might also confer resistance to second-line drugs. If resistance happened on a wide scale it might become necessary to screen all new patients starting on ART for resistance to determine which drugs to start them on. Testing for resistance was expensive and a technologically challenging exercise. Freezing AIDS funding could in the long term turn out to be a very costly mistake.

I felt that it was essential to highlight these issues and warn about the grave consequences of denying life-saving therapy to new patients.

By the time the financial crunch was over it would be too late for millions of people.

Turning Patients Away

"Many very ill patients are still turning up at our outpatient clinic daily, insisting that they have nowhere else to go," our worried clinic manager, Dr Fiona Kalinda, lamented. "Please advise what we can do." It was almost a year since my last lobbying mission to Washington during which I had appealed for full release of PEPFAR funds so that we did not get to this precarious stage, but the budget, at least for Uganda, remained frozen.

I asked my deputy, Dr Cissy Kityo, to check and establish the numbers of very sick patients being turned away from our ART clinics. On 12 March 2010, she reported that up to 200 new very ill patients were being turned away from eight of our treatment centres per week. The actual numbers in need of treatment were much higher but could not be ascertained because they were being turned away at the gates and only the very sick, who were the only ones counted, were allowed in. We realised that some were no longer showing up because we had put notices up to inform people that we had no drugs for new patients.

Only a few years earlier, there had been national campaigns to get people tested for HIV. The majority of those being turned away were those who had responded to this campaign and who had been assured that AIDS was no longer a death sentence. Lured by the promise of treatment, hundreds of thousands of people in Uganda and millions in Africa queued up for tests. Healthcare providers had to go back on their word. Once again, they had a gruesome task to perform, breaking the bad news to their patients, which many had thought was all behind them. They braced themselves to stand by and watch while patients they had been following up for years, and to whom they promised drugs, died.

All HIV-positive people, irrespective of whether they were on treatment or not were encouraged to join Post-Test Clubs, which were linked to treatment centres. The clubs were educational centres in which AIDS preventive messages were communicated. Adherence, which is vital for a successful outcome, was also the key area of regular discussion, as were other topics such as development of income-generating skills. Some of the patients became so knowledgeable that they acquired the title "expert patients". These became members of the "faculty" and participated in educating newly diagnosed patients. Whenever the need arose, volunteer club members served as assistants to our healthcare providers. Many would be found in villages following up their fellow patients to ensure adherence to therapy, disseminating preventive messages, and encouraging people to go for HIV testing. Most of our post-test club members had long ceased to regard themselves as an AIDS problem. They were instead part of its solution, but all of a sudden they were being informed that they were on their own. I recall one irate club leader, coming to my office to protest. She came accompanied by two fellow club officials who were similarly affected.

"You promised that treatment would be available to us when we need it," she said, hardly controlling her anger. "We are registered with your clinic, and have been coming here regularly for the last five years. How is it possible that you are now turning us away when time for the treatment that you promised us has come?"

She did not realise, or if she did, as I suspected, she ignored, the fact that I was equally disappointed. I felt like I had lied to them. "But this is not what you promised us when you encouraged us to test for HIV," the irate woman retorted when I tried to explain to her the new PEPFAR standpoint. "Eight months ago, my CD4 cells fell below 200, and I fear I might die if I am not immediately started on therapy," she said. "Where are the ARVs that you promised me?"

It was difficult to know how to handle this problem. Should we close the care clinics in which we followed up infected patients who were not yet in need of ARVs? If we did, what would be the fate of thousands of patients whom we had registered? What about hundreds of healthcare providers we had hired to take care of them? Should we dismiss them right away or should we wait a while to see what might happen — something like a stay of execution? Should we stop the testing programme? If we continued to test new patients what should we say to those that tested positive? We hadn't thought we would ever have to tell patients again that there was nothing we could do for them, and to go home and die, the words that President Bush said "patients should never have to hear in the era of miraculous medicines".

I devised a plan to help out the very poor who could not afford treatment from private clinics. I asked our staff to go over the clinic registers and databases, and fill the treatment places available through attrition, including those who had died or were permanently lost to follow up. I was then forced to do what I had thought neither I nor other healthcare providers would ever have to suffer again. We had to choose among the desperate patients and say who was to live and who would be left to face his or her own fate. This was not the first time that we played God. It had been almost routine in the nightmarish pre-PEPFAR times, as I described in *Genocide by Denial*. However, this time round, I did not have to go through an agonising exercise of trying to find a humane way of going about this dreadful task. I had learnt that there was no humane way of doing it.

I looked up an old memo that I had sent to the staff in early 2002. I found that I did not have to reinvent the wheel. The same old message would do to instruct staff on how to deal with the new crisis: "Please do not turn away poor pregnant HIV-positive women. They should be given top priority. Then after them you may consider the other poor patients who are too sick to join the long queues in the few clinics that still have treatment slots."

Way back in 2002, the second priority, after pregnant women, were children. Fortunately, we still had enough drugs for all the children, thanks to the Clinton Foundation HIV/AIDS Initiative (CHAI) working in partnership with UNITAID which were supporting treatment for paediatric AIDS.

UNITAID is an international drug procurement facility that was launched in September 2006 by Brazil, Chile, France, Great Britain and Norway. Its mission was to reduce the prices of expensive drugs and diagnostics for HIV/AIDS, tuberculosis and malaria, and to make these products more accessible to developing countries. UNITAID had developed an innovative financing mechanism described as sustainable, predictable and able to provide long-term support to developing countries to better respond to these three diseases. It relied to a considerable extent on levies on plane tickets.

Despite assurances of sustainability, CHAI in 2009 gave notice that it would soon be winding up. When I first heard this news I could not believe that a critical humanitarian initiative, and moreover for children, could simply be wound up after such a short time. It would be difficult to say to an orphan child, that the programme that kept him or her alive had ended, and now the child was on his or her own. It then looked like a matter of time, before I sent out the 2002 communiqué to our staff again. However, I still hoped that it would not come to this, that humanity would win out and reverse this threat to the innocent children.

It did not take long to fill the slots that we identified among our patient database. Yet the numbers in need of treatment still rose. The death rate among those we started on treatment was very low, thanks to the powerful effect of ARVs and the expertise of our staff. The small numbers of deaths were those who had presented themselves too late, who had generally died within the first month or so after initiation of therapy. We did not have many slots, and certainly not enough to meet the big demand.

In earlier days, when PEPFAR programme was still trying to enrol as many patients as possible so as to meet the targets set by President Bush, some new organisations with limited experience had been enlisted. They were given minimum targets to meet but were finding it difficult to realise the numbers within the time limit. Some resorted to "raiding" our clinics, enticing our patients with food supplements and other inducements which our programme did not provide because we put all our resources into treating patients. My instruction to our staff was that they should always check whether the new organisations were able to provide the same care and drugs, and if they were, to help them take as many of our already stabilised patients as possible, especially those that lived close to where these organisations were operating. We saw this as an opportunity to reach others still in urgent need of ARV therapy as replacements. But when the patient ceilings were announced the new organisations immediately stopped recruiting new patients. Instead, they started referring some of them back to us, when we had no slots for new patients. Exhausted patients would tell us of their unsuccessful rounds and long waits at various PEPFAR clinics around town trying to find any that would accept them.

Despite the warning not to take on new patients, I could not bear turning away pregnant women. I just could not send a mother and the new life she carried to their deaths. I asked my staff to do all they could to find them slots in other organisations and if they failed, to accept them at the JCRC. Although my centre could not afford it, I felt I had a moral responsibility for their welfare. As expected, it did not take long before the numbers went through the roof. Soon, a dreaded warning letter arrived, stating that:

It has been clearly communicated to JCRC to stop enrolling new patients. We seek confirmation from JCRC that PEPFAR funds have not been used to procure drugs or provide ART services for any new patients since Dec. 2008. JCRC will not be responsible for any costs associated with enrolment of new ART patients ... and we have reports that JCRC continued to enrol new patients...

The warnings were not only from PEPFAR, but also from other sources, including some Ugandan colleagues. In various ways they warned that I should desist from advocating for AIDS treatment for Africa.

"You must realise that the Bush Programme is no more, and if you are not careful, you will lose the grant your own organisation has been getting. I can't even reveal to you how unhappy they are with your lobbying," one senior colleague from Makerere University, who claimed to be highly connected in international circles, warned.

Yet, all I aspired to achieve was a respite for my AIDS patients. I merely acted with a sense of urgency because the carnage was once again mounting, right in front of me, bringing back the bad memories of the 1990s and early 2000s. Silence would cost lives—lives that could be saved.

"Now I am truly besieged," I thought, "I am being stopped from treating patients, on the one hand, and on the other being blocked from trying to plead for help on their behalf!" This was a classic Catch 22. As a physician who had been trying to help AIDS sufferers for over two decades and knew very well that denying treatment to critically ill patients would result in death, I was being pushed into a situation I could not endure on ethical grounds.

This was not the first time that I was compelled to speak out, and receiving similar warnings. I remember being asked to sign a gag commitment before attending a UNAIDS drugs access meeting in Geneva. I had insisted on doing the right thing then, and I intended to continue pointing out what needed to be done to save lives.

Wishful Thinking

When I was invited to testify to the US Congressional Subcommittee on Africa, I felt I was obliged to go, in spite of the threats that I had to keep silent. With the support of AIDS Healthcare Foundation (AHF) and other humanitarian organisations, I left for Washington once again.

On Thursday 11 February 2010 I made my presentation to the US House Committee on Foreign Affairs, Subcommittee on Africa and Global Health. Testifying with me was actress Debra Messing, who also served as Population Services International (PSI) Ambassador, Joanne Cater DVM, and Norman Hearst MD, from University of California, San Francisco, who had a short experience of working in Uganda and was for that reason considered an HIV/AIDS authority on Uganda and Africa.

Dr Hearst's presentation took me by surprise, though most of what he said was not new. I had heard the same rhetoric many times in the 1990s, even from professional colleagues. However, I was dismayed to find that the same old, ineffective and discredited remedies, that had demonstrably failed to make any impact on the AIDS disaster in Africa, were being raised again.

Hearst attributed Uganda's success in reducing the HIV rates in early 1990s only to A and B – Abstinence and Being faithful – and left out the 'C' for condoms. He explained that the HIV infection rate in Uganda was rising again and attributed this negative trend to HIV testing, availability of condoms, and ARVs. He referred to his earlier testimony to Congress, explaining that his views on condoms, like those of religious zealots, were not new. "The main emphasis of my testimony was the solid scientific evidence behind the A and B of the ABC strategy for AIDS prevention ...and to make clear that it wasn't just some sort of plot by the religious right," he said.

He warned of the danger brought about by condom promotion, and his fear that prevention (A and B) money may be siphoned off for treatment.

"...we cannot treat our way out of this epidemic," he cautioned.

He dismissed all the established and emerging evidence that treatment also has a preventive role.

"Don't be fooled. Prevention is prevention; treatment is treatment," he said, adding that any overlap was just "wishful thinking" by Africans.

He expressed his displeasure with a compassionate statement attributed to Eric Goosby quoted in The Wall Street Journal namely that PEPFAR would not turn away anyone in need of treatment. "Such statements only breed resentment when it becomes impossible for us to make good on those words." To all of those who advocated increased funding to cater for increased numbers of AIDS patients who would without access to treatment suffer and die, he had one simple, uncompromising message; "We need to say, in a clear, unapologetic way, because we have nothing to apologise for, how much we can contribute." In other words, promise the "wishful thinking Africans" nothing. By so doing, you immunise yourself from any moral responsibility when the AIDS carnage worsens.

Actress Debra Messing, on the other hand, gave a moving testimony full of compassion and hope. She talked of her visit to AIDS and economically devastated Zimbabwe. "What I saw in Zimbabwe was that …. PEPFAR, the Global Fund to Fight AIDS, Tuberculosis, and Malaria, and other donors, as well as the Zimbabwean government, is paying off in dramatic ways."

Messing, who became involved in fighting HIV after her acting teacher died of AIDS in 1993, concluded her touching presentation by saying: "I urge your ongoing robust support for PEPFAR and the Global Fund so that we can halt the spread of HIV and comprehensively expand access to HIV prevention, care and treatment."

After the session, I embraced this great humanitarian actress. It was the first time, and likely the last, that I could hug an actress! It was a sweet and rare opportunity but if you ever get the chance to embrace an actress, choose a humanitarian one, because they bring pleasure to many people, and save lives at the same time. There cannot be a better choice as PSI ambassador than she is.

I made my presentation before the two starkly contrasting submissions summarised above. I started my testimony the truly African way by first acknowledging and thanking our benefactors. I said that by increasing ARV drugs access to millions of patients, PEPFAR had transformed a tragic situation in Africa. "These people –their mothers, husbands, wives and children – got a chance to live. This is a chance they simply would not have had without the humanitarian donation from the American people," I told the meeting.

Then I went to address the main issues. I expressed fear that the impressive progress achieved in AIDS care, treatment and prevention faced a grave threat because of level budgeting. Yet right from the beginning, it was understood that the AIDS crisis would need increased funding for the foreseeable future before it was finally stabilised and ultimately controlled. I illustrated the still dire situation based on the latest UNAIDS data which showed that only 44% of the over 7 million people in immediate need of ART in Sub-Saharan Africa, were getting it. Every year patients in need of ARVs were increasing and were projected to exceed 14 million out of over 23 million PLWHIV in the medium term.

I explained that the numbers in immediate need of treatment were in reality much higher because countries in Africa were still starting treatment late based on the discredited old level of CD4 200, instead of the new WHO recommended level of CD4 350. Resource constrained African governments feared that if the new criterion was adopted, the numbers in immediate need of ARVs would overwhelm their already overburdened health systems.

Meanwhile, emerging data seemed to support the concept of 'Test and Treat' (T and T) for adults irrespective of CD4 level. T and T was already a well established standard of care for newborns and infants, following scientific evidence that delayed treatment for HIV-infected babies was associated with high mortality.

New and compelling evidence indicated that treatment could also be part of a wider preventive strategy. Studies in discordant couples had demonstrated that if the infected partner is treated with ARVs, there is a high degree of protection of the uninfected partner. New evidence suggests that if there was lowering of viral load at community level by treating a critical number of infected people, the rate of HIV would also fall. Although a number of studies to verify this were still continuing, it was already abundantly clear that ARVs were effective for HIV prevention.

I also described other requirements including needs for laboratories, clinic spaces, and human resources which are vital for successful control of the HIV epidemic in Africa. I quoted UNAIDS data which indicated that the epidemic was still spreading at an alarming rate. Meanwhile, for every two patients started on therapy, five new ones, mainly females, were infected. This meant that the epidemic in Africa was increasingly becoming feminised because of gender issues and inequitable access to care and treatment. In the previous year, there were an estimated 1.9 million new infections in Sub-Saharan Africa. Therefore preventive initiatives in Africa needed to be strengthened by adopting and funding new strategies, including male circumcision, and targeting emerging vulnerable groups especially women for assistance "This brief glimpse of a grim and still deteriorating AIDS situation in Africa is not commensurate with a frozen budget. On the contrary, it calls for urgent intervention by increasing funds, mainly for treatment and prevention of HIV," I said.

I explained that the flat-lined budget had already led to some worrying trends. The most heartrending was that of care providers being forced to turn away desperate patients daily. Meanwhile, lack of new funds forced many African countries to continue using the toxic high dose Stavudine based treatment combinations, which WHO had removed from the list of recommended first-line AIDS drugs.

I told the committee the story of an HIV-infected woman who was breastfeeding her HIV-negative child because she could not afford formula milk. She came to our clinic having been turned away from a number of others in Kampala. She knew that every day she breastfed her baby without being on treatment greatly increased the chances of her child getting infected, but she had no alternative. As we were trying to find her a treatment centre we were repeatedly told that they were turning away similar cases. But this was not the only serious case I had come across. I had encountered patients unable to access therapy, including pregnant women resorting to desperate and dangerous measures, including sharing drugs with family members, ignoring the good counselling they had received advising against this dangerous practice.

Sometimes someone received therapy while family members with similar needs did not. We had learned that it is virtually impossible to have a successful public sector AIDS treatment programme if some people could access free therapy and others not. Studies carried out at JCRC had found that inequitable access compromised the quality of ART programmes and fuels resistance to ARV drugs. Patients who develop resistance to simpler and low-cost first-line drugs would need more expensive second-line therapy. Such a situation would make the current cost of ART therapy seem very low by comparison, especially if HIV resistant strains started spreading within the community. However, I pointed out that this unfortunate situation was not inevitable if timely action was taken.

I commended President Obama's resolve to extend PEPFAR beyond HIV/AIDS, TB, and malaria to encompass wider Global Health

Initiative (GHI) goals. The new plan included "orphan diseases", so called because donors and pharmaceutical companies tended to ignore them. Yet these mainly tropical diseases were exacting a big toll as they wreaked havoc on the people of Africa. However, I pointed out that the main requirement for successful integration of these diseases into the AIDS treatment plan was to ensure sufficient funding, with new money. It should not be at the expense of HIV/AIDS, which continued to need increased support because the problem was still escalating.

I also suggested some innovative ways that could be incorporated for cost-effective integration of these diseases in the PEPFAR programme. These included joint funding support for critical facilities like laboratories and clinics, which could be shared for diagnostic, monitoring, logistics and treatment of these and as many other diseases and health conditions as possible. This suggestion envisioned widening the scope of training syllabuses for healthcare providers and community support groups to cover the whole spectrum of common diseases. In consideration of insufficient trained manpower in Africa, multitasking of staff could be prioritised so that the same staff would provide care and treatment for all prevalent diseases, especially in rural areas, where most of the population lived. To succeed, this strategy would require some incentives, including salary top-ups for public sector workers, especially those in remote and underserved rural areas.

I used my institution as an example to demonstrate how AIDS treatment has contributed to health-systems strengthening. I talked of the miserable situation way back in the early 1990s, when our staff and their relatives were dying of AIDS. The surviving staff were spending a lot of time attending funeral ceremonies of their colleagues, parents, siblings and other close relatives. Our trained staff were dwindling. The turning point was brought about by PEPPFAR, when all sick staff members and their relatives who needed treatment got it. My institution then started working smoothly.

I emphasised that the time of recession necessitated decisive action to ensure that the grip on AIDS was not relaxed, because the treacherous virus had not gone in recession too. The AIDS epidemic called for long-term commitment to help poor countries to cope with the huge numbers of PLWHIV that still constituted a state of emergency. But this did not mean that we were wanton wishful thinkers advocating for limitless aid, like Dr Hearst intimated in his submission. African governments realised that the ultimate responsibility for their citizens' heath was primarily theirs and that they needed to play an increasing role in the management of AIDS in their countries. However, almost all African health systems were still too weak to cope with the enormous task alone. The catastrophic AIDS crisis had further strained and increased the vulnerability of their fragile systems. They therefore needed continued support and adequate time to build up the necessary capacity in the public sector to eventually take over the work started by PEPFAR. Otherwise, to freeze support at this time, or a hurried handover of this still developing initiative, without allowing time for systematic capacity building, would just break the system, and set the programme back.

A number of journalists from major US newspapers including, *The New York Times, The Boston Globe* and *Newsweek* were interested in my testimony. They sent journalists to check the facts on the ground in Uganda and their stories were published as headline news. Surely the situation could not be ignored anymore, neither by donors nor by our own governments in Africa.

My testimony prompted the sly man who claimed close association with high level international contacts to return. Talking in whispers as if spies were listening behind the curtains, he warned: "Why do you care so much? Now, everyone is not only angry with you, they are livid," he added.

But two months later, something really exciting happened. We were delighted by the news that the ban on treatment of new patients had been lifted. It was the best news, especially for our despairing AIDS patients, some of whom were already preparing for their own funerals. I had to ask my clinic manager to repeat the news. "PEPFAR officials came to the clinic. They said we do not need to turn away new patients anymore," she said.

This timely relief was the work of many caring people and humanitarian organisations who have championed the fight against HIV/AIDS. Ultimately, our heartfelt thanks were to the American people for the gift of PEPFAR, and timely action that averted another round of AIDS carnage.

My sincere hope is that this was not mere postponement of a crisis, but rather an unwavering commitment to fight AIDS all the way through the tough times that still lie ahead, until the ultimate goal of a world without AIDS is achieved.

Epilogue

The End of AIDS

A question that people keep asking me over and over again is whether it is true that an AIDS cure has been found. I always reply that if a cure had been discovered, nobody would ask me that question.

AIDS, the monster disease, has killed millions, tormented individuals, tortured families, and anguished communities across Sub-Saharan Africa and beyond. Throughout the 1990s its victims filled virtually all hospital beds, overflowing on to the floors and into the corridors. Meanwhile, bodies piled up in mortuaries as grave-diggers worked overtime. The scourge orphaned millions of children across Africa. The devastation caused headlines all over the world for almost three decades. Its toll in monetary terms is staggering with billions of dollars having so far been spent on research, care and treatment programmes. Billions more have been used on trials to develop vaccines and other preventive measures. With such an ominous reputation and a fortune having been spent, it is virtually impossible that a cure that would put an end to all this mayhem could be introduced by stealth.

The day an AIDS cure is announced it will take over the news. This event will take its place as an epic scientific breakthrough, and would remain the talk of the town for months if not years. Millions infected with HIV or those living in fear of it around the world will be dancing. Not to be carried away, all we have as I write in 2012 are ARVs, which are the next best thing to a cure. When used properly, ARVs have been proven to restore a visibly ailing AIDS patient to good health, the so-called Lazarus syndrome. Indeed, the treatment is so effective that some lay people mistake it for an AIDS cure. We now know that ARVs are also highly effective in preventing transmission of HIV if used properly.

An AIDS cure remains a dream that most HIV-affected and infected people are praying for. It would mean not having to take ARV drugs every day, with all its inconveniences and side effects. ARV drugs remain expensive and in short supply, and unless the poor are assisted to access them, they remain beyond the means of the majority in dire need. That is part of the reason why people desperate to save their own lives continue to be easily taken in by conmen promising fake cures or healing prayers.

The reality is that all available ARV drugs have so far failed to completely clear the virus from the body. The treacherously elusive HIV "cleverly" escapes their effect by inserting its genetic code into human cells, especially the CD4 cells, which are crucial for a body's defence against infections. HIV-infected CD4 cells produce billions of HIV particles before they die, which go on to attack and similarly destroy numerous other cells. ARV drugs disrupt this replication process, and reduce the amount of HIV in a person's body to such extremely low levels that it may not be detectable by a test known as PCR RNA or more commonly, as viral load test-although the common HIV test always remains positive. But some other HIV-infected cells behave differently. Among them are the so-called "resting" CD4 cells that remain dormant for a long time with the HIV genetic material inside them. These can be compared to an undercover agent or a saboteur known as a 'sleeper' who is planted in an adversary country with instructions to remain quiescent and hidden, passing for an ordinary law-abiding citizen and waiting for the instruction to launch a surprise attack. Current ARV drugs cannot remove HIV's genetic material from such cells, even after many years of treatment. The infected person may look and feel well, but he harbours HIV-infected sleeper cells, ready to escape from these "hiding" places, also referred to as "reservoirs" or "sanctuaries", to quickly start replicating again, causing the same terrible symptoms. This is one of the main reasons why current drugs are not able to cure AIDS. Newer drugs that interfere with the integration of HIV genetic materials into the cells have recently become available, but they are also not able to completely eliminate or remove HIV genes from all resting cells.

As detailed above, claims of AIDS cures started soon after the frightening epidemic was recognised early in the 1980s. Since then, numerous so called "AIDS cures" have been prescribed to frantic patients. In many cases this has made a bad situation worse, as duped or unsuspecting patients suffered toxic effects or just wasted their meagre resources on useless concoctions. Worse still, some sufferers met with premature deaths because of poisonous concoctions. Among those that I helped to stop, contained a wide range of toxins including hydroxybenzene, herbs mixed with industrial solvents, pharmaceutical products in disproportionate doses, disinfectants and unhygienic preparations.

Frustratingly, even after the PEPFAR programme had increased access to effective ARV drugs in Uganda, I continued to see many patients die needlessly. They were victims of peddlers of bogus cures, who convinced them to stop taking ARVs, claiming that they had superior and safer alternatives. Unfortunately, by the time many of them realised that they were being conned it was often too late. I also met a number of people who were told by quacks and fake pastors that they could stop treatment and freely resume unprotected sex because they had been cured of AIDS. The whole unpleasant business is a tragedy that continues today albeit with less frequency. I am glad that I helped to expose a number of conmen and threw out numerous fake concoctions and drugs. Luckily the retaliatory threats by some of these con artists did not materialise. Fortunately, not everybody who were trying to find cures were conmen. Many, including Rouchy, Lionel, Van Grouch, Lu Weibo, and Okot were ethical scientists trying to find a solution to a serious problem. The world needs many more of these, and much fewer of the other type.

Meanwhile, a search for a cure continues. Scientists are pursuing various approaches. Some research has focussed on fighting the resting cells harbouring the HIV virus, or rather trying to "provoke' them into becoming active (reveal themselves) and start producing HIV copies. It is during active reproduction – the infective circle stages – that HIV is most vulnerable to ARV drugs, but the elusive virus has to date lived up to its reputation. It appears that there are other HIV sanctuaries or other mechanisms that have made it possible for HIV to remain "invisible" to the currently available drugs. However promising research continues.

There are other grounds for optimism, or at least grounds to build dreams on. There is a small number of people (about 3%) who seem to have natural resistance to the full-blown HIV disease. These are often referred to as long-term survivors. Though infected they do not readily progress to the AIDS stage. These patients are suspected of having a natural immunity to the disease. When their blood was tested, it was found that many had neutralising antibodies that, when mixed in a test tube with the virus of other patients, cleared it in more than 90% of cases. Unfortunately, as was found in the case of Nairobi's commercial sex workers, unlike other diseases, antibodies against HIV do not necessarily always protect someone against the disease. The fact that they seem to be protective in some patients raises the question as to whether a therapeutic agent or vaccine can be made to mimic their special kind of protective antibodies to protect other patients. With the STEP study disappointment still vivid, we cannot take anything for granted.

Despite numerous setbacks and despair by some scientists that "a cure may never be found", the search continues. The pessimistic remarks remind me of the comments in the early 1990s, when it was openly stated that AIDS treatment would never be found. It did not take long to prove them wrong!

There has been at least one documented case of a "suspected" cure, which did raise real hope. German scientists announced in 2008 that they had successfully cured a man of HIV infection by giving him a bone marrow transplant, using cells from a donor with a rare genetic mutation known as Delta 32, which confers resistance to HIV infection. Almost two years after the transplant they reported that they could not find any trace of HIV in the recipient's body. However, soon after a debate started as to whether this could ever be a feasible method of HIV treatment. It would meet with severe technical and safety challenges. However it also promised the prospect of future research on gene therapy for a possible role in AIDS treatment.

As of 2010, for every two new patients started on ARVs, five new ones get infected. Evidently, the threat still hovers and the situation will inevitably deteriorate unless the world's governments and donors make an irrevocable long-term commitment to address the still blazing killer plague by embracing and implementing all the scientifically proven preventive and treatment strategies. The world's governments' and donors' commitment to increasing funding as the need for treatment escalates has, however, been tested and found wanting. Unless the elements of this dire equation change, the epidemic will be much more difficult to bring under control.

But, for the first time in the 30 years of escalating AIDS epidemic, there is a real opportunity to end the scourge. Scientific evidence in support of this new hope emerged from landmark results of the discordant couples study by the HIV preventive Trials Network coded HPTN 052 trial, which released its results in May 2011 (Chapter 3). This unique study compared clinical outcomes and rates of transmission within couples in which one partner was HIV positive and the other was HIV negative (discordant couples). The findings were so striking that research on delayed ART initiation was stopped four years ahead of schedule due to evidence of overwhelming benefit of early initiation of therapy. Specifically, the trial found that early initiation of ART in HIV-positive individuals reduced the transmission risk to the HIV-negative partner by a staggering 96 percent! It was also found that early treatment significantly reduced cases of extra-pulmonary tuberculosis in the HIV-positive partner.

This study has clearly demonstrated that effective HIV treatment is also powerful HIV preventive armament especially when started early.

These findings point to a better and more effective way of managing the AIDS epidemic. This reinforces calls by many scientists and activists for serious consideration of the concept of Test and Treat (T & T), instead of the current practice of waiting for sufferers to first reach a set level of immunological decline. As for discordant couples, T & T should be the standard practice. Many people would find tolerance of what happens as newly diagnosed patients wait, including increased morbidity, mortality and the spread of HIV, totally unacceptable.

Furthermore, the studies provided compelling evidence in support of increased government and donor funding support for HIV/AIDS treatment and calls for expedited progress towards universal access. The benefits of universal access, besides the millions of lives that would be saved, include the millions of new HIV infections that would be prevented. The exciting new research findings point to a new way forward. It is time to change our approach to the management of the epidemic by adopting new treatment and preventive strategies using ARVs as a key component. In the absence of an AIDS cure or an effective vaccine, this would be an effective measure that would break the back of the ever-escalating HIV epidemic, and for the first time, bring it under control.

Obviously, this necessitates increased funding support in the short to medium term. But there is no doubt that the long-term benefits would more than compensate for the initial high investment in early treatment and universal access to ART. Otherwise, the current practice of funding treatment for only a small proportion of patients out of the many in urgent need of therapy, while many more keep getting infected, is just like mopping the floor while the main tap flows.

Timothy Ray Brown, who had been living with HIV for more than 12 years, became the first person to be considered as cured of HIV after receiving a blood stem cell transplant in 2007. Although biologist continue to debate whether he is truly cured because of questionable HIV signals reportedly found in his tissues. However Brown who remains well is an inspiration to scientist in search of a cure.

"I don't want to be the only person in the world cured of HIV. I want a cure for everyone", Brown said; adding that he hopes his personal survival story would inspire HIV sufferers that a cure is possible.

At this time, nobody disputes the fact that finding an AIDS vaccine and a cure remains a formidable scientific challenge, but the very ethos of science is to overcome such challenges.

It is now clear that we need not wait for a cure or vaccine to be discovered first. On the eve of the 2011 United Nations High-level Meeting on AIDS, Mark Harrington, a long term AIDS activist, hit the nail on the head:

> The global response to AIDS is at a turning point and we call upon all governments, donors, international agencies, researchers, implementers and civil society to act on this evidence and end the AIDS epidemic now.

End it, we must.

Acknowledgements

First of all, my sincere thanks go to all HIV-infected or affected people, (although many of them remain anonymous) whose life stories illustrating the complex issues associated with HIV/AIDS are embodied in this book. I especially thank all patients who volunteered for the trials, which helped me and my colleagues to expose the many quacks who sought to exploit their plight and eventually led to the time when effective ARV therapy became available.

I would like to acknowledge the very important roles played by my colleagues at the JCRC, as well as the Centre's collaborating scientists and researchers from many parts of the world. Special thanks go to humanitarian organisations and individuals who have worked to alleviate the HIV/ AIDS scourge and their continuing struggle to find a solution.

I also take this opportunity to pay tribute to the late Dr Catherine Othieno, a young Ugandan scientist, in recognition of her contribution to the start of Africa's pioneer HIV vaccine trial.

I acknowledge with gratitude all those people who provided me with information and records of important past events reported in this book, and others, including Arthur Gakwandi, Mukotani Rugyendo, Anthony Canavan and Arthur Ndimbirwe, who read the manuscript and made useful suggestions. I thank Fountain Publishers for the great work done in editing and shaping this book.

I am indebted to the readers of my previous book, *Genocide by Denial*. Their concern and enthusiasm were an inspiration in writing this follow-up book.

Finally, I thank my immediate and extended family for their encouragement in writing this book

Bibliography

1. Abayomi Sofowara 1993: *Medicinal Plants and Traditional Medicine in Africa*. (Ibadan: Spectrum Books limited)

2. A Cure for AIDS: HIV and AIDS information from AVERT. org, 2010 www.avert.org/cure-for-aids.htm - accessed 10 March 2011.

3. Ambika, Ahuja and Casey Michael, "Volunteers. Associated Press, 2009: Key to success of Thai vaccine Trials" (Nearly 16,000 Thais ignored rumours and stigma in groundbreaking trial); www.msnbc.msn.com/id/33046118/.../health-aids/, 23 February 2011.

4. Among Barbara, "Ugandans make it big as fake witchdoctors in South Africa, The big story", *Sunday Vision,* 5 December 2010, Pages 12-13.

5. Barnes Fred, "Bush's Achievements - Ten things the President got right.", The Weekly Standard, 19 January 2009, Volume 014, No. 17

6. Berkley S.F. and W.C. Koff, 2007: "Scientific and policy challenges to development of an AIDS vaccine." Lancet. 370:94–101.

7. Boston Globe, 11 Apr 2010 'US seeks to rein in AIDS program' - The Boston Globe www.boston.com/news//04//US seeks to rein in AIDS program.

8. Brannon Heather, 'The History of smallpox: the Rise and fall of a disease' (Updated September 2004). dermatology.about.com/cs/smallpox/a/smallpoxhx.htm Smallpox.

9. Cao H, P et al, (15 March 2003). "Immunogenicity of a recombinant Human Immunodefficiency Virus (HIV) – Canarypox Vaccine in IV-Seronegative Ugandan Volunteers.", JID 2003: 187

10. Centers for Disease Control and Prevention, "How effective are latex condoms in preventing HIV?", www.cdc.gov/hiv/pubs/faq/faq23.htm.

11. Chun T. W. et al, 28 Oct 1999 "AIDS: Re-emergence of HIV after stopping therapy", Nature 401(6756)

12. Nullis, Clare, 13 Jan 2009 "PEPFAR: Bush's bright legacy in Africa" Associated Press, 10:43:00 AM

13. Clinton Health Access Initiative (CHAI): [In 2006, CHAI entered into a partnership with the international funding.] www.clintonfoundation.org/.../clinton-hiv.../access-programs

14. COMMENTARY: The failed HIV Merk vaccine study: a step back or a launching point for future vaccine development? By Sekaly R P. Exp Medicine 2008 Jan 21, 205(i) 7-12

15. Congressional Hearings- Foreign Affairs Subcommittee on Africa and Global Health: www.pepfarwatch.org/about_pepfar/congressional, hearings

16. CONRAD (2010, July 20): "Microbicide gel: Reduced risk of HIV and herpes infections in women, study shows." Science Daily, retrieved 10 January 2011 from http://www.sciencedaily.com / releases/2010/07/100719142444.htm.

17. Dobson Mary, 'The extraordinary stories behind history's deadliest killers (Published by Quercus 2007).

18. Green, Edward, Vinand Nantulya, Rand Stoneburner, and John Stover: "What happened in Uganda? Declining HIV prevalence, behavior change and national response." Editor; Janice H. Hogle. Contributors: Lessons learned - case study. 2002.

19. FDA Consumer, October 1987 issue, "Defrauding the Desperate: Quackery and AIDS" www.quackwatch.com/01QuackeryRelatedTopics/aids1987.html: Accessed 10 March 2011.

20. Female praying mantis eats male after mating: www.youtube/watch ,

21. Flight, updated 2011, Feb 17 Collette, Eradicating the scourge, 'The story of man's victory over smallpox is one of determination, scientific endeavor and vaccination on a global scale.' www.bbc.co.uk/history/british/empire_seapower/smallpox_01.shtml

22. Garber E. G. et al (August 1991), "The use of ozone-treated blood in the therapy of HIV infection and immune disease: a pilot study of safety and efficacy", AIDS 5(8)

23. Goldacre Ben. 2008. *Bad Science*, Published by Fourth Estate.

24. Hayden Erika, Jan.14, 2009. "PEPFAR, Bush's Legacy: An Unlikely Champion.", Nature 457, 254-256.

25. Huzicka I. (March 1999), "Could bone marrow transplantation cure AIDS?: review", Medical Hypotheses 52(3).

26. Howard Brian Clark (14 June 2012) The man who was cured of AIDS. IOL news. www.iol.co.za

27. IOL news (15 September 2007), "'These few pills will cure your Aids'" By Chiara Carter and Lennox Oriver.

28. Kaiser Daily " NIH Report Opens Debate on Effectiveness of Condoms against STDs," July 20, 2001.

29. Kinsman F. J. "Pragmatic Choices: Research, politics and AIDS control in Uganda." http://dare.uva.nl/document/110229 accessed 11 Jan 2011

30. Kruger Jeffrey, January 2005. Penguin USA, Splendid Solution: Jonas Salk and the Conquest of Polio. [biography of the man who discovered the vaccine for one of the world's most horrible diseases]

31. Mahoney Gene, Interview with Dr David Rasnick. www. purewatergazette.net/rasnickinterview

32. McNeil Donald G, "AIDS Vaccine Trial Shows Only Slight Protection.", New York Times October 20, 2009.

33. McNeil D.G: 13 November 2008. "Rare Treatment is Reported to Cure AIDS Patient", New York Times.

34. McNeil Donald, September 27, 2009. "If AIDS Went the Way of Smallpox.", New York Times.

35. McNeil Donald G. In Uganda, AIDS War Is Falling Apart –NY Times. com. Published May 9, 2010. www.nytimes.com/2010/05/10/world/ africa/10aids.html

36. Merck press release: Vaccination and Enrollment Are Discontinued in Phase II Trials of Merck's Investigational HIV Vaccine Candidate, 21.09.07, http://www.merck.com/newsroom/press_releases/research_ and_development/2007_0921.html

37. Mugerwa, et al, "First trial of the HIV-1 vaccine in Africa: Ugandan experience 26 January 2002.", BMJ 2002, 324 : 226: 10.1136/ bmj.324.7331.226

38. Mugyenyi Peter, 2008. *Genocide by Denial*, Kampala: Fountain Publishers Ltd.

39. Mugyenyi Peter, "HIV Vaccines: The Uganda Experience.", Elsevier Science Publication 2002.

40. 'Revamping PEPFAR Causes Concern in Africa' Newsweek 27 Apr 2010 www.newsweek.com/.../aids-programs-hit-setbacks-in-africa.html

41. News of the World (13 November 2005), "I'm first in world to be cured of HIV"

42. Carol Natukunda, October 10, 2008. 'Religious Sect Stores Dead Bodies' New Vision,

43. New Vision 26 Mar, 2008 President Museveni orders cult probe. Rakai-based religious organisation, Sserulanda. New Vision Online, www. newvision.co.ug.

44. Nordqvist Christian, "Medical Bush's AIDS Treatment Program Saved 1.2 Million Lives In Africa", News Today, http://www. medicalnewstoday.com/articles/145376.php

45. Kihura Nkuba, 'Polio vaccine genocide in Uganda' A talk given at the National Vaccine Information Center's Third International Public Conference on Vaccination November 7-9, 2002 - Arlington, Virginia. www.whale.to/a/nkuba_h.html

46. "Preparation for PAVE- A prospective cohort study of the seroincidence of HIV-1 infection in High risk military recruits in Uganda" approved on February 20, 1995.

47. Sagot-Lerolle, D. et al, 19 June 2008. "Prolonged valproic acid treatment does not reduce the size of latent HIV reservoir"

48. Simpson, Victor I. and Winfield Nicole: "Vatican: Condom use less evil than spreading HIV.", Associated Press, Tue Nov 23.

49. Sekaly Rafick, Pierre, Université de Montréal, CR-CHUM, Institut National de la Santé et de la Recherche Médicale U743, Montréal, Québec H2X1P1, Canada

50. Sky News "Aids Victims Risk Lives" (18 September 2007)

51. Teen sex abstinence study sparks controversy. Study, led by Buzz Pruitt at Texas A&M University. www.newscientist.com/.../dn6957-teen-sex-abstinence-study-sparks-controversy.html Accessed 9 May 2011

52. 17 Nov 2008. STEP study shows HIV vaccine from Merck does not protect against HIV infection. The Lancet www.thelancet.com

53. The New Vision (Uganda daily Newspaper): "Government to pay Sh500 million for doctor's death.", 2 September 2009

54. Tibomanya P.: "Kitovu home care based services." (Kitovu Hospital Report 1992)

55. Warren, Mitchell, October 2009 "An AIDS vaccine is now more than a dream", www.hvtn.org/media/news.html.

56. Watson J (2006), "Scientists, activists sue South Africa's AIDS 'denialists'"., Nat. Med. 12 (1): 6. doi:10.1038/nm0106-6a. PMID 16397537.

57. Groundbreaking trial results confirm HIV treatment prevents transmission of HIV, WHO/UNAIDS joint press release www.who.int/entity/hiv/mediacentre/trial_results/en/index.html. Accessed 15 May 2011.

58. Yang Q.E. July 2004 "Eradication of HIV in infected patients: some potential approaches", Med Sci Monitor. 10(7)

Indexes